To Dr. Kurt Benisch,

With deepest ad[illegible]ion, respect, and appreciation for all you have done. Thank you for enabling the rest of us to understand and contribute. Thanks for your spirit of humor! ☆

Your friend,

Ora Fraga Petersen

Handbook of

Placental Pathology

Second Edition

Handbook of Placental Pathology

Second Edition

Ona Marie Faye-Petersen MD
Associate Professor of Pathology and Obstetrics and Gynecology
Head, Microdissection Laboratory
The University of Alabama at Birmingham
Birmingham, Alabama
USA

Debra S Heller MD
Professor of Pathology and Laboratory Medicine,
and of Obstetrics, Gynecology and Women's Health
Director of Pediatric Pathology
UMDNJ – New Jersey Medical School
Newark, New Jersey
USA

Vijay V Joshi MD, PhD, FRCPath
Director Emeritus, Consultant
Connecticut Children's Medical Centre
Pediatric Pathology
Hartford Hospital
Hartford, Connecticut
USA

Taylor & Francis
Taylor & Francis Group
LONDON AND NEW YORK

First published in the United Kingdom in 2006
by Taylor & Francis,
an imprint of the Taylor & Francis Group,
2 Park Square, Milton Park
Abingdon, Oxon OX14 4RN, UK

Tel.: +44 (0) 20 7017 6000
Fax.: +44 (0) 20 7017 6699
E-mail: info.medicine@tandf.co.uk
Website: http://www.tandf.co.uk/medicine

British Library Cataloguing in Publication Data
Data available on application

Library of Congress Cataloging-in-Publication Data
Data available on application

ISBN10: 1-84214-232-1
ISBN13: 9-78-1-84214-232-5

Distributed in North and South America by

Taylor & Francis
2000 NW Corporate Blvd
Boca Raton, FL 33431, USA
Within Continental USA
Tel.: 800 272 7737; Fax.: 800 374 3401
Outside Continental USA
Tel.: 561 994 0555; Fax.: 561 361 6018
E-mail: orders@crcpress.com

Distributed in the rest of the world by
Thomson Publishing Services
Cheriton House
North Way
Andover, Hampshire SP10 5BE, UK
Tel.: +44 (0) 1264 332424
E-mail: salesorder.tandf@thomsonpublishingservices.co.uk

Composition by Parthenon Publishing
Printed and bound by T. G. Hostench S.A., Spain

Contents

Preface to the Second Edition

It has been estimated that about 20% of placentas from deliveries are submitted to pathology departments in the United States. Hence, pathologists in all types of practice receive large numbers of these specimens. Training in pathology often does not address this organ in great detail, and many pathologists who do not have a special interest in the placenta are at a loss. However, the importance of placental findings is indisputable. The placenta can shed light on conditions relating to the current pregnancy outcome, as well as be predictive of future pregnancies. The placenta has a major role to play in medicolegal litigation as well. The few texts that are currently available are greatly detailed, and do not take the needs of the busy surgical pathologist into account. This book was designed to fill that need, while also being of interest to placental pathologists, obstetricians, neonatologists, as well as trainees in these specialties. As such, the original format was retained, aiming at being easy to read and follow. Furthermore, we wanted to give updated data, introduce recent concepts and expand on aspects of etiopathogenesis and clinical features relevant to placental pathology, and hence new sections were added as well. The original photographs have been entirely replaced by a new set of digitized images and diagrams. The number of gross and microscopic photographs has been increased. It is our hope that this book will find an equal home on the workbench of the practicing pathologist, the desk of the trainee, and the reference shelf of all practitioners who deal with aspects of the delivery of a healthy newborn.

Ona Faye-Petersen
Debra S Heller
Vijay Joshi

Preface to the First Edition

The seeds of this book were sown when, about 4 years ago, I started signing out placentas in large numbers for the first time in my career. In order to prepare for the task and approach it in a systematic manner, I started reading monographs, book chapters, and articles on the subject. I prepared a short write-up on placental pathology for my surgical pathologist colleagues. As I continued signing out placentas at the rate of about 1400 per year, and began seeing variants of common placental lesions and different types of uncommon and rare placental lesions, I felt the need to organize the process of signing out in a more systematic way. That led to the preparation of this handbook, which should serve as a concise yet comprehensive guide for general surgical pathologists in carrying out gross and microscopic examination of placentas and preparing reports systematically, expeditiously, and with better understanding of placental pathology. I believe that it should also be useful to trainees in pathology, obstetrics and gynecology, and neonatology, as well as to practicing clinicians in these specialities.

It is estimated that about 20% of the placentas from about 5 million births occurring every year in the United States are submitted to the surgical pathology laboratory. (It appears that in some countries, many of the placentas that are not sent to the surgical pathology laboratory are used for preparation of albumin, immunoglobulins, and collagen.) Thus pathologists working in all types of hospitals are likely to get placentas in their laboratories. The single-author and multiauthor monographs on placental pathology published in the past several years are excellent and comprehensive. However, they are not oriented to the needs of busy surgical pathologists, clinicians, and trainees in various specialties. On the other hand, the chapters on placental pathology in various textbooks of pathology and its subspecialties are not sufficiently comprehensive for their needs. This handbook occupies an intermediate position. In the opening section of the book, the normal structure of the placenta is briefly described. Common gross and microscopic lesions of the placenta are briefly discussed and adequately illustrated. These sections will help both the trainee and the practicing physician to develop a better understanding of and a systematic approach to placental pathology. The subsequent sections describe and illustrate the primary disorders. Besides the pathologic features, pathogenesis and clinical significance are described in every section for better understanding of various lesions. Tables that summarize the features of various lesions are suited for quick reference by the side of the microscope while one is signing out a case. In addition, pertinent original and recent references are cited at the end of the book. These references should serve as the source of more detailed discussion of various topics. Those who wish to keep up with the literature on the placenta need to review not only pathology journals but also obstetrics journals and the journal *Placenta*. This book, which represents an attempt to fulfil the practical needs of practicing and trainee physicians, is largely based on material that has been published by various investigators. However, wherever indicated, I have given my own views and related my own experience. I hope that the readers will find the book helpful.

Vijay V Joshi
Greenville, NC

Authors' acknowledgments

The quality of the contents and the assembly of this book would have been impossible without the contribution of numerous individuals.

First, we would like to thank Ms Veronica Owens, Ms Linda Plunkett, Ms Lee Ann Brown, Ms Tara Allen, Mr James ('Bo') Moreno, and Mr E. Scott Young of the University of Alabama (UAB) Surgical Pathology service and Mr Thurman Richardson and Mr David Stephens of the UAB Autopsy Pathology service for the overwhelming majority of the gross photographs used in this manual. Their efforts are truly appreciated since the gross examination is so critical to a meaningful evaluation of the placental specimen.

Stephanie Reilly, MD, a UAB pathologist and colleague of Dr Faye-Petersen, also contributed to the case material used in this book. We are also especially thankful for the superior artistic talents of the medical illustrator, Mr David Fisher. He patiently transformed pencil drawings and ideas into the wonderful illustrations now available in this book. We would also like to thank Ms Kristina Woodley who scanned many, many projection slides of gross and microscopic images and provided unflagging, cheerful, and expert artistic support. We are also very grateful for the secretarial assistance provided by Ms Julie Mahaffey, of UAB. Ms Mahaffey helped enormously with the final assembly of the manuscript. Ms Ginger Goodall also deserves thanks for her secretarial support in the early stages of the book's construction. We would particularly like to express our deepest appreciation to Frederick T. Kraus, MD for his review of the entire manuscript. Finally, we would like to extend our sincere gratitude to Mr Oliver Walter and Mr Nick Dunton and their editorial staff at Taylor & Francis Medical Books for their assistance with and support of this book and their unified efforts to ensure its publication.

Ona Faye-Petersen
Debra Heller
Vijay Joshi

Individual acknowledgments

There are many outstanding individuals, colleagues, and friends in Pediatric and Perinatal Pathology, who have continued to inspire me over the years. Space precludes me from thanking them all, but they are remembered with gratitude. However, I would very much like to thank J. Bruce Beckwith, MD and Dagmar K. Kalousek, MD for really opening the doors to a field that has fascinated and challenged me for so long. I would also like to thank Robert W. Bendon, MD, for his generosity, special wizardry, and professional support, and Raymond W. Redline, MD for his unfailing expertise and colleagueship.

Ona Faye-Petersen

I thank William Pastuszak MD, Martin Berman MD, Mark Ludwig MD and my other colleagues in the Departmant of Pathology at Hartford Hospital, Hartford, CT, who during the last phase of my career have provided unstinted support for my academic activities.

Vijay Joshi

1

Introduction

The placenta (derived from the Latin word translating as 'flat cake') provides oxygen, nourishment, and protection to the fetus. It also has excretory and endocrine functions. Numerous hormones such as human chorionic gonadotropin, progesterone, estrone, estradiol, estriol, and human placental lactogen are secreted by the placenta. Thus, the trophoblast contributes significantly to the hormonal milieu during pregnancy. Examination of the placenta in cases of poor pregnancy outcome and certain maternal disorders provides documentation and information useful to the obstetrician and neonatologist. Pathologic lesions of the placenta can be broadly classified into four types depending on their clinical relevance:

(1) Lesions responsible for fetal or neonatal morbidity and/or mortality (infarction, infection, abruption, etc.);

(2) Lesions related to premature delivery (chorioamnionitis, abruption, etc.);

(3) Lesions that are likely to modify immediate management of the mother (e.g. hydatidiform mole);

(4) Lesions that may recur in future pregnancies (thrombi, villitis of unknown etiology, maternal floor infarction, etc.).

The placenta has not been a particularly favorite subject of surgical pathologists for a variety of reasons. There seem to be too many of them, the terminology is different from other surgical pathology terminology, the yield of information is low for the volume of specimens, and information obtained is less likely to have a one-to-one correlation with that particular newborn's situation than is a usual surgical specimen. There are also issues of cost to consider. On the other hand, the placenta can sometimes provide exceedingly useful information relating to perinatal morbidity and mortality, or subsequent pregnancy outcome. With the increase in medical malpractice suits against obstetricians, the placenta is often an important component of the defense. A placental finding that indicates significant prior compromise will be supportive in defending against a suit for failure to intervene appropriately during labor.

Both the American College of Obstetricians and Gynecologists, and the College of American Pathologists, are supportive of the value of placental examination[1,2]. The purpose of this handbook is to make placental pathology comprehensible to the practicing surgical pathologist, trainee, and obstetrician who deal with placentas, and would like to be more comfortable with their interpretation.

2

Development of the placenta

After repeated mitotic divisions, the zygote, composed of the fused male and female pronuclei, transforms into a 32-cell ball of blastomeres or a *morula* (from Latin word *morum*, mulberry) by day 4 postfertilization. The morula then begins to take on fluid, blastomeric segregation and compaction occur, and a fluid-filled cavity develops within the morula, changing it to a *blastocyst*. The blastomeres of the blastocyst form an outer shell of cells, now called *trophoblast* (from the Greek, *trophe*, meaning nutrition), and a localized, inner cell mass, the *embryoblast*. The side of the blastocyst with the inner cell mass is called the embryonic pole. The blastocyst emerges from its covering of zona pellucida, and is thereby enabled to attach tightly to the endometrium on about day 6. The site of attachment is at the embryonic pole, and, upon implantation, the trophoblast cells at the embryonic pole rapidly proliferate and differentiate into an outer, leading layer of *syncytiotrophoblast* and an inner, proliferating mass of *cytotrophoblasts*. These broad solid trophoblast columns invade the endometrium, which, due to progesterone from the corpus luteum, has become decidualized, and additional cytotrophoblast differentiation into an intermediate type occurs. Invasion (implantation) enables the conceptus to derive nourishment from the endometrium. Before implantation is completed, the embryoblast differentiates into a bilaminar embryo, composed of *epi*blast and *hypo*blast. On about day 6–7, epiblasts nearest to the site of implantation (i.e. the dorsal epiblast) differentiate into *amnioblasts*. The amnioblasts proliferate, become decohesive, and fluid collects between them; the amnioblast is split and forms a small space, the amniotic cavity, by about the end of day 7. Thus, amnioblasts cover the epiblast, line the newly formed amniotic cavity, and separate the embryo from the trophoblast. Simultaneously, the trophoblasts invade the decidual interstitium and its blood vessels (capillaries and spiral arterial vessels); this vascular invasion results in blood extravasation and the formation of decidual blood lakes. At about day 9, the invading trophoblast also develops *internal* sites of cellular decohesion that progress to form lacunae; these become filled by maternal blood of the lakes. These lacunae then progressively enlarge and coalesce to form a network of blood-filled channels, the early intervillous spaces. These, the lacunar-lake formations, represent the beginning of the uteroplacental circulation as the maternal blood drains back into the maternal circulation via maternal veins. In addition, during the second week of development, the bilaminar embryonic disk exhibits an *extra*embryonic extension at its lateral aspects, the *extraembryonic mesenchyme*. Also, the invading fingers of syncytiotrophoblast have formed a radiating but spherical shell around the embryo and the amnion. The invasive syncytiotrophoblast projections gain a central, conical component of cytotrophoblast between days 11 and 13 and become the primary stem villi. The primary villi, which lie

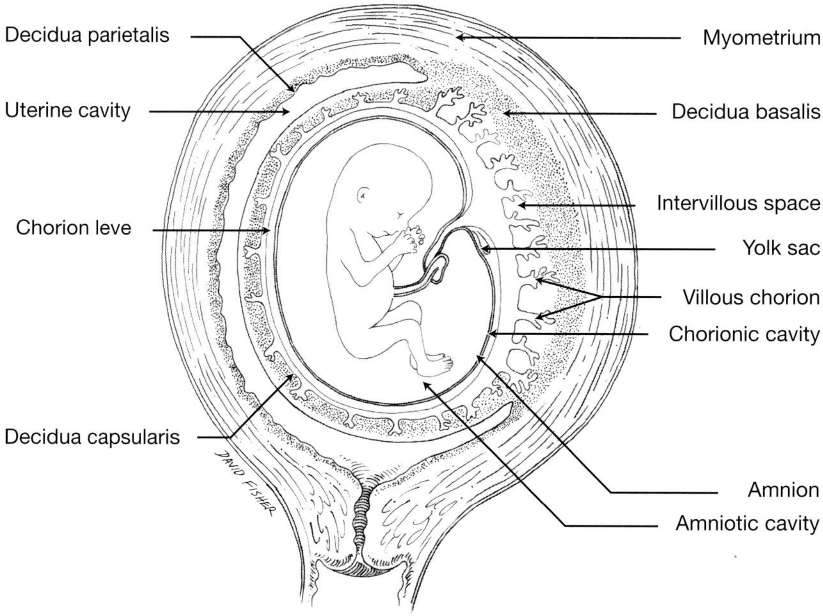

Figure 1 Diagram of fetus *in utero*. Representation of an intrauterine singleton pregnancy at about 16 weeks of gestation. In this illustration, some license is taken, since the amnion is shown as still *separate* from the chorion; this is done to illustrate the process of apposition of the amniotic sac to the chorion and to accentuate the interposition of the yolk sac between the amnion and the chorion. (Normally, the amnion and chorion are fully apposed by 12 weeks.) However, as is true at this stage of gestation, the chorion is shown fused to the decidua capsularis, and the fetal sac is not yet large enough to obliterate the uterine cavity

within blood-filled lacunae, in turn become infiltrated by protrusions of the extraembryonic mesenchyme, which has come to line the shell of the radiating trophoblast villous projections, and become secondary villi. The innermost core of extraembryonic mesenchyme within each secondary villus then gives rise to villous blood vessels, changing them to tertiary villi. By the end of the third week, the vessels of the tertiary villi become connected through channels in the extraembryonic chorionic plate and root of a connecting stalk to those vessels of the *intraembryonic* mesenchyme of the embryo proper. Thus, the extraembryonic mesenchyme develops into the vascular chorion plate of the placenta and the vascular cores of the chorionic villous tree. Due to the folding of the embryo during the 4th week, the chorion forms a sac whose projections vascularize the villous cytotrophoblast and its syncytiotrophoblast covering. The embryo and its amniotic sac thereby lie suspended within this chorionic sac via the connecting stalk of vessels; this connecting stalk develops into the umbilical cord and contains the allantois (a ventral, tubular extension of the developing cloaca in the embryo), the yolk sac (the ventral extension of the primitive endodermal canal) and its tiny vascular supply, and two umbilical arteries and two veins. Later, the right umbilical vein disappears and the umbilical cord begins to lengthen. Up to about 8 weeks, chorionic villi cover the entire chorionic sac, but with growth of the sac, there is compression atrophy of the villi along the decidua capsularis. This compressed and atrophic chorion is called the chorion leve, or smooth chorion, and constitutes the free membranes. The villi along the decidua basalis rapidly proliferate, forming the chorionic plate and villous chorion (chorion frondosum), which constitute the placental disk. The amniotic sac enlarges faster than the chorionic sac, resulting in fusion of the amnion with the chorion leve, by about 12 weeks of gestation. The chorioamnion, in turn, fuses with the decidua capsularis (Figure 1). By about 18–20 weeks of gestation, progressive enlargement of the fetal sac results in obliteration of the uterine cavity as the decidua capsularis fuses with the decidua parietalis of the opposite uterine wall. At 20 weeks of gestation, the dome of the uterus is typically palpable at the level of the maternal umbilicus; thereafter, uterine size, as measured by fundal height above the umbilicus, increases by about 1 cm/gestational week.

3

Structure of the placenta

The placenta consists of the placental disk, the extraplacental free membranes, and the umbilical cord. The fetal surface of the disk is the chorionic plate (Figure 2), and the cotyledons and basal plate constitute the maternal surface (Figure 3). The fetal surface, the chorionic plate, is covered by amnion, and normally the cord is inserted here. The free membranes are normally inserted at the margins of the disk. On microscopic examination, the following structures are noted:

(1) Placental disk: from the fetal to the maternal surface (Figure 4);

(a) Chorionic plate (fetal surface) (Figure 5): amnion, chorion, subchorionic fibrin, larger branches of umbilical blood vessels in the chorion, and smaller branches in the stem villi;

(b) Placental parenchyma (Figure 6): stem villi with smaller branches of the umbilical

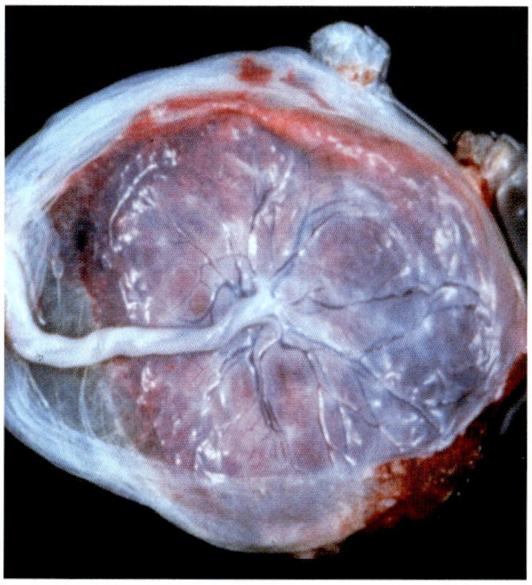

Figure 2 This placental specimen is from a spontaneous, uninfected, previable delivery at 20 weeks of gestation. The fetal surface of the placenta has a normal bluish tinge, is translucent, and shiny, the vessels of the umbilical cord split and ramify evenly over it, and the membranes attach at the placental margin

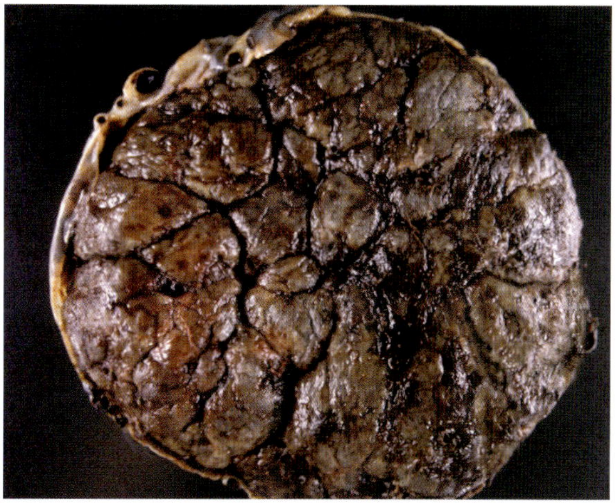

Figure 3 The maternal surface of this trimmed placenta shows numerous demarcating cotyledons. (The upper left margin of the placenta also shows cut ends of velamentous segments of an abnormal umbilical cord insertion; velamentous cord insertion is discussed in a later section in this manual)

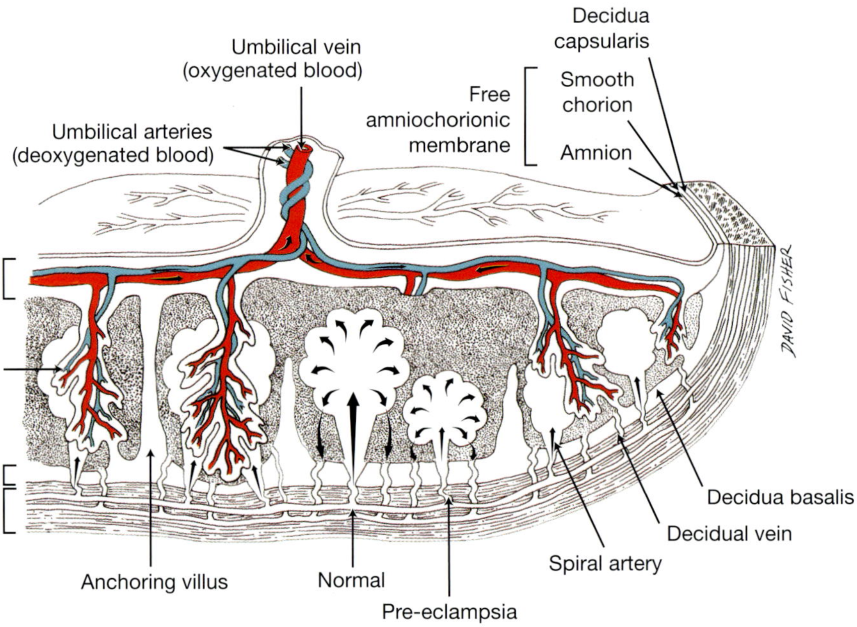

Figure 4 Cross-section of the mature placenta. The three-vessel umbilical cord consists of two arteries (carrying deoxygenated blood away from the fetus to the placenta) and a single vein (carrying oxygenated blood from the placenta to the fetus) and inserts onto the chorionic plate, which, like the cord, is covered by amniotic epithelium. The cord vessels branch within the chorion, then divide and further branch to provide the vasculature of the chorionic villous tree that is covered by villous trophoblast. The capillaries of the terminal villi contribute to the formation of vasculosyncytial membranes that enable villous transfer of oxygen and nutrients from and waste to the blood in the maternal space. The blood circulating in the maternal space is enclosed in an extravillous trophoblastic shell that is further bordered by a complex interface of fibrin and fibrinoid, maternal lymphocytes, and decidual cells. Open-ended, low-pressure, dilated, physiologically transformed arteries allow blood to enter the maternal space. The blood returns to the maternal circulation via open-ended veins. Poor adaptation of placental bed arteries, such as occurs in pre-eclampsia, may restrict blood flow to the maternal space, as pictured in this illustration, and impair placental development and function, as described in the text

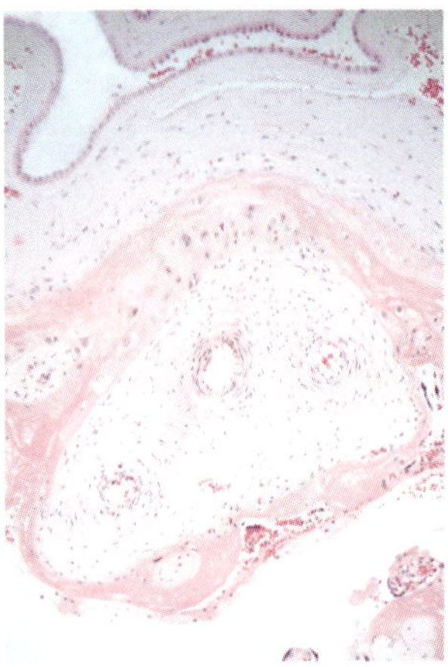

Figure 5 Chorionic plate. The amnion, chorion, and a cross-section of a large primary stem villus are included in the field

blood vessels, intermediate villi, and terminal villi, and the intervillous space;

(c) Placental septa and extravillous trophoblast cell islands (Figure 7): during embryogenesis most of the trophoblast contributes to the development of the villi; however, the extravillous trophoblast forms other chorionic portions of the placenta, i.e. the chorionic plate, chorion leve, septa, and cell islands. The septa arise from the basal plate and subdivide the placenta into grossly detectable cotyledons; the septa are identifiable as irregular grooves on the maternal surface. (As a point of clarification, a

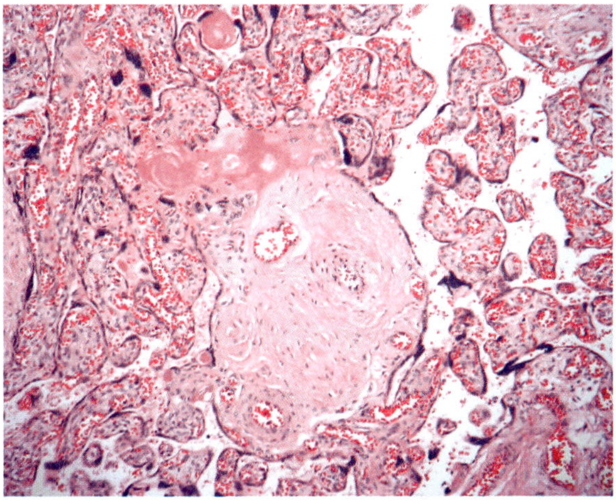

Figure 6 Placental parenchyma. A stem villus (in center), mature intermediate villi (upper and lower right), and numerous terminal villi are seen. Focal aggregates of perivillous fibrinoid and terminal villi with syncytial knots, histologic topics addressed subsequently in the text, are also present

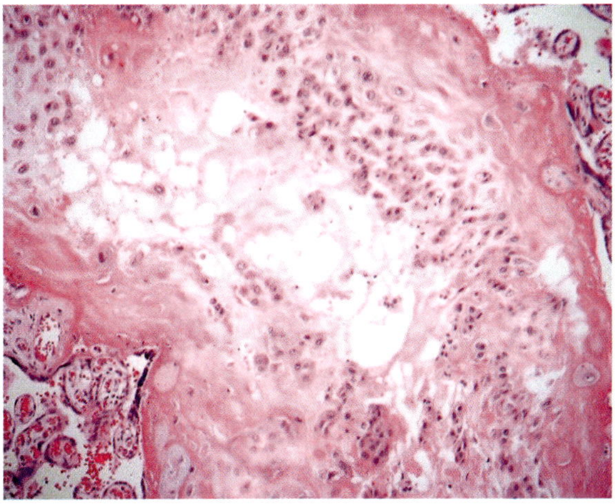

Figure 7 Septum containing extravillous trophoblast

cotyledon, therefore, does not actually correspond to a true, functional unit of the placenta, since a single cotyledon may be supplied by a number of decidual arteries.) The septa rarely reach the fetal surface and contain extravillous trophoblasts (the so-called 'X' cells and intermediate trophoblasts) and a few decidual cells. Cell islands, composed primarily of extravillous trophoblast, fibrinoid, and possibly a few decidual cells, are connected to the villous tree or chorionic plate;

(d) Basal plate (Figure 8): fibrin, extravillous trophoblast cells, decidua basalis, and maternal blood vessels.

(2) Membranes (Figure 9), from the fetal to the maternal surface: amniotic epithelium and connective tissue, potential space, chorion (composed of extravillous trophoblastic cells and involuted villi), attached fused decidua capsularis and parietalis, and maternal blood vessels within the decidua. The remnant of the yolk sac can be seen as a yellowish firm or calcified, oval, flattened nodule, a few millimeters in diameter, usually near the placental margin, but it can also be seen nearer to the cord insertion.

(3) Umbilical cord (Figures 10–12): surface epithelium, two arteries, one vein, and Wharton's jelly. Embryonic remnants may also be seen on occasion (see section on 'Embryonic remnants of the umbilical cord' in Chapter 11).

FIBRIN (FIBRINOID) IN THE PLACENTA

This eosinophilic, amorphous material, normally seen as patches on the villous surfaces, aggregates in the maternal space, and as clumps and laminations along the roof and floor of the placenta, and is one of the most prominent substances visualized in gross and microscopic examination of the placenta. It has been called 'fibrin', but this term 'fibrin' generally refers to the product of coagulation in blood vessels (i.e. acute thrombi). While the intervillous space is a vascular space of sorts, it differs because it is lined by villous trophoblast (i.e. epithelium). In addition, coagulation within the maternal space does not simply reflect activation of the *maternal* clotting cascade. 'Maternal space fibrin' also appears to include admixtures of trophoblastic secretions and products of

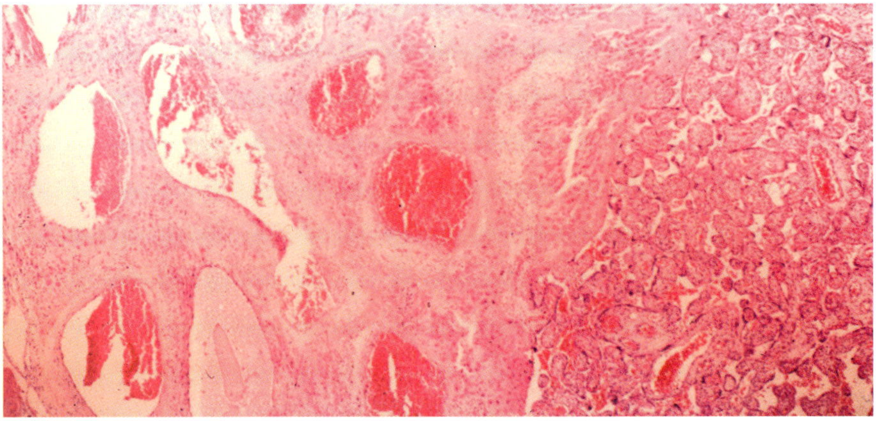

Figure 8 Basal plate showing physiologically remodeled maternal arteries in the decidua

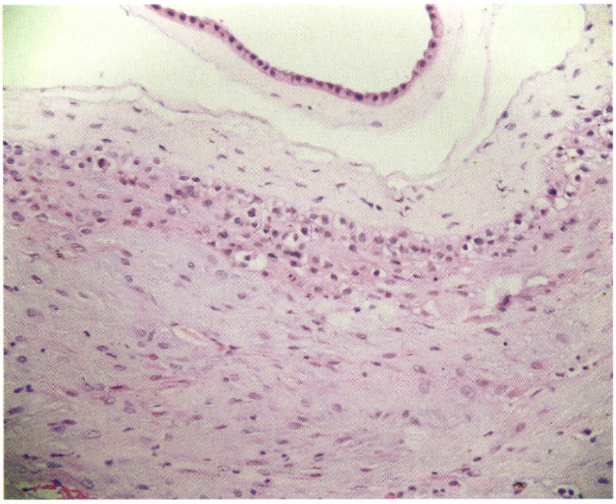

Figure 9 Free membranes. A section from the membrane roll shows the amnion, chorion, and attached decidua capsularis

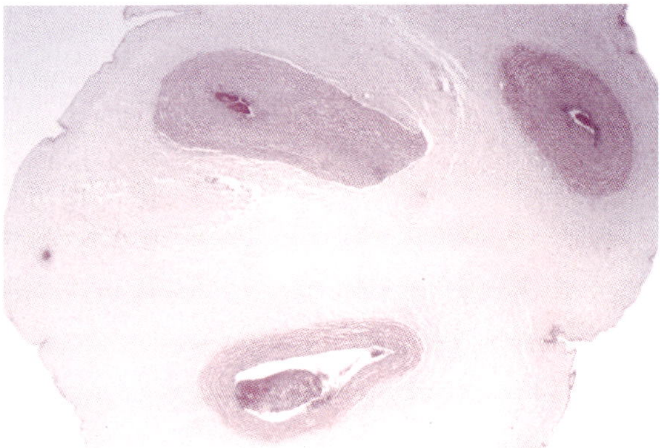

Figure 10 The umbilical cord contains two arteries and a vein. A vitelline vessel and other embryonic remnants are described in a subsequent section

cellular degeneration, hyaluronic acid, sialic acid, immunoglobulins, and albumin, etc., and it has different immunocytochemical staining characteristics and electron microscopic features from routine fibrin thrombi. Thus, some investigators have proposed that the term '*fibrinoid*' be used to distinguish this material. However, 'fibrin' and 'fibrinoid' continue to be used interchangeably in the literature, likely reflecting resistance to, or confusion over, use of the term 'fibrinoid'[3,4].

We submit that the more appropriate term for this material is 'fibrinoid', because it is likely that abnormalities in fibrinoid production are associated with pathology, and because two types of fibrinoid have been identified[5]:

(1) '*Fibrin-type fibrinoid*', consists of a meshwork of fibers with fibrin-type cross-striations, and, while primarily derived from maternal blood, it is not identical to intravascular fibrin and may contain fetal blood and other components. It is found in areas facing maternal blood, such as the perivillous surfaces, the subchorionic region, and the floor of the basal plate. It may also coat 'matrix-type fibrinoid' depositions.

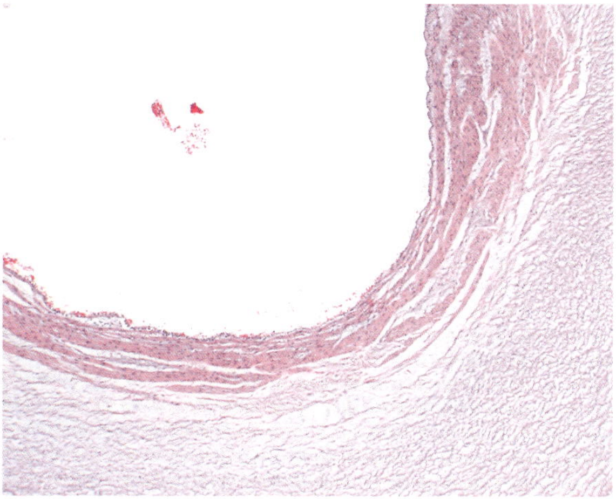

Figure 11 The umbilical venous musculature and the immediate subendothelial layer region are less compact-appearing when compared with those within the umbilical arteries. This looser arrangement of the subendothelial fibers is a very helpful feature in distinguishing the vein from an artery, especially when the vessels are dilated and/or when only one artery is present

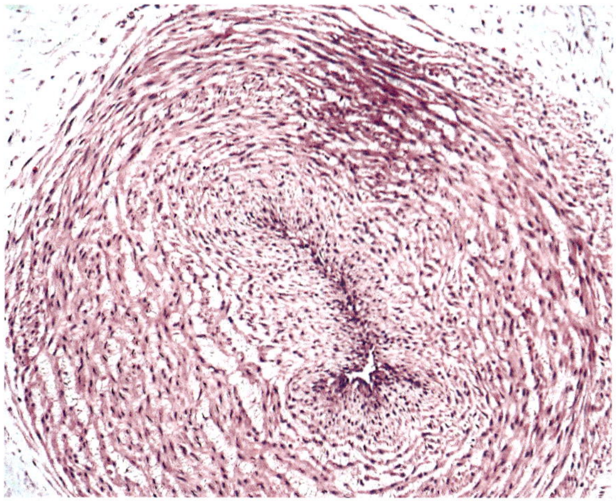

Figure 12 The umbilical arteries have a two-layer muscular wall. They have an internal elastic lamina, but, unlike the intrafetal systemic arteries of which they are extensions, they lack an external elastic lamina

(2) *'Matrix-type fibrinoid'* is mostly composed of extracellular components such as collagen IV, laminin, tenascin, fibronectin isoforms (e.g. oncofetal fibronectin), heparan sulfate, and embedded extravillous cytotrophoblast cells. Matrix-type fibrinoid is found on extravillous columns and villous tips. Furthermore, villous trophoblasts may, even in late gestation, transform to become extravillous trophoblasts and lose their polarity, and are believed to secrete matrix-type fibrinoid. At the interface with decidua, matrix-type fibrinoid may also include decidual interstitial factors.

Fibrinoid is, therefore, a normal component of the developing and mature placenta and also of its repair[4–6]. It is also likely that it has a protective role. It probably serves to sequester the fetoplacental allograft from maternal immune surveillance[7], and act as an antigen sponge barrier. It probably also contributes to the control of villous transport and helps to limit the invasion of trophoblasts at the basal plate[5].

The following localizations of fibrinoid are seen in both the normal and the abnormal placenta (in abnormal placentas, deposition is present in excessive amounts and may be of relatively abnormal compositional ratios, for the site):

(1) *Subchorionic fibrinoid* This has also been referred to as *Langhan's stria* as it forms a discontinuous layer on the inferior surface of the chorionic plate (Figure 13). It may form firm patches or plaques that are visible from the fetal surface, and shows laminations upon gross and microscopic examination. It is seen in about 20% of term placentas[3]. Deposition is related to turbulence and stasis of the maternal blood as it changes direction in the subchorionic zone. A moderate amount is of no clinical significance. While its composition of a fibrin-type fibrinoid is shared by the pathologic lesion subchorionic thrombohematoma (see section on 'Breus' mole' in Chapter 8), its thin, flat appearance and relatively small size distinguish it from the characteristic mass of subchorionic thrombohematoma.

(2) *Perivillous fibrinoid* Also referred to as *Rohr's fibrinoid* by some authors[8], perivillous fibrinoid is seen on gross examination in approximately 22% of term placentas[3] and on

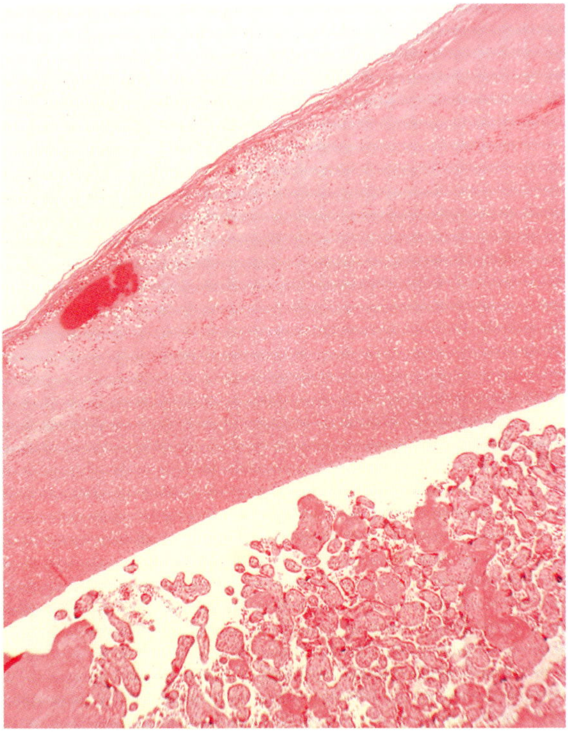

Figure 13 Subchorionic fibrinoid (Langhan's stria)

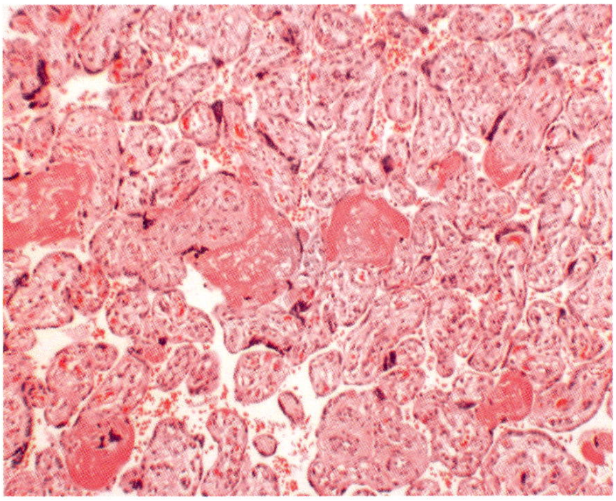

Figure 14 Perivillous fibrinoid (Rohr's fibrinoid)

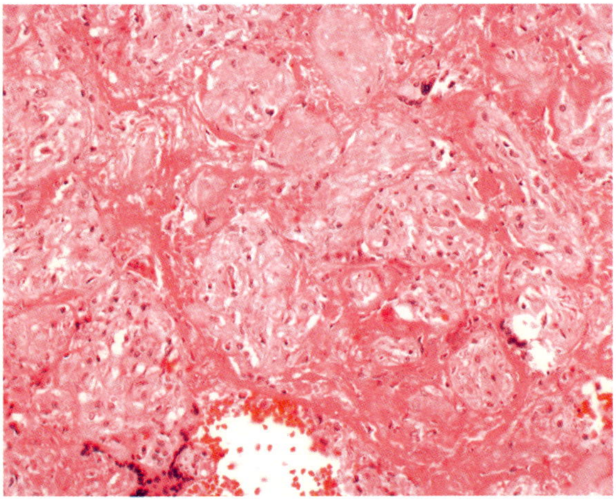

Figure 15 Much more extensive perivillous fibrinoid deposition

histologic examination of virtually all placentas (Figure 14). The foci vary from a few hundred micrometers to a few millimeters. Microscopically, individual villi may show patchy surface deposits to a more extensive layer of fibrinoid that may meet that of neighboring villi and form a mesh-like network in the intervillous space. Entrapped villi may be histologically unremarkable, or show early degeneration and loss of syncytiotrophoblast, or more advanced degeneration with stromal fibrosis and hypovascularity (Figure 15). Perivillous fibrinoid is generally fibrin-type fibrinoid and shares circulatory factors implicated in the formation of subchorionic fibrinoid, including hypoxia and acidosis. *Massive* perivillous fibrinoid deposition is a distinctly pathologic condition associated with fetal growth restriction, intrauterine fetal demise, neonatal morbidity, and a high recurrence risk in subsequent gestations (see section on 'Maternal floor infarction/massive perivillous fibrinoid deposition' in Chapter 10).

(3) *Intravillous fibrinoid* This is also called '*fibrinoid necrosis of the villi*'. It may replace villi partially or completely (Figure 16), and normally involves about 3% of the chorionic villi in a term placenta, but its detection is affected by microscopic sectional thickness. Its pathogenesis remains enigmatic, but immunologic and degenerative changes in the villi (particularly of

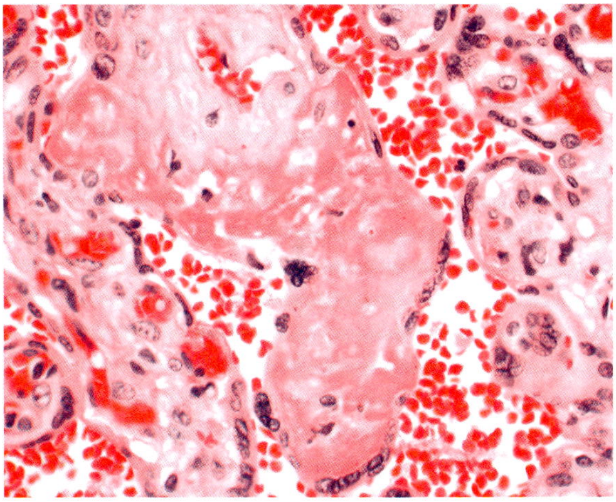

Figure 16 Intravillous fibrinoid ('fibrinoid necrosis of the villi')

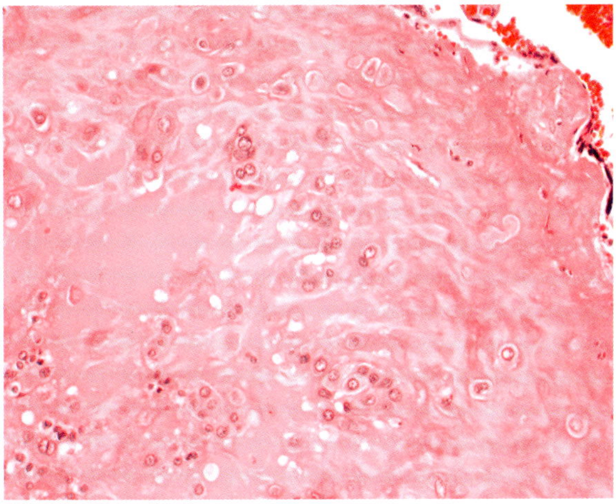

Figure 17 Fibrinoid in cell island

the cytotrophoblast) have been implicated in its pathogenesis. Antigen–antibody reactions in the villous stroma have been suggested as immunologic factors. Studies of the composition of intravillous fibrinoid, observations of its formations in rhesus (Rh) immune disease and a proportional relationship between anti-D antibody titer and the incidence of intravillous fibrinoid necrosis, and elution of immunoglobulin G (IgG) and the presence of complement, all support an immunologic etiology. However, its presence should not be taken necessarily to represent an immune-mediated attack on the trophoblastic tissue[3].

(4) *Fibrinoid deposit in cell islands and septa* Degeneration of and secretion by the extravillous cytotrophoblast has been implicated in the genesis of fibrinoid in this location (Figure 17). It is matrix-type fibrinoid.

(5) *Intervillous fibrinoid* This is also referred to as '*intervillous thrombus*' since it is usually a grossly visible 2–5-cm thrombus in the intervillous space. Villi are absent within the focus of the intervillous fibrinoid (in contrast to perivillous fibrinoid deposition). Careful histologic examination reveals the presence of nucleated erythrocytes, and evidence strongly supports a fetal origin of these red blood cells. The intervillous thrombus is an admixture of maternal and fetal blood components and represents a site of fetal blood extravasation or hemorrhage from the villi into the maternal space[3,4,9] (Figure 18).

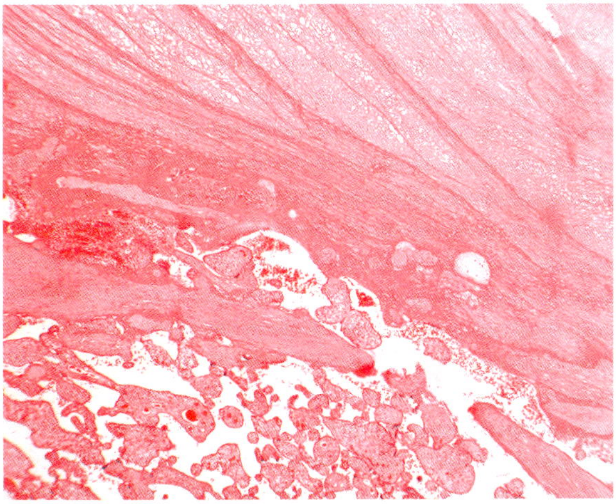

Figure 18 Intervillous fibrinoid thrombus

(6) *Superficial fibrinoid of the basal plate* This is also known as *Rohr's stria* and consists of a homogeneous or lamellar layer in the superficial aspect of the basal plate. It forms a discontinous layer of variable thickness and is

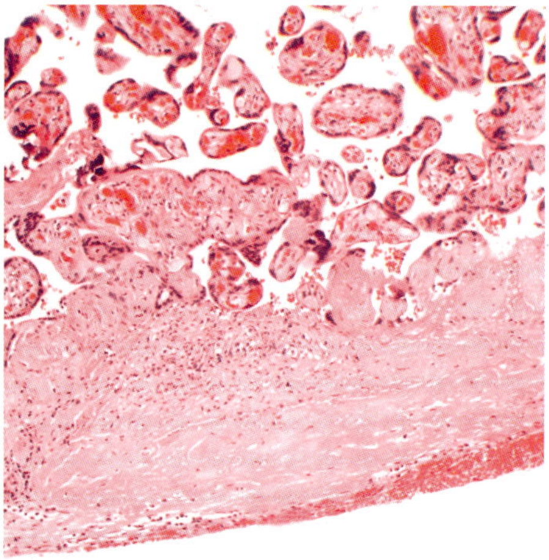

Figure 19 Uteroplacental fibrinoid of deep basal plate (Nitabuch's membrane)

probably derived from maternal fibrinogen at the basal plate. However, it may include some elements of decidual cellular degeneration. Its location and content are mostly compatible with fibrin-type fibrinoid, but some matrix-type fibrinoid may be included in its composition.

(7) *Uteroplacental fibrinoid of the basal plate* This is commonly called *Nitabuch's membrane*, and is a continous, membranous compaction of eosinophilic fibrinoid, in the basal plate at the maternofetal junctional zone (Figure 19). It is usually not grossly visible, but microscopically, it may be up to 100 μm in thickness. Decidual cells just peripheral to Nitabuch's membrane form irregular planes of separation of the placenta from the maternal tissue[3,4,8]. It is composed of both fibrin-type and matrix-type fibrinoid. As noted above, fibrinoid may help to limit chorionic villous infiltration of maternal tissue and serve in a protective role against allograft rejection. Immunologic mechanisms are favored in the pathogenesis of Nitabuch's membrane, because of both its location and its composition[4].

4

Examination of the placenta in the clinical setting

The placentas from all deliveries should be examined grossly in the clinical setting. Gross abnormalities such as incompleteness of the maternal surface, retroplacental hemorrhage, premature separation, abnormal adherence, cord hematoma, rupture of vasa previa (exposed fetal vessels from membranous cord insertion when coursing over the cervical os, meconium staining, etc.) should be noted and recorded. The length of the cord should be measured, as the full cord is often not sent to the pathology laboratory. Sampling of the fresh placenta for cytogenetics, placental cultures in cases of suspected infection or premature labor, and freezing of placental tissue in cases of possible metabolic disease may also be performed in this setting. In special cases of concern, the pathologist can assist in these preparations if informed and in receipt of the specimen promptly. Placentas meeting the indications (see below) for full examination by the pathologist, which will include further gross and microscopic evaluation, can then be sent to the laboratory. Institutional policy varies as to whether all placentas are sent or selected placentas are sent to pathology. Ideally, they should be sent to the pathology laboratory fresh; however, in some institutions, this is not feasible, and placentas are received in 10% formalin. Fresh placentas may be stored at 4°C for a week, allowing time to determine whether a neonatal issue dictates a laboratory placental examination[10].

5

Clinical data to be sent to the pathologist: how can the obstetrician ensure optimal/meaningful pathologic examination?

In an ideal world, all specimens sent to pathology would have adequate clinical information to evaluate each case appropriately. Information about the pregnancy should be given, including the mother's age, parity, week of gestation, and any problematic issues relating to the prenatal course or course of labor, such as oligohydramnios or fetal compromise, any significant maternal diseases, diagnostic or therapeutic interventions on the fetus or placenta during the pregnancy, and any abnormalities of the fetus/neonate. Information of significance includes history of trauma, substance abuse, sexually transmitted disease, pertinent maternal serological studies, signs and symptoms on admission (e.g. preterm labor, premature rupture of membranes with duration), peripartum complications such as infections, abnormalities of fetal heart rate tracings, pertinent ultrasound findings such as position, any anomalies, oligohydramnios or polyhydramnios, any infant karyotypic, structural or metabolic abnormalities, method of delivery, cord complications, total cord length if short, and vessel number. If premature separation was noted clinically, it should be described. This is particularly appreciable at cesarean section, where the percentage of placental separation can be assessed. Common obstetrical abbreviations and methods of fetal evaluation are listed in Tables 1–4. A variety of antepartum evaluations may have been performed to determine fetal well-being. Fetal movement assessment by the mother, contraction stress testing, which evaluates the fetal heart rate with contractions, non-stress testing, which evaluates the appropriate fetal heart acceleration with movement, uterine artery Doppler velocimetry, or fetal pulse oximetry may be employed. The biophysical profile described by Manning and colleagues[11] is a non-stress test combined with an ultrasound scoring system of antenatal fetal well-being, with a maximum score of 10 for five parameters. A normal score is $\geq 8/10$, with 6/10 equivocal, and 4 or less an abnormal score[1]. Placentas may be evaluated prior to delivery by ultrasound, and a grading system may be applied (grade III being a mature placenta), although no good correlation has been shown with fetal lung maturity[12]. The normal aging process of the placenta includes calcifications, on which the grading system is based. Increased calcification has also been noted in mothers who smoke cigarettes, or who have thrombotic orders and are under prophylactic therapy with aspirin or heparin[12]. At birth, the infant is also evaluated. The Apgar score, described by Virginia Apgar[13] (Table 3), is assessed at 1 min, 5 min, and sometimes again at 10 min. The 1-min score is a good indicator of the need for immediate medical intervention, while the 5-min score is prognostic of the longer-term welfare of the infant, with a score greater than or equal to 7 being a good indicator of survival. Placentas that are sent for pathological evaluation can be considered to fall into one of three categories: maternal issues, fetal issues, or placental issues (Table 5).

Table 1 Common obstetrical abbreviations

Gravida, G	gravidity, number of times pregnant	IUGR	intrauterine growth restriction
AFI	amniotic fluid index	IUFD, DIU	intrauterine fetal demise, death *in utero*
AFP	α-fetoprotein	LMP	last menstrual period
AROM	artificial rupture of membranes	NRFHR	non-reassuring fetal heart rate
BPD	biparietal diameter	NST	non-stress test
BPP	biophysical profile	Para, P	parity, the outcomes of pregnancy, usually listed as numbers of full-term, premature, abortions, living (FPAL)
CPD	cephalopelvic disproportion	PPROM	premature prolonged rupture of membranes
C-hyst	cesarean hysterectomy	PROM	prolonged rupture of membranes
CST	contraction stress test	PTL	preterm labor
EDC	estimated date of confinement (due date)	SGA, AGA, LGA	small, appropriate, or large for gestational age
EFW	estimated fetal weight	SROM	spontaneous rupture of membranes
EGA	estimated gestational age	VBAC	vaginal birth after cesarean
FHR	fetal heart rate		
GBS	group B streptococcus		
HELLP	hemolysis, elevated liver enzymes, low platelets		

Table 2 Fetal biophysical profile performed over 30 min[1,11]

Variable	*Normal = 2 points*	*Abnormal = 0*
Fetal breathing movement	at least one 30-s episode	none or none long enough
Fetal movement	at least 3	2 or fewer
Fetal tone	at least one active extension with flexion or hand open and close	slow or absent
Fetal heart rate (NST)	at least 2 accelerations above baseline of 15 s duration	fewer than 2 such accelerations
Amniotic fluid volume	at least one 2 x 2-cm pocket of fluid	pockets of fluid smaller than 2 x 2 cm

NST, non-stress test

Table 3 Apgar scores. Adapted from reference 13

	0	*1*	*2*
Heart rate	absent	< 100 beats/min	> 100 beats/min
Respiratory effort	absent	weak	vigorous, crying
Reflex irritability to catheter	none	grimace	active sneeze, cough, etc.
Muscle tone	limp	flexed arms/legs	active
Color	blue	normal except blue extremities	normal

Table 4 Clinical signs of potential fetal compromise

Late decelerations, variable decelerations with ominous features, absence of accelerations, abnormal baseline, abnormal variability, sinusoidal pattern on fetal heart tracing (normal fetal heart rate 120–160 beats/min, bradycardia < 110 beats/min, tachycardia > 160 beats/min)

Biophysical profile < 6/10

Apgar < 7 at 5 min

pH < 7.2

Non-reactive non-stress or positive stress test

Meconium (may be present in uncompromised fetuses)

Oligohydramnios

Polyhydramnios

Table 5 Indications for placental examination[2]

Maternal indications	*Fetal indications*	*Placental indications*
Diseases such as SLE, diabetes, chronic hypertension, collagen vascular disease	intrauterine fetal demise or perinatal death	small or large placenta
Poor reproductive history	intrauterine growth restriction	abruption
Pregnancy-specific conditions such as pregnancy-induced hypertension/ pre-eclampsia/eclampsia/HELLP, oligohydramnios, polyhydramnios	low birth weight, < 10th centile, or high birth weight, > 95th centile	infarction
Chorioamnionitis, infection, fever	postmaturity > 41 weeks	thrombi
Substance abuse	premature delivery ≤ 34 weeks (consider between 34 and 37 weeks)	velamentous insertion, vasa previa
Multiple bleeding episodes	indicators of clinical compromise: cord pH < 7.0, 5-min Apgar < 6, ventilator needed, severe anemia	amnion nodosum or other gross lesion
Other maternal conditions such as severe anemia, seizures	hydrops	abnormal shape, e.g. succenturiate, circumvallate, or bilobiate
Clinical concern of exposure to infection during pregnancy, such as HIV, syphilis, CMV, primary herpes, toxoplasmosis, rubella	seizures	incomplete disk
Oligohydramnios, polyhydramnios	isoimmunization	abnormally long or short cord (< 40 cm or > 70 cm)
Poor reproductive history	multiple gestation including vanishing twin after first trimester	premature rupture of membranes
Suspected abruption	admission to NICU	suspected placenta accreta
Instrumentation with concern for injury	abnormalities in pH, Apgar, heart tracing, etc.	mass
Maternal trauma	meconium	abnormal color or odor
Prolonged (> 24 h) and/or premature rupture of membranes	suspected or confirmed sepsis	cord lesions, such as thrombosis, true knot, single umbilical artery
Other maternal conditions	congenital anomalies	excessively short (< 35 cm) or long (> 75 cm) cord
	suspected or known metabolic disease	abnormal cord insertion, e.g. velamentous
	thick meconium	vasa or placenta previa
	other fetal disease or abnormality	other placental abnormality

SLE, systemic lupus erythematosus; HELLP, hemolysis, elevated liver enzymes, low platelets; HIV, human immunodeficiency virus; CMV, cytomegalovirus; NICU, neonatal intensive care unit

6

Indications for pathologic examination

Placentas are submitted to the pathology laboratory for three categories of reasons; fetal, maternal, and placental. The purpose is to evaluate for current fetal or maternal disease, to provide prognosis for the current pregnancy and future pregnancies, to evaluate the effect of maternal disease on the pregnancy, and for legal considerations. Placentas should all be examined in the delivery room. Major indications for submission of placentas to pathology are listed in Table 5 in the previous chapter[2]. This list is not all-inclusive, and any clinical concern should lead to more intensive placental evaluation.

7

Pathologic examination of the placenta: retention of the specimen and surgical pathology report

Placentas may be received either fresh or fixed, depending on institutional practice. Fresh placentas can be stored in a refrigerator, kept at 4°C, for at least a week; therefore, placentas can be held for this period and thereby enable a later pathologic examination should an indication for such examination arise. Fresh tissue has the added advantage of providing material for cultures, genetic and metabolic studies, and electron microscopy. Placentas from pregnancies with blood-borne diseases such as maternal human immunodeficiency virus (HIV) or hepatitis should be well-fixed prior to handling. Adequate fixation of a placental specimen can only be achieved if it is immersed in a truly adequate amount of formalin and in a container large enough to prevent its deformation.

GROSS EXAMINATION

Gross examination should include notation of the following features:

(1) Abnormalities of placental shape or configuration, such as a succenturiate lobe;

(2) Abnormalities of placentation, such as extrachorial (circumvallate, circum-marginate) or membranous placentation;

(3) Abnormal cord insertion, e.g. velamentous;

(4) Abnormalities of the umbilical cord, such as color, edema, hemorrhage with or without hematoma formation, trauma, torsion, stricture, false and true knots, length (remembering that the entire length is frequently not submitted to the pathologist), number of vessels;

(5) Free membranes, including site of rupture (shortest distance to the disk), translucency, color, amniotic bands, amnion nodosum, fetus papyraceus, etc. The site of rupture can provide an approximation of the site of placental implantation. A very short distance from the rupture point to the disk would indicate a lower-lying placenta, and vice versa.

Three-dimensional measurements of all lesions should be recorded, as well as an estimation of the percentage of the placenta involved in a process such as infarction. The completeness or lack of completeness of the maternal surface should be noted. Appropriate photography of lesions should be utilized.

The umbilical cord and free membranes should be removed prior to weighing the placenta, for the trimmed weight, upon which placental weight tables are based. Providing the trimmed weight also promotes consistency across institutions. Fox and colleagues have shown that formalin fixation for 24 h increases the placental weight by 7.67%; hence, fresh weight = fixed weight × 0.929[14]. If the placenta is weighed in the fixed state, this should be noted in the report.

After trimming and weighing the placenta, the fetal surface is inspected for translucency and color of membranes, presence of lesions such as amnion nodosum, subamniotic or subchorionic hemorrhage, thrombosed fetal vessels, or surface cysts. In fused twin placentas, the dividing membrane should be evaluated for degree of translucency, and vascular anastomoses should be evaluated (see section on 'Twin placentas' in Chapter 15).

The maternal surface is inspected for completeness, tears, calcification, plaques, adherent blood clots and whether or not there is parenchymal compression associated with such a clot.

The disk is then sliced at intervals of 0.5–1.0 cm from the maternal to the fetal surface, the slicing stopping short of the chorionic plate to maintain orientation and integrity of the placental disk, to evaluate for gross parenchymal lesions such as cysts, intervillous thrombi (round or oval soft dark lesions), subchorionic fibrin plaques (whitish, firm), perivillous fibrin (firm to hard, white, yellowish or brownish), recent infarct (dark-red firm, triangular, more palpable than visible), or older infarcts (firmer brown to yellow to white). Areas of pallor may correspond to the chorionic villous distribution of a thrombosed fetal stem artery. Punctate, yellowish foci of necrosis may represent an intrauterine infection with *Listeria*, syphilis, or herpes virus.

SECTIONS FOR HISTOLOGIC EXAMINATION

The number of sections taken varies among institutions, but it is more critical that the appropriate areas be examined. If multiple pieces are packed into a cassette, often the full surface of a placental section, or a full cross-section of umbilical cord, is not obtained. At a minimum, three sections should be submitted for histological examination. One cassette would then contain two membrane rolls (Figure 20), with the point of rupture at the center, and two cross-sections of umbilical cord, one from the fetal end and one from the maternal end. This may take more than a single cassette. Two additional cassettes should each contain a full-thickness (maternal to fetal surface) section from different central portions of the placenta, away from the periphery. Peripheral placental tissue is less well perfused than central tissue, and the finding of ischemic changes in peripheral placental tissue is not always representative of placental function as a whole. If the histology laboratory cannot consistently obtain good sections with three cassettes, more should be considered. Additional sections should most certainly be submitted in order to document lesions. The pathologist should divide a sample section of placenta, if its transmural dimension exceeds the dimensions of the cassette and, therefore, cannot be submitted as a full-thickness section in a single cassette. We recommend submitting such a divided sample in two consecutive cassettes. However, sections may be submitted with one cassette containing two fetal surface sections, one with larger fetal vessels and one with smaller vessels, and one cassette with two maternal surface sections with complete basal plate. There is ample evidence that a shave section, taken *parallel* to the maternal surface, greatly increases the detection of decidual vasculopathy, decidual infiltrates, and myometrial fibers, and the authors strongly recommend this simple practice[15,16]. When grossly undetected lesions are

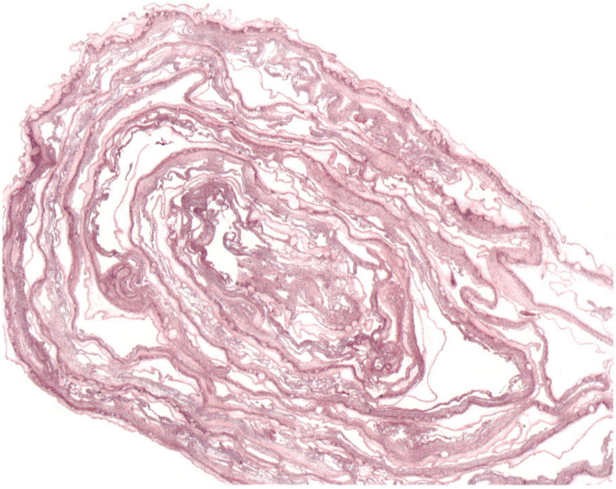

Figure 20 Membrane roll, low-power view. These sections optimize the area that can be evaluated on a single slide

discovered during microscopic examination, then the submission of additional sections becomes necessary in order to evaluate the extent of the lesions and their potential clinical significance. Finally, since the placenta is a blood-laden tissue, it is especially important to ensure adequate fixation of the tissue samples, prior to histologic processing.

SURGICAL PATHOLOGY REPORT

The usual patient demographics and clinical history should be included. A sample gross examination template is shown in the Appendix. Numerous descriptive terms and/or pathologies are listed for each of the major aspects of the gross placental examination. They are included as potential options from which the pathologist can simply select those most applicable for his/her given specimen and potential pathologies to include or exclude, accordingly, in order to reduce risks of underappreciation or inadvertent omission of potentially significant features. This approach has appreciably aided trainees in pathology, in our experience. The microscopic examination can be thought of in terms of compartments, for convenience, making sure to address the umbilical cord, membranes, chorionic villi, and decidua. The inclusion of a microscopic description, in the surgical pathology report, prior to the final diagnosis, is at the discretion of the pathologist. We recommend that a pathologist's comment should be included that relates the placental findings to the *known* clinical history of the mother, intrapartum events, and/or the fetus/infant. We strongly recommend that such information be sought if not provided[17].

RETENTION OF SPECIMENS

Fixed wet tissue, slides, and blocks should be retained according to regulatory requirements and institutional policy as it applies to surgical pathology tissues.

8

Gross abnormalities of the placenta: lesions due to disturbances of maternal and of fetal blood flow

Patchy or isolated gross lesions of the placenta can be categorized as those primarily resulting from disturbances of maternal blood flow to or within the placenta and those primarily resulting from disturbances of fetal blood flow to the placenta (Table 6). It should be noted that many of the lesions addressed in this chapter and in Chapter 9 on 'Histologic lesions of the placenta' exist in the normal placenta (Table 7). Those abnormalities that affect the placental disk as a whole, or are more likely to show a more extensive involvement, such as maternal floor infarction/massive perivillous fibrinoid deposition, are dealt with in Chapter 10.

As stated in the earlier section on 'Fibrin (fibrinoid) in the placenta' in Chapter 3, the maternal space is a unique milieu, and fibrinoid is a complex material whose composition reflects varying admixtures of maternal, trophoblastic, and fetal blood components. Fibrinoid production, therefore, is a complex process because, in addition to the components named in the aforementioned section, there is also mounting evidence that the villous and non-villous cytotrophoblasts elaborate their own separate, unique class of protease activators, inhibitors, and receptors of thrombogenesis/thrombolysis. These molecules are important in early trophoblastic invasion of the decidua, but they also appear to be expressed later for additional roles in a kind of trophoblastic 'paracoagulation complex'. The molecules bear some structural similarities to the elements of the classic, hematologically based cascade, and they also show activity profiles which indicate that they interact with each other and with elements of the maternal system[18–23]. Their properties and patterns of trophoblastic cellular surface expression and elaboration provide supportive evidence that they probably act to maintain the fluidity of the maternal space so critical for maternofetal exchange[24,25].

Figure 21 is a composite representation of the various placental lesions associated with abnormalities of either maternal or fetal blood flow, and supplements the discussions of these entities and the differences among them, which follow.

LESIONS DUE TO DISTURBANCES OF MATERNAL BLOOD FLOW

Perivillous fibrinoid deposition

Gross features These lesions are firm to hard, irregularly outlined, but usually sharply demarcated, and yellowish-white, nodular aggregates. They are most frequently seen at the placental margin and are usually only a few millimeters in maximal dimension. (Larger deposits usually represent intervillous hematomas (see later in this chapter) and displace villi, rather than coating them.)

Table 6 Normal range of gross and microscopic lesions of the term placenta

Feature	*Normal range*
Subchorionic fibrinoid	present in 20% of term placentas
Intervillous fibrinoid (thrombus)	present in 36% of term placentas
Infarct(s)	present in 25% of term placentas (involving < 5% of parenchyma)
Grossly demonstrable perivillous fibrin	present in 22% of term placentas (histologically demonstrable perivillous fibrin present in virtually all placentas)
Stromal fibrosis	seen in ~ 3% of villi at term
Syncytial knots	seen in 11–30% of villi at term
Vasculosyncytial membranes (VSM)*	uncommon until 32 weeks; increase rapidly after 32 weeks; at term 20% villi show VSM
Thickened trophoblastic basement membrane	seen in ~ 3% of villi of term placentas
Cytotrophoblast†	20% villi at term show inconspicuous, flattened cells
Fetal artery thrombosis	seen in 4.5% of term placentas
Obliterative endarteritis	seen in 10% of term placentas

*VSM deficiency: VSM in < 5% villi; †cytotrophoblastic hyperplasia: prominent cytotrophoblast in > 20% of villi at term; VSM and cytotrophoblast numbers detected depend upon 5-μm section thickness

Table 7 Gross lesions of the placenta

Lesions due to disturbances of maternal flow to or through the placenta
Perivillous fibrinoid deposition
Subchorionic fibrinoid plaque
Massive subchorial thrombosis/thrombohematoma (Breus' mole)
Basal intervillous thrombus
Intervillous lakes
Retroplacental hematoma
Marginal hematoma
Maternal surface infarction
Chorionic villous infarction
'X cell' or chorionic cysts
Lesions due to disturbances in fetal blood flow to the placenta
Intervillous thrombus (including Kline's hemorrhage)
Fetomaternal hemorrhage (major)
Subamnionic hematoma
Fetal arterial thrombosis

Histology These foci are lamellar, eosinophilic, amorphous deposits surrounding or partially covering villi, and superficially are fibrin-type fibrinoid; they may cover islands of matrix-type fibrinoid or encase clusters of villi[5] (Figure 22). The underlying syncytiotrophoblast degenerates and progressively disappears; there is villous fibrosis, vascular obliteration, and cytotrophoblastic proliferation.

Incidence It is reportedly seen in 22% of term placentas[3], but some investigators submit that it is present and multifocal in virtually all mature placentas[4]. Perivillous fibrinoid deposition is nonrandom[6], occurring at sites of de-epithelialization with apoptosis and syncytiotrophoblast injury, and increases with gestation, especially on the surfaces of stem villi; it is uncommon to find significant amounts prior to 32 weeks of pregnancy. It is markedly increased in maternal floor infarction/massive perivillous fibrinoid deposition (see Chapter 10), and increased in placentas with maternal

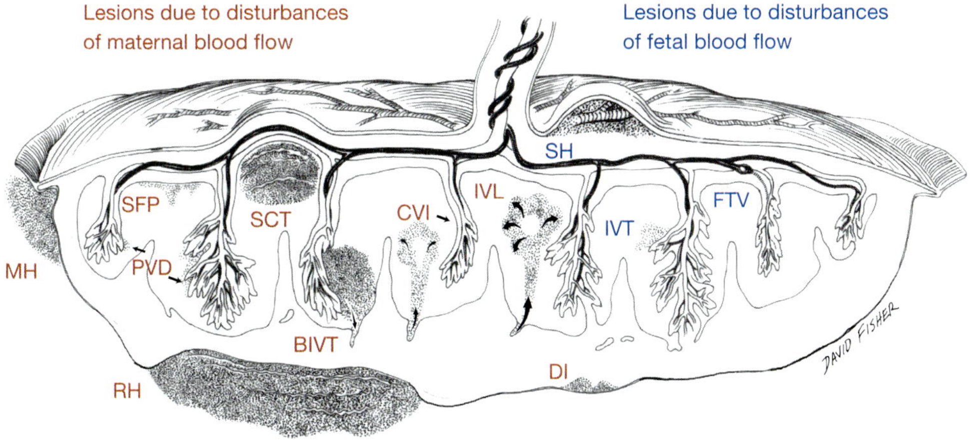

Figure 21 Lesions due to disturbances of maternal and fetal blood flow. This composite illustrates the various lesions resulting from disturbances in either maternal (labeled in red) or fetal (labeled in blue) blood flow. However, intervillous thrombi (IVT), while initiated by disturbances in fetal blood flow, incorporate maternal blood components, since they extend into the maternal space (See text for full discussion of these entities). Maternal: MH, Marginal hematoma; SFP, subchorionic fibrinoid plaque; PVD, perivillous fibrinoid deposition; RH, retroplacental hematoma; SCT, subchorionic thrombus; BIVT, basal intervillous thrombus; CVI, chorionic villus infarction; IVL, intervillous lake; DI, decidual infarction. Fetal: SH, subamnionic hematoma; IVT, intervillous thrombus; FTV, fetal thrombotic vasculopathy

thrombophilia[26] and ischemia. Large portions of the villous tree embedded in fibrinoid have been called '*Gitter infarcts*'[27], and are abnormal.

Pathogenesis Fibrinoid deposition occurs due to eddy currents and stasis within the intervillous space that presumably leads to hypoxia. The normally relatively hypoxic zones of the placenta, the subchorial and basal strata, and the marginal zones are the sites that normally exhibit perivillous fibrinoid deposition. (Thus, routine sampling of the margin is rarely informative.) Perivillous fibrinoid also replaces gaps left by loss of damaged syncytiotrophoblast; exposure of the basement membrane and its collagen and laminin components initiates clotting.

Significance Since placentas have a good reserve capacity, loss of ≤ 30% of the villous population and lesions of moderate distribution may not have any effect on fetal oxygenation or growth or be of clinical significance. However, larger areas of involvement may be associated with fetal loss[3,8], and caution should be exercised particularly in cases in which the placenta is small for the period of gestation and/or if the placenta shows injury by more than one lesion. In these instances, the cumulative effect of multiple injurious processes that include perivillous fibrinoid deposition, fetal thrombotic vasculopathy, prominent chronic intervillositis, and other lesions, addressed in subsequent sections, may result in fetal demise or postnatal manifestations of neurologic damage in the infant[28,29].

Excessive amounts of fibrinoid effectively encase individual villi and villous clusters and impede villous transport. When massive, they can create abnormal channels and baffles that interfere with normal blood circulation in the maternal space and can contribute to villous ischemia. Moreover, by increasing the diffusion distance for maternal oxygen, fibrin-type fibrinoid deposition may stimulate extravillous trophoblastic transformation and exacerbate the deposition of matrix-type fibrinoid[5]. Excessive perivillous fibrinoid is associated with perinatal morbidity, including fetal intrauterine growth restriction, and perinatal mortality.

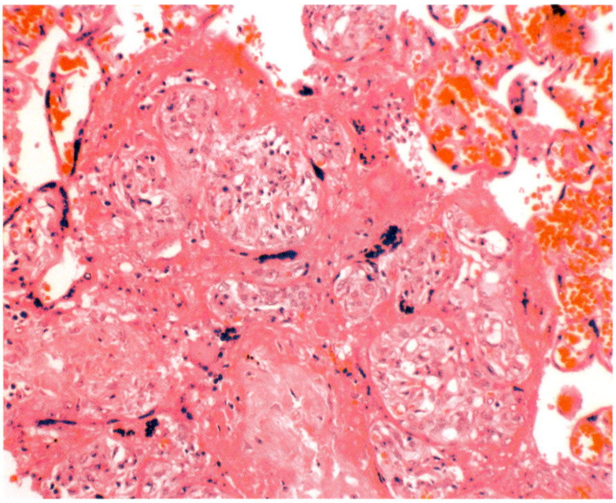

Figure 22 Perivillous fibrinoid encasing clusters of villi; see also Figures 14 and 15

Subchorionic fibrinoid plaque

Gross features These lesions appear as firm to hard, white-yellow, laminated plaques in the subchorionic area (Figure 23). They can be several centimeters in greatest dimension and protrude, like inverted pyramids, into the parenchyma below. Often they may exhibit transmural extension, from the subchorion to the maternal surface. Fresh thrombus may be seen at their borders with the placental parenchyma.

Histology Laminated fibrin-type fibrinoid is seen under the chorionic plate. No villi are included, since the fibrinoid is deposited in plaques against the trophoblastic monolayer covering the undersurface of the chorion (Figure 23). At their deep aspects new thrombus can be seen, becoming converted into fibrinoid.

Incidence As can be inferred from the above discussion, subchorionic fibrinoid deposition increases with gestation. It is seen in ~ 20% of mature placentas.

Pathogenesis Turbulence, stasis, and eddy currents in the deflected blood in the subchorionic space have been implicated as the etiologic factors.

Significance The lesions have not been identified to be of clinical significance, but they are noted to be increased in maternal cardiac disease[4].

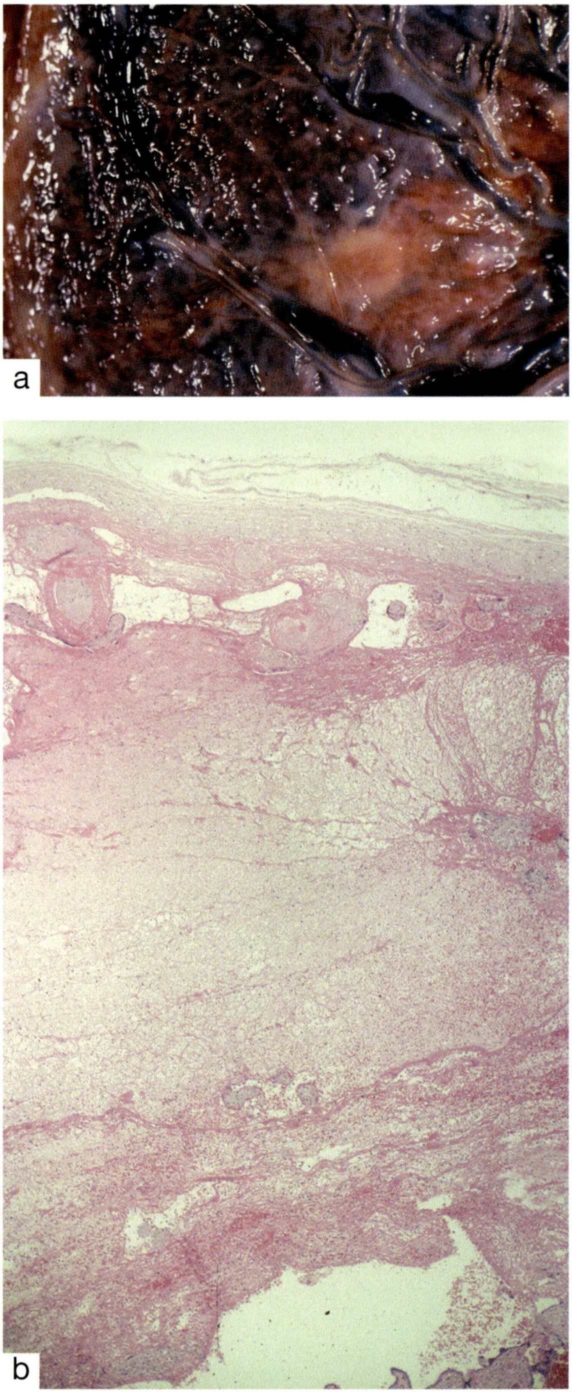

Figure 23 (a) Subchorionic fibrinoid plaque. (b) This subchorionic fibrinoid plaque shows displaced chorionic villi at its perimeters and a few entrapped villi in its deeper, right aspects

Subchorial thrombosis/ thrombohematoma (Breus' mole)

Gross features This lesion is a large nodular protuberance on the fetal surface that is due to thrombus formation in the subchorionic zone. As can be inferred from the discussion of subchorionic fibrinoid above, the subchorionic zone is a site where the maternal (intervillous) blood is deflected against the underside of the chorionic plate and eddies. Thus, virtually all placentas have small amounts of fibrinoid accumulations and these become increasingly detectable in third-trimester placentas. However, deposition of subchorionic fibrinoid is a chronic process progressing slowly during the pregnancy, whereas subchorial thrombohematoma represents a more acute event, resulting in a large to massive coagulum that involves a large portion of the subchorionic zone. It generally undergoes liquefaction hemolysis and color change from dark red (acute thrombohematoma) to brown red, laminated, and progressively organizing and more chronic mass with pale white-yellow areas (Figure 24) to one with a brown-greenish color of distinctly old lesion (Figure 25). A Breus' mole (coagulated mass) can be so large that it is detectable by prenatal ultrasonography as a protuberance bulging from the fetal surface.

Histology The lesion consists of thickly laminated fibrin admixed with erythrocytes. No villi are present in the lesion. It should be distinguished from the *subamnionic hematoma*, which lies *between* the amnion and chorion and is due entirely to *fetal* blood extravasation (see section on 'Lesions due to disturbances of fetal blood flow').

Incidence It is difficult to assess their true incidence, but Shanklin and Scott[30] found thrombohematomas in 1 : 1200 placentas from gestations of 25 or more weeks' duration. They are also more commonly seen with Monosomy X[4] and are associated with maternal thrombophilia[31].

Pathogenesis The etiopathogenesis remains unknown. Breus (1892) first recognized these as large 'sacculations' of blood and thrombus, on the fetal surface, associated with missed abortions. He interpreted these 'sacculations' to be postmortem artifacts (i.e. subchorionic diverticuli that resulted from continued maternal pressure in the intervillous space pressing against the shrinking amniotic cavity of a dead fetus and creating protrusions on the fetal surface). However, they were later recognized to be non-artifactual and prenatal formations, in the series studied by Shanklin and Scott[30], and associated with infant death in the neonatal period. While many of the maternal subjects in the series had other diseases, including diabetes mellitus and hypertension, no

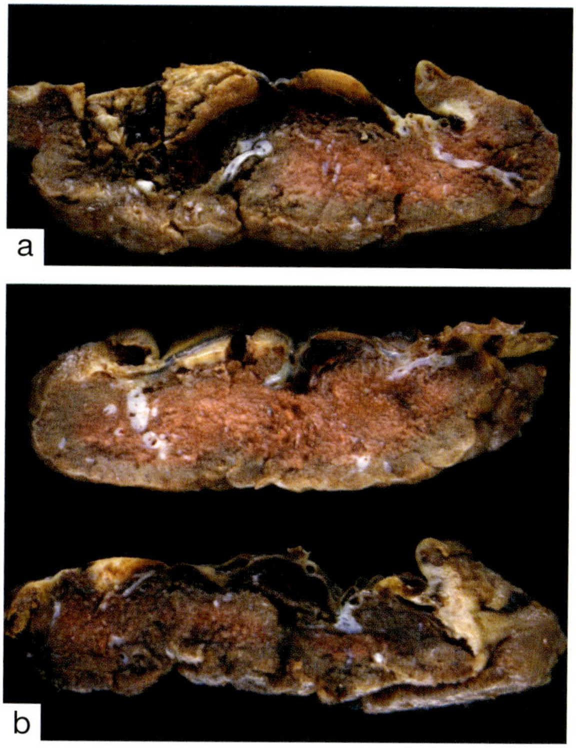

Figure 24 (a) This transmural placental section shows a massive subchorionic Breus' mole with a prominent superficial organized component and a deep transition to a fresher component. There is some compression and distortion of the subjacent chorionic villous tissue, with some ischemia. The left side of the large thrombohematoma has been further sectioned to reveal a central zone of liquefaction. (b) This shows additional transmural sections of the same placenta and areas of both chronic thrombohematoma and more recent extension with fibrin lamination. Note that the chorionic plate vessels lie atop each protuberance of the thromobohematoma

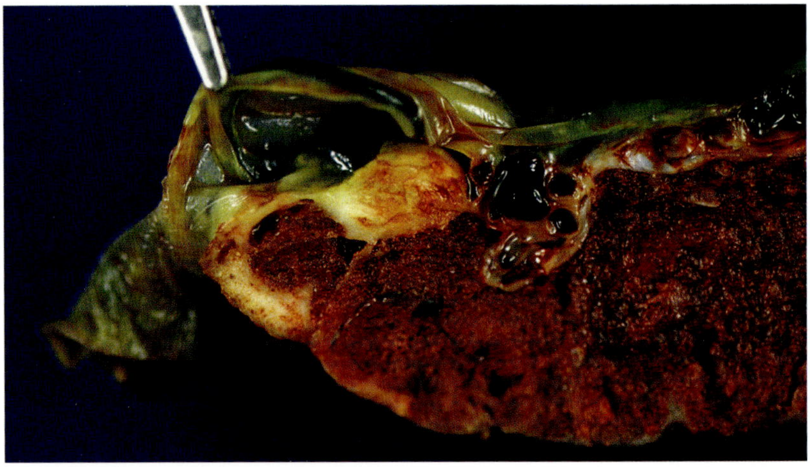

Figure 25 This old, subchorionic thrombohematoma is marginal (see sections on 'Marginal hematoma' and 'Extrachorial placenta' for comparison) and largely degenerated, consisting of a subchorionic saccular cavity filled with thin greenish fluid. The roof of the sac is coursed by chorionic plate vessels, which, microscopically, were in a hemosiderin-laden chorionic stroma. The uneven floor of the cavity was made up of densely laminated fibrinoid with foci of dystrophic mineralization

particular underlying etiopathogenesis for Breus' mole was identified. Benirschke and Kaufmann[4] include them in their discussion of subchorionic fibrin masses; perhaps in some cases they begin as plaques but progress to protrude into the amniotic cavity. Recently, maternal hypercoagulability has been identified as a likely pathogenic component[31].

Significance Their significance remains unclear. Some investigators consider their presence to be of no particular clinical significance. However, other studies have identified them as risk factors for perinatal morbidity and mortality. If near the cord insertion site, they may result in some compression and compromise of the cord vasculature[4]. Heller and colleagues[31] have suggested that a Breus' mole may be a *forme fruste* of an underlying maternal thrombophilic condition.

Basal intervillous thrombi

Gross features The basal intervillous thrombus may be acute, red, soft, and ovoid, or show laminations. With age, its color changes to pale pink or tan-white, and its texture becomes firm. Basal intervillous thrombi are usually 2–5-cm lesions that widely separate the parenchyma of the villous tree. They are commonly mistaken for infarctions (see section on 'Chorionic villous infarction'), but differ in that they are not granular and do not actually involve villi, but merely displace them. Grossly, except for their characteristic, basal, and paraseptal (intercotyledonary) distribution, they may be difficult to differentiate from the more common, *central* intervillous thrombi that more often contain *fetal* erythrocytes and represent sites or sequelae of fetomaternal extravasations and hemorrhages (see section on 'Lesions due to disturbances of fetal blood flow').

Histology Basal intervillous thrombi are characterized by fibrin/fibrinoid lamellae admixed with essentially non-nucleated (maternal) erythrocytes that show degenerative features. Aging thrombi may show denser lamination and progressive lysis of entrapped erythrocytes, but intervillous thrombi do not exhibit fibroblastic ingrowth or collagen deposition. Chronic thrombi may contain scattered maternal hemosiderin-laden macrophages. The underlying decidua may show necrosis.

Incidence Scattered lesions are seen in normal, mature placentas as incidental findings, but are increased in conditions of placental bed ischemia, such as hypertension and pre-eclampsia (Figure 26a),

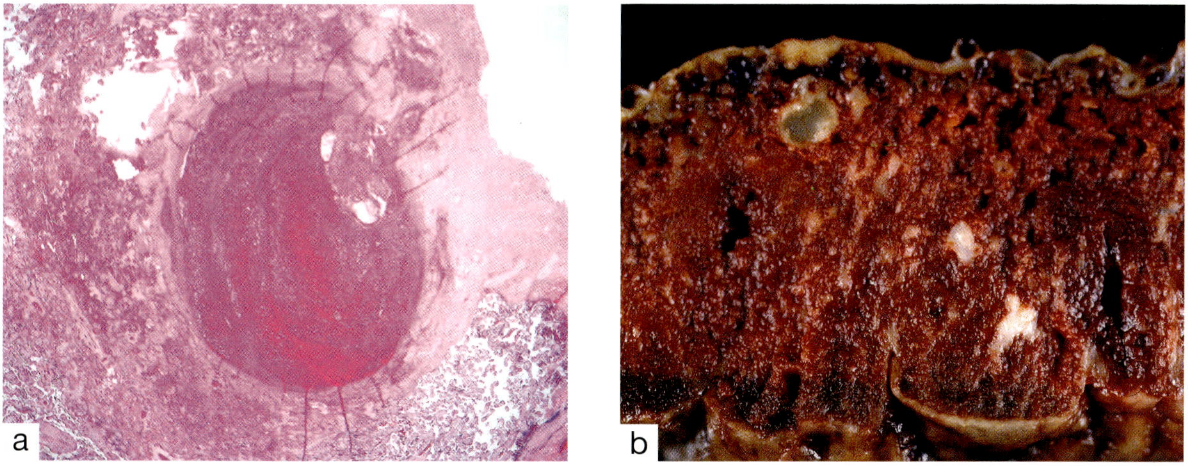

Figure 26 (a) This low-power section from a third-trimester placenta from a gestation complicated by pre-eclampsia demonstrates an acute, basal intervillous thrombus that displaces adjacent ischemic and infarcted chorionic villi. The underlying decidua shows infarction. Basal intervillous thrombi in these settings may not be adjacent to septa. (b) Several lower to mid-parenchymal intervillous lakes ('holes') are present in this transmural placental section. In addition, a small, extravillous trophoblastic cell cyst, seen as a simple, whitish-yellow cavity in the subchorionic parenchyma, is present (see section on 'X cell cysts')

and in maternal floor infarction (see section below) and maternal thrombophilias.

Pathogenesis While there is debate as to whether these lesions are truly separate from those that include fetal blood (see section on 'Lesions due to disturbances of fetal blood flow'), most are believed to be the result of *thrombosis of decidual veins* that drain the placental bed[4].

Significance In isolation, or in limited number and size, they are not significant. When observed frequently on cross-section in the basal region, they should be considered indicators of maternal vascular disease and/or venous thrombosis.

Intervillous lakes

Gross features These are manifest as 'holes' in transmural sections and are normal findings that reflect 'jet sites' from decidual arterioles. These hollow-appearing foci are surrounded by red to dark-red blood (Figure 26b).

Histology Foci are variably detectable microscopically, depending upon post-delivery interval, compression of the parenchyma, drainage of the maternal space with storage, and sectioning. They may show relative loss of erythrocytes in the maternal space or simply be evidenced by deviation of the chorionic villous tree.

Incidence They are commonly seen in third-trimester placentas.

Pathologic significance They are not truly pathologic lesions, but they may cause concern, to the unfamiliar.

Retroplacental hematoma

Gross features The lesions may involve variable portions of the maternal surface. The site of the hematoma, and percentage of the surface it occupies, should be estimated. Many hematomas may be small and are more easily demonstrated in serial sections of the placenta. The hematoma may compress the overlying parenchyma, which may show chorionic villous infarction. The fresh, acute hematoma is soft, bright red, and can easily be separated from the maternal surface (Figure 27). Thus, an acute hematoma may become detached during delivery or transport of the specimen to the laboratory, and the detached clot may not be sent to the laboratory. Within approximately 24 h of the formation of the hematoma (and/or its ongoing formation), it may compress the maternal surface and basal parenchyma (Figure 28). The presence of a shallow, crater-like depression on the maternal surface bordered by congested chorion villous parenchyma, therefore, is a finding highly suggestive of a site of a previous retroplacental hematoma, even in the absence of an accompanying portion of blood clot. Part, or the entirety, of a blood clot, when submitted, may have contours similar to that of the crater and fit snugly within the cavity. In some cases, however, a large amount of loose blood clot accompanying the specimen may be the only clue to the presence of retroplacental hematoma (RH). Older hematoma is red-brown to brown and firm, it is adherent to the maternal surface, and, depending upon its duration of presence, produces a depression or frank crater. The chronic hematoma shows peripheral 'organization' consisting of brown-red to golden brown to tan-white, compact laminations with alternating layers of gelatinous blood and a dry, friable texture. In its most central aspects, the hematoma remains dark red and unorganized. The maternal surface is deeply hollowed, its cavity containing portions of the multinodular organized hematoma. The overlying, compressed placental parenchyma shows progression from chronically infarcted (pale, firm, and granular) chorionic villous tissue in areas immediately adjacent to the hematoma, to recently or acutely infarcted (congested, compressed and hemorrhagic tissue) chorionic villous tissue in better-preserved, generally more distant areas. The chronic hematoma may also exhibit superimposed and superficially dissecting, acute hematoma. The chorion of the free membranes and fetal plate may show hemosiderosis. A massive chronic RH, demonstrating many of these features, is shown in a composite view in Figure 29. In contrast to the chronic hematoma, the acute RH may not produce any depression on the maternal surface or delimited region of parenchymal hyperemia. A large amount of blood clot, accompanying the specimen, may be the only clue to the presence of RH.

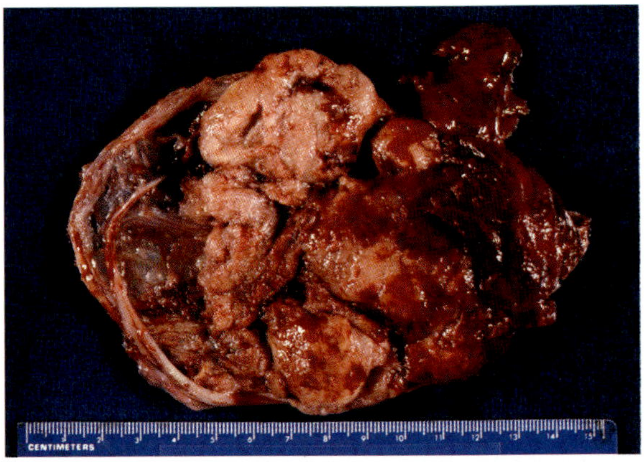

Figure 27 A fresh, soft bright-red retroplacental hematoma is seen on the maternal surface of this placenta from a 28-week gestation. The mother presented with abdominal pain and passage of bright-red blood per vaginam

However, acute RH should be distinguished from an incidental, simple blood clot on the maternal surface. Incidental clot is usually thin, localized, and easily removed, and produces no depression on the maternal surface and is not associated with chorionic villous infarction or membranous insertional abnormalities.

Histology The features are 'age-dependent'. However, for obvious ethical reasons, there is no controlled study of the onset of clinical placental abruption with the generation of a definitive, correlative time-line of histopathologic change of aging (period of intrauterine duration) of RH. Forensic pathology has provided some understanding of the changes, but not all RH is due to trauma, the timing of the traumatic event does not necessarily coincide with the onset of RH, and clinical abruption may not be evident in at least one-third of cases of RH. In addition, pathologic dating of the RH is difficult, since organization of a RH is different from organization of intravascular thrombus; there is no fibroblastic ingrowth and the center may remain essentially unaltered for a long time. In the acute RH, a few to sometimes numerous and laminated peripheral strands of fibrin can be seen, together with a peripheral polymorphonuclear leukocyte reaction in the overlying basal plate. Erythrocytes can be aggregated or pale, or exhibit lysis. Acute formations may exhibit no ischemic chorionic villous histopathology, or intravillous hemorrhage[32] and non-specific decidual features. 'Recent' hematomas may show hemosiderin-laden macrophages in the maternal space and solidification of the laminations. The adjacent chorionic villi show recent to chronic infarction with ghost-like remnants of degenerated villi and intervillous thrombi. Preserved chorionic villi may show fetal normoblastemia. Decidual necrosis with hemosiderosis is often prominent[3,4]. However, it must be stressed that there are also no published criteria of discrete features that distinguish the classification of the 'acute' from the 'recent' RH; there is considerable histopathologic overlap, and light microscopic findings may reflect both sampling- and time-dependent factors.

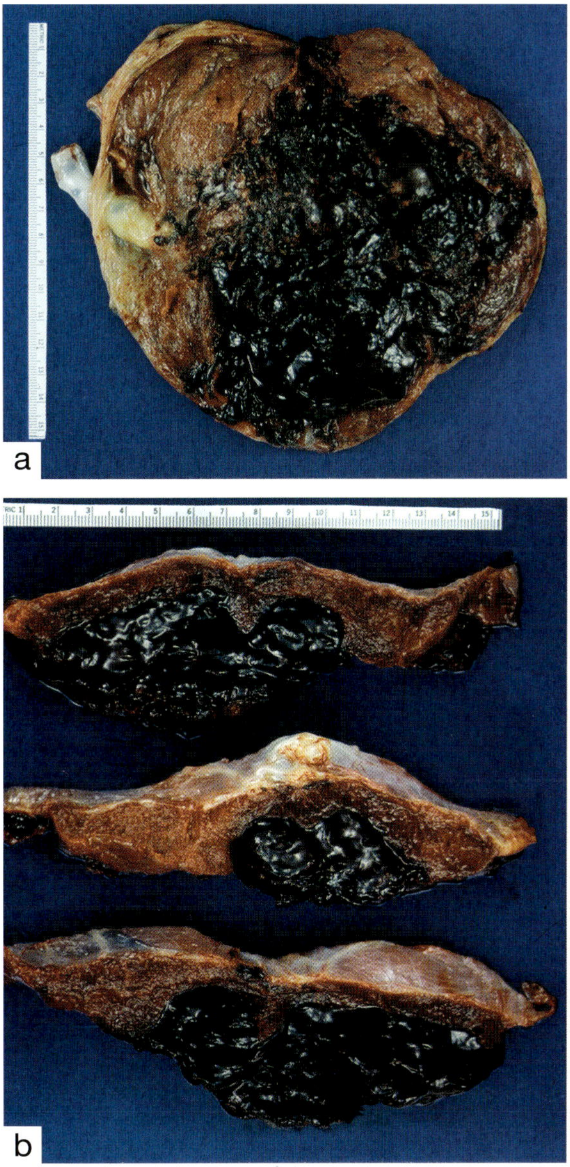

Figure 28 These views demonstrate a massive, acute retroplacental hematoma (RH) that caused a marked crater-like depression on the maternal surface (a). Serial sections show its depression of the basal to mid-zonal parenchyma (b). Note the darker-red coloration of the clot compared with that of the RH in Figure 27

Incidence RH is seen in 4.5% of all placentas[3]. The incidence is higher in placentas from gestations complicated by pre-eclampsia, hypertension, and thrombophilias. However, RH is an *anatomic* diagnosis and shows only partial overlap with the occurrence of the *clinical* condition of placental abruption. Therefore, it is important to underscore that abruptio placentae (AP) is a *clinical* diagnosis based on findings that include uterine enlargement, maternal hemorrhage and/or shock, and the clinical impression of premature separation of the placenta from its site of implantation; the term is usually reserved for normally implanted placentas (and distinguished from bleeding associated with placenta previa and vasa previa). AP occurs in about 0.5% of deliveries[33]. RH is present in only about 30% of cases of clinically diagnosed AP and, conversely, the presence of RH is accompanied by the clinical syndrome of abruption in only about 35% of cases. Nevertheless, some correlations exist: AP is more common among preterm (5.1%)[34] than among term deliveries (0.3%)[35], and RH is also more commonly identified in preterm placentas. Part of the clinicopathologic correlative discrepancy likely reflects the variation in criteria used for the diagnosis of AP, since it may be especially difficult to detect in its earliest stages. AP may result in dissection of blood around the placental margin and behind the membranes, and the onset of vaginal bleeding and abdominal pain. AP may also result in a concealed collection of blood progressively dissecting the decidua basalis, but remaining sequestered within the uterus by partial retention of the placental margin, preservation of its membranous

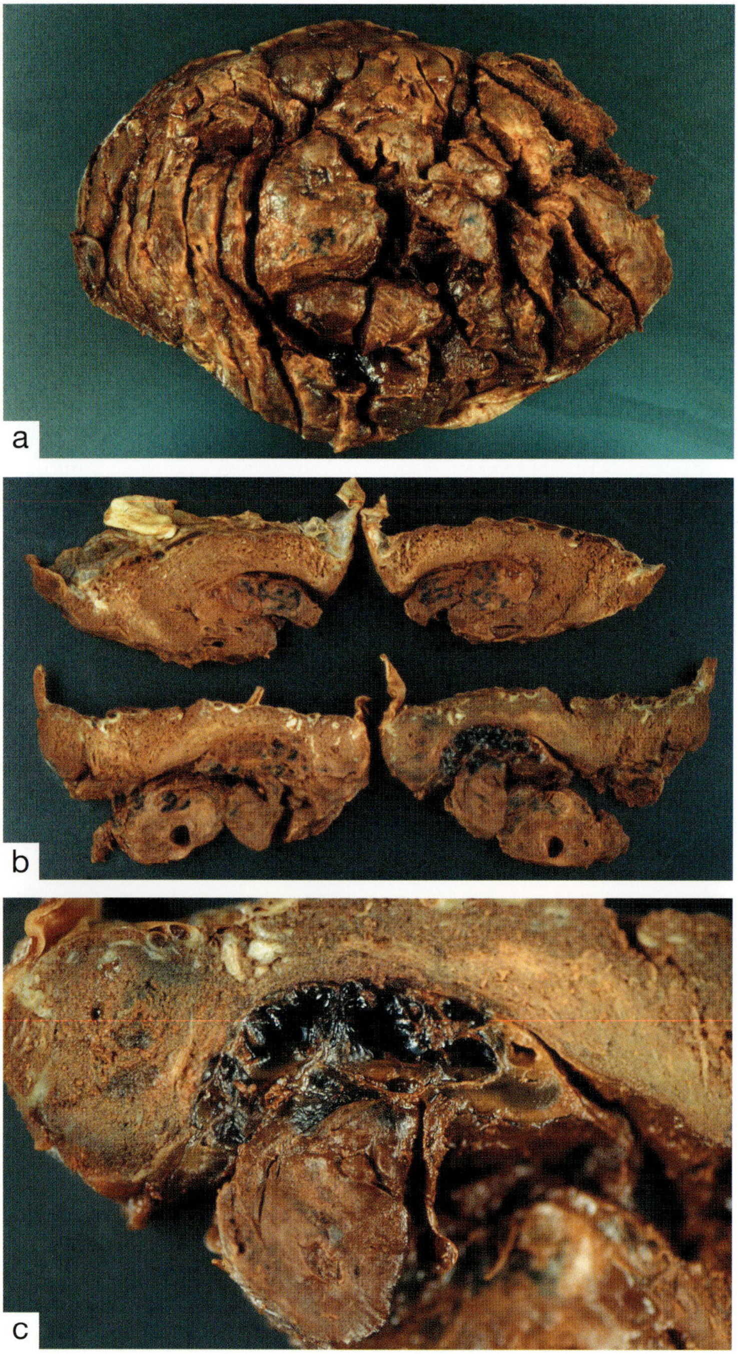

Figure 29 This 880-g placenta was delivered vaginally with a live-born, but intrauterine growth-restricted infant at 36 weeks, following note of a large retroplacental hemorrhage (RH) on prenatal ultrasonography approximately 5 weeks before delivery. (a) A massive chronic, yellowish-brown and tan, nodular RH replaces the majority of the maternal surface. (b) Representative serial sections show extensive compression of the parenchyma, its cavitation, and the massive size of the multinodular clot. (c) A closer view of one section shows a central pocket of liquefaction in the hematoma, closest to the compressed edge of decidua and parenchyma that has remained unorganized. It is bordered by infarcted chorionic villous tissue above and variably organized clot alongside and below

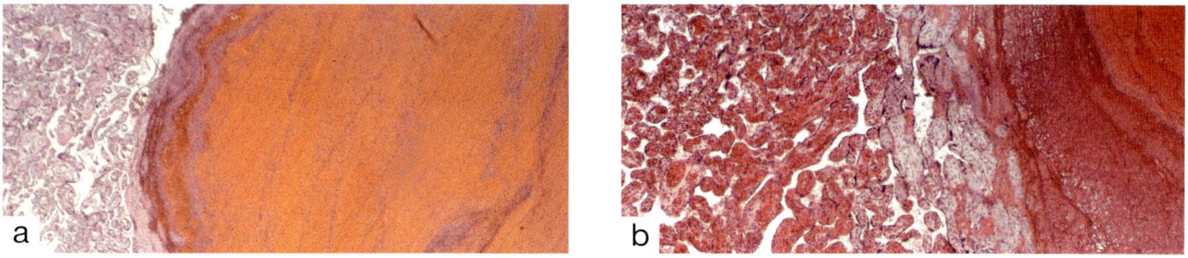

Figure 30 Histopathology of acute retroplacental hemorrhage may include a portion of hemorrhage/hematoma with a leading edge of fibrin laminations with or without maternal neutrophilic reaction, compressed decidua, and acute villous compression and crowding (a), and/or features of acute chorionic villous ischemia and acute intravillous hemorrhage (b), which may be a manifestation of villous reperfusion injury

attachment, or blockage of the blood's passage from the uterus, by the vertex position of the fetal head[33]. An acute abruption may leave no pathologic imprint on the placenta if most of the blood has been passed via the vagina, or if insufficient time has elapsed for the hematoma to adhere to, or produce a depression in, the maternal surface. Conversely, as noted above, a large mass of acute blood clot, received with the placenta, may be a clue to the prior, *in situ* presence of an acutely formed hematoma.

Pathogenesis The cause is unknown, but it is generally agreed that RH is due to the rupture of maternal decidual arterioles. It occurs when the arteries are diseased, as in toxemia of pregnancy or hypertension, but it is also seen when the arteries are histologically normal. This absence of arteriopathy may reflect sampling, but it is virtually impossible to demonstrate ruptured arteriole(s) because of the distortion of the decidua. A number of risk factors are associated with clinical abruptio placentae. Thus, the incidence of RH is increased in gestations complicated by maternal pre-eclampsia, hypertension, cigarette smoking, cocaine abuse, abdominal trauma, increased inferior vena caval pressure, preterm premature rupture of the membranes, sudden intrauterine compression, short umbilical cord, uterine anomaly, retroplacental uterine leiomyoma, chorioamnionitis[3,4,36,37], and maternal thrombophilia[33,38–45]. In addition, prior marginal hemorrhage and dissection, with repair, may explain why RH is also more commonly associated with circumvallate placentas (see section on 'Extrachorial placentas' in Chapter 10). RH is also associated with unexplained increased mid-trimester levels of maternal serum β-human chorionic gonadotropin (β-hCG)[46]. Ethnicity is a risk factor for AP: African-American and Caucasian women have a greater risk than do Asian or Latin-American women[33]. Furthermore, some risk factors are additive; women with hypertension who develop superimposed pre-eclampsia are twice as likely to have a placental abruption. Abruption at *term* is associated with non-vertex presentation, fetal intrauterine growth restriction, polyhydramnios, multiparity, multiple gestations, and advanced maternal age[47].

Significance A small RH, although it may be accompanied by infarction of the overlying placental parenchyma, is generally of no significance, since there is considerable placental reserve, especially in the otherwise healthy term placenta (losses of up to 30% of villous exchange area, due to cessation of blood flow to the intervillous space, in a healthy placenta, may not have any clinical significance if the remaining parenchyma has normal blood supply[48]). In contrast, a small RH affecting a diseased placenta, such as one with hypoxic changes from placental bed underperfusion (i.e. pre-eclampsia), may result in pathologic compromise of chorionic villous function. Thus, the correlative clinical significance of RH will vary among cases in which there is placental disease and antecedent events, including the occurrence of a small, prior RH that later becomes complicated by superimposed acute hematoma formation. RH involving between 20 and 40% of the maternal surface, in a diseased placenta, has been considered clinically significant in terms of deprivation of the oxygen supply to the fetus. RH involving > 40% of the maternal surface in a healthy placenta is associated with fetal morbidity or demise[3,4]. From the clinical point of view of fetal well-being, rupture of the maternal arterioles, and separation of chorionic villi from the maternal blood supply and chorionic villous infarction, are the most significant aspects of RH. Placental abruption, especially when severe, is associated with a high rate of perinatal mortality (22–35%) and is seen in 12–24.2% of cases of third-trimester stillbirth[36,37,49]. Placental abruption is also associated with a 9% rate of cerebral palsy in live-born infants[49]. The actual volume of blood lost and the initiation of a consumptive coagulopathy are major concerns for the mother's well-being. Finally, a follow-up study, by Nagy and colleagues[50], of intrauterine hematomas ultrasonographically detected during the first trimester revealed that a *retroplacental* position correlated with increased risks for adverse maternal and neonatal complications, and rates of operatively assisted vaginal and cesarean section deliveries. Risks of development of pregnancy-induced hypertension and pre-eclampsia; placental abruption and placental separation abnormalities; preterm delivery; fetal growth restriction, distress, and meconium passage; and neonatal intensive care admission, were all found to be significantly elevated.

Marginal hematoma

Gross features A marginal hematoma (MH) is crescent-shaped, reflecting its relationship to the placental margin, and may extend for some distance over the maternal surface. On section, it has a triangular configuration at the lateral angle of the placenta; its base lies on a plane with the maternal surface, and its sides are respectively formed by the lateral edge of the placental parenchyma and the reflection of the fetal membranes. MHs are usually acute and delimited, but some affect more than a quadrant of the placental perimeter, and a circumferential MH has been described[51]. Generally, if no grossly appreciable loss of the distinct border between the lateral placental margin and the limits of the hematoma is present, then the MH is likely incidental. Figure 31 shows sections of acute marginal hematoma. Large MHs, and those with early organization, marginal adherence, rim width of a centimeter or more, or medial dissection or chronic changes, are more likely to be associated with significant antenatal or intrapartum events. A recent or chronic MH may produce a depression at the adjacent lateral margin. The cut surface of chronic MH reveals laminated, friable, yellowish-brown and/or calcified thrombohematoma with blurring of the lateral border of the placenta; it may also show a superimposed, acute component. Histology should be pursued when thrombosis at the placental angle cannot be distinguished from passive or incidental accumulation of blood in this anatomic crevice.

Histology If acute, the mass is largely composed of erythrocytes, with interspersed coagulum and variable numbers of leukocytes. The hematoma is likely to be of little clinical significance if medially bordered by an intact lateral placental margin that separates the hematoma from the chorionic villi and hematoma that shows minimal fibrin deposition. Histologic examination of the lateral placental margin is key, since thrombosis or disruption of the large lateral decidual veins, decidual necrosis, and hemorrhagic dissection of the decidua, intervillous space, or subchorial or retromembranous zones are more likely to correlate with a pathologic gestational or intrapartum event/process. A chronic MH shows hemosiderin deposition, organized thrombus, dystrophic mineralization, chorionic villous infarction of the adjacent parenchyma, and/or features of circumvallation (plica formation) of the fetal membrane insertion.

Incidence Reported incidence has ranged from 0.74 to 1.9%[3], but in the authors' experience, MHs are encountered more frequently (10–20% of serially examined placentas), possibly due to the relatively greater numbers of patients with complicated gestations and preterm labor and delivery who are admitted to academic centers.

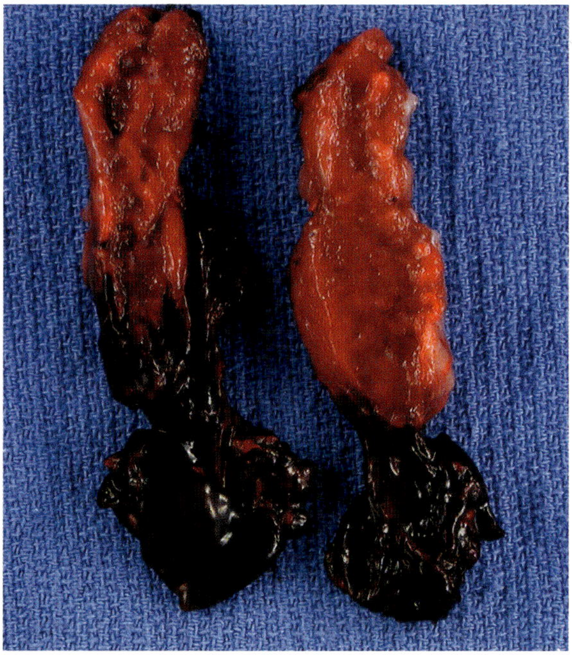

Figure 31 These sections demonstrate the importance of thorough sampling in cases of marginal hematoma (MH). The section on the right does not show dissection by the hematoma into the villous parenchyma whereas the section on the left does. The triangular configuration of the soft acute MH was disrupted with specimen manipulation, but such manipulation does not artifactually induce dissection

Pathogenesis and significance The pathogenesis and significance of the MH remain debated issues. Some placental pathologists submit that acute third-trimester MH is of doubtful significance to the fetus[3], and is often incidental (personal communication). However, Harris and colleagues[52] noted that over half of the placentas delivered of women with idiopathic premature labor without antepartum bleeding showed marginal adherent clot, with fibrin deposition and lamination, polymorphonuclear infiltration, and marginal decidual necrosis: gross and histologic criteria of acute antepartum peripheral placental separation. These authors suggested that the separation was of uterine venous origin and had a role in the process of preterm labor, but they were unclear as to whether marginal hematoma formation was a causal event. Precipitous delivery, sequelae of concentrated oxytocin induction, and marginal placental abruption, as well as preterm labor and delivery, may all be associated with acute MH formation. Clinically, MH is referred to as 'subchorionic hemorrhage' or 'periplacental hemorrhage'. However, the clinical use of the term 'subchorionic hemorrhage' in these cases is *not* synonymous with the pathologic term, *subchorial thrombohematoma* (see above section on 'Breus' mole'), because the clinical use refers to a margin-associated hematoma, not a central, subchorionic thrombohematoma in the maternal space. Early gestational subchorionic hematoma noted by ultrasonography has been detected in 1.8–4.92% of women with threatened abortion (recurrent bleeding)[53,54]. Outcome appears to be related to initial size and progression of the lesion. Small and/or decreasing size did not result in spontaneous abortion in the series of 406 women with threatened miscarriage, conducted by Stabile and colleagues[54], whereas initial large size, progressive enlargement, and onset of maternal pain (irrespective of placental marginal elevation, gestational period, or maternal age or parity) were poor prognostic signs associated with adverse outcome (71%) in the study by Abu-Yousef and associates[55]. Subchorionic hematoma may completely disappear within a few months and/or contribute to the formation of an extrachorial placenta[53]. Since adverse antenatal events may be associated with MH formation, it seems prudent to report the presence, dimensions, type of adherence, cut surface appearance, and any extent of dissection of an MH, and to submit sections for histologic evaluation.

Maternal surface infarction

Gross features These are firm, pale to whitish areas on the maternal surface, and, as such, are focal lesions of the maternal surface decidua. Small patches of pale tan to whitish decidua can be normally seen in mid- to late third-trimester placentas from uncomplicated gestations, since the placenta is a naturally senescent organ. In late third-trimester and post-term placentas, the foci may also be calcified and appear as punctate, gritty nodules (Figure 32a and c). They are usually only a few millimeters in diameter and scattered over the maternal surface.

Confluent areas or a more extensive distribution, with brown to yellowish discoloration or prominent mineralization, however, should be regarded as pathologic and potentially clinically significant (Figure 32b). The extent of involvement by these lesions should be estimated as a percentage of the total maternal surface and pathologic sites sampled for histology. In the authors' experience, infarctions involving 25% or more of the surface are more likely to be associated with maternal conditions resulting in underperfusion of the placental bed (unpublished observations).

Histology The decidua shows non-specific bland necrosis sometimes with a leukocytoclastic component or microcalcifications. Thrombi or arteriolopathic changes are other pathologic features. Hemosiderosis indicates chronic decidual hemorrhage that is most likely due to chronic ischemic infarction; its presence should be assessed in the context of placental weight, chorionic villous features, any accompanying decidual arteriolopathy, and the extent of decidual necrosis (Figure 32b).

Significance and pathogenesis As stated above, patchy and punctate decidual necrosis is a feature of normally occurring degenerative involution and senescence, late in gestation. However, these sites are increased in number and extent in arteriolopathy associated with maternal pre-eclampsia, hypertension, diabetes mellitus, sickle cell hemoglobinopathy, cigarette smoking, and cocaine abuse.

Chorionic villous infarction

Gross features Infarcts are more commonly seen in the basal and marginal aspects of the placenta, since they are the sequelae of ischemia. Their gross (and microscopic) appearance may reflect acute or more long-term conditions of inadequacy of blood flow to and within the maternal space. Often they are adjacent to areas of maternal surface infarction, described above. An acute infarction is variably shaped, but is generally a roughly triangular (with its base towards basal plate), fairly well-demarcated region of increased plethora a few millimeters or centimeters in

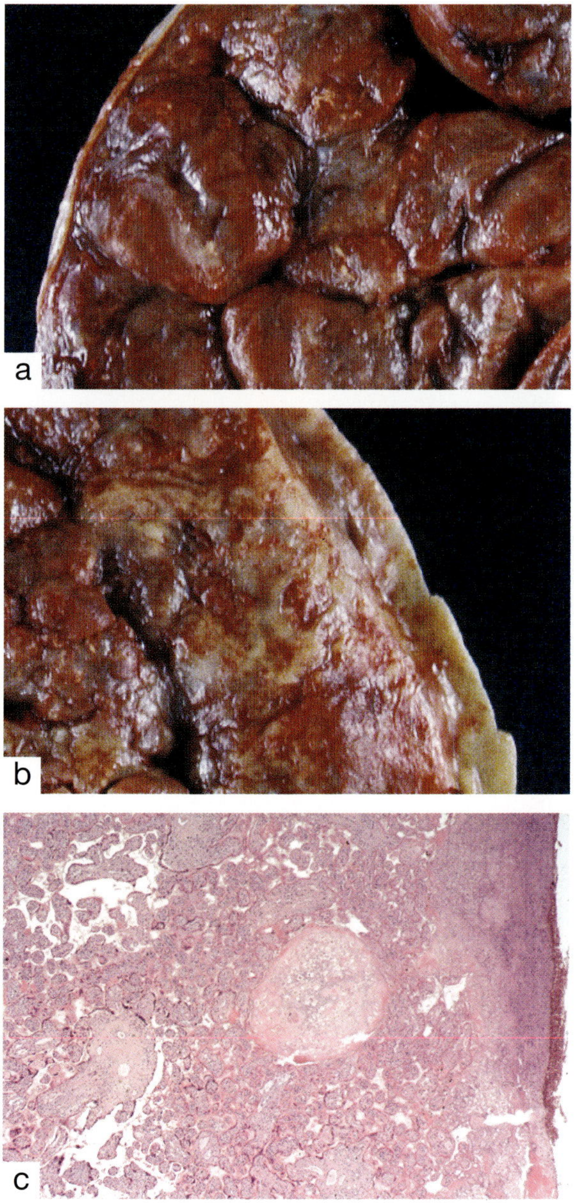

Figure 32 (a) This composite shows scattered punctate infarcts that are present as yellow-white lesions on the maternal surface of this term placenta. (b) When these lesions are increased in number and dimension, they may form confluent plaques. (c) Punctate infarcts are characterized by foci of bland decidual necrosis with leukocytoclastic features and chorionic villous ischemia and/or early necrosis, as shown. Plaques belie more extensive lesions of decidual infarction and chorionic villous parenchymal infarctions.

size. In the fresh state, sites of acute infarction may be difficult to appreciate visually, and are more easily detected with palpation, which reveals a relative firmness in the affected parenchyma. (Acute infarctions are also more easily detected after fixation.) Over time, acute infarctions tend to be more distinctly wedge-shaped and pale. With increasing age, the sites of infarction become progressively firm and delimited, and exhibit a brown-red coloration; by about 10–14 days, they become yellow-white, and acquire a smooth and waxy texture[3]. More long-standing infarctions are typically very firm, well demarcated, white to yellowish, and may also be gritty, due to dystrophic mineralization (Figure 33). The sites and types of infarctions within the basal, subchorial, and middle zones of the placenta should be documented, as well as an estimate of the total percentage of the parenchymal volume they affect.

Histology Acute chorionic villous ischemia is typified by acute congestion and dilatation of villous capillaries and intravillous extravasation and hemorrhage. These features, together with chorionic villous 'crowding', are the histopathologic correlations of sites of gross plethora and firmness. Chorionic villous crowding, or the close approximations of the terminal villi, in part reflects a reduction in intervillous blood volume that normally keeps the villi separated. These features may precede or overlap with loss of syncytial cell nuclear staining and nuclear pyknosis and karyorrhexis. The trophoblasts become an eosinophilic and sometimes smudged villous border, and the stroma starts to show endothelial karyorrhexis, with stromal capillaries containing ghost-like outlines of hemolyzed erythrocytes. Recent infarcts show overlapping features with acute infarction, but more loss of tinctorial quality and distinction of the chorionic villous architecture, capillary luminal loss, and greater crowding and compaction. Acute to recent infarctions are likely accompanied by the release of fetal plasma constituents, and perivillous fibrinoid becomes deposited in the central aspects of the infarct. A mild reactive *peri*villous infiltrate of neutrophils may be seen at the periphery of an infarct; these are evidence

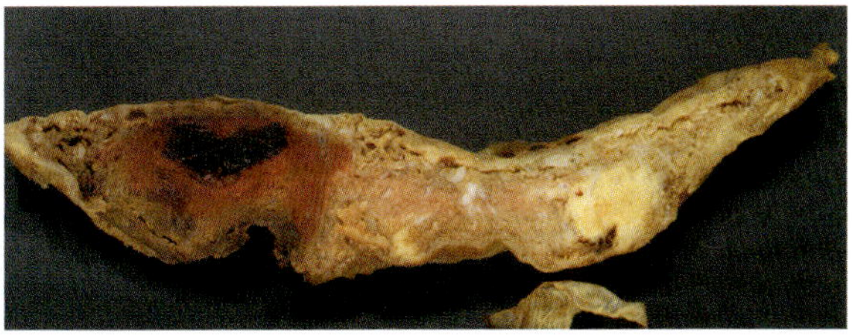

Figure 33 Fixation highlights demarcation of the large paramarginal red-brown recent chorionic villous infarction in this section, and its upper zone of intervillous thrombosis, and also clear distinction of the two, yellow-white, basal chronic chorionic infarctions, to its right. The larger chronic infarct also shows a superimposed acute component, evidenced by the dark red-brown congested tissue in its basal periphery. (The most basal villi are most vulnerable to ischemic insult.) A focus of relatively more congested chorionic villous tissue is seen in the left marginal basal aspect of the section as well

that contact with maternal blood brings a non-specific influx of maternal neutrophils, most likely due to chemotactic factors released upon chorionic villous damage and infarction. This inflammatory response should not be confused with infectious intervillositis[56] or villitis of unknown etiology (see 'Villitis' section in Chapter 10). Figure 34 shows several features of chorionic villous ischemia and infarction. Chronic changes are typified by the presence of eosinophilic ghost-like outlines of individual villi, with little or no detectable residual nuclear basophilia. The compacted mass of eosinophilic, necrotic, ghost-like remnants of the villous tree show central, thin deposits of fibrinoid; there is no evidence of maternal circulation reaching these intervillous spaces. The perimeter of the infarct may show small and variably distributed infiltrates of reactive, neutrophilic inflammation. Villous stromal shrinkage, sclerosis, and dystrophic micromineralizations of the chorionic villous basement membranes occur, but fibrosis and true organization of the infarct do not. The stem villi supplying the affected villi may become sclerotic.

Incidence About 25% of normal term placentas contain infarcts affecting < 5% of the parenchymal volume. The frequency is increased in conditions of placental bed underperfusion, and extensive infarcts are present in 60–70% of placentas delivered from

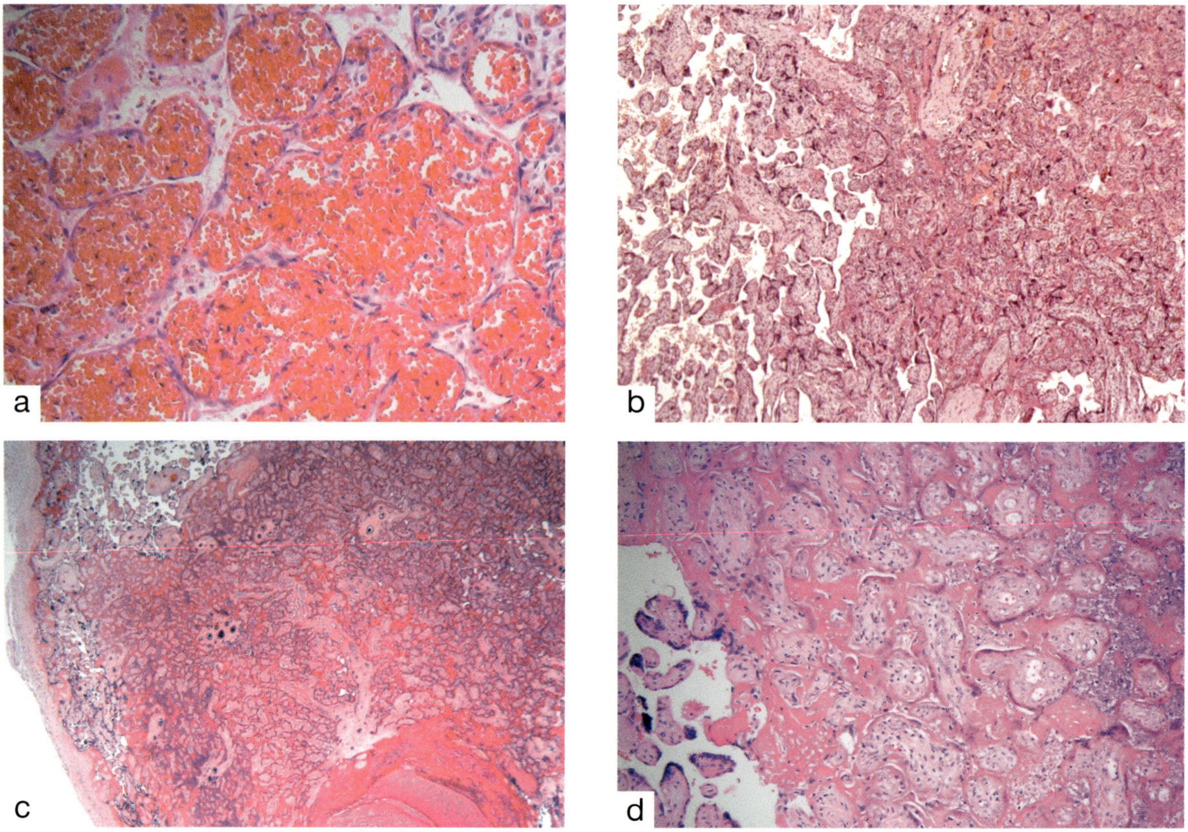

Figure 34 Microscopic features of acute chorionic villous infarction. (a) Acute chorionic villous ischemia can be evidenced, as it is here, by villous crowding, increased syncytial knotting, and congestion and signs of early infarction with intravillous hemorrhage, which itself may be a feature of reperfusion injury. (b) This low-power view of acute chorionic villous ischemia shows transition to a region of villous crowding with increased syncytial knotting and perivillous fibrinoid deposition. (c) This low-power photomicrograph shows a defined acute basal chorionic villous infarction. The lateral borders are more distinct, reflecting the lowered but continued perfusion of the maternal space by the neighboring decidual arterioles. In contrast, recall that the most basal chorionic villi are normally less well supplied, and their relatively greater crowding and syncytial knottings, in this setting of added infarction, reflects this. Perivillous fibrinoid is seen within the infarct, as is intervillous basophilic karyorrhexis. Chorionic villi demonstrate degenerative change (see (f)). Chorion villous infarction contributes to local release of thrombogenic mediators and also to altered blood flow patterns in the maternal space. A basal intervillous thrombus is present in the lower right aspect of the image. (d) Higher-power images of the infarct edge show perivillous fibrinoid, and eosinophilic smudging of the villous syncytiotrophoblast and loss of villous architecture. (e) As described in the text, a reactive neutrophilic response can be seen at the peripheral aspects of some lesions of acute chorionic villous infarction. (f) This field shows a high-power view of eosinophilic degenerating villi of the infarction shown in (c) and (d). With time there is progressive loss of villous cytologic detail in the infarct, until only shrunken, back-to-back arrangements of eosinophilic to mineralized ghost-like outlines of the villi remain

patients with severe disease[3]. Infarctions of varying age are more typical of pre-eclampsia, due to its variable distribution, age, and severity of arteriopathy.

Pathogenesis The oxygen supply of the chorionic villi is obtained from the blood in the maternal space. The viability of the chorionic villi and thereby of the fetus is dependent on adequate oxygenation and fluidity of the intervillous space. The oxygen is supplied from blood delivered to the maternal space by gaping, open-ended terminations of decidual arterioles. However, due to this 'open' pattern of circulation, this oxygenated blood becomes admixed with deoxygenated 'venous' blood already present within

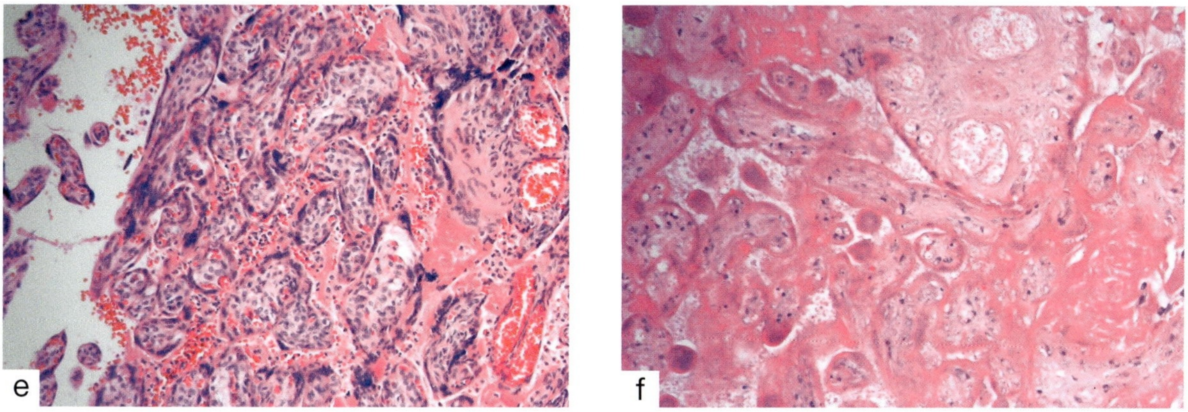

Figure 34 *Continued*

the intervillous space. Occlusion of the arteriolar terminus or lack of physiologic conversion of deciduomyometrial arterioles results in diminished blood flow and oxygen supply in the maternal space. If sufficient numbers of the placental bed arterioles are compromised, and the compromise persists or worsens, significant portions of the chorionic villous tree are ischemic and become infarcted when sudden occlusion of the arterioles, due to thombosis, occurs.

Significance In a normal term placenta, chorionic villous infarction affects < 5% of the parenchymal volume. However, according to the discussion of RH above, sufficient chorionic villous tree branching and terminal villous development is present, such that loss nearly a third of the total terminal villous surface area can be tolerated, at term, provided that the blood supply to the remaining villous tree is uncompromised[48]. A diseased placenta (i.e. one with less villous tree development, impaired function, or thrombosis of the fetal vasculature of the tree) may only be able to withstand loss of 15–20% of the villi[3]. Overall, central placental parenchymal infarction is more significant than marginal infarction, since the marginal placenta is normally relatively less well perfused. (The placental margin presumably has less collateral blood supply and less physiologic change in the arteries[57]). Therefore, central infarction implies loss of greater numbers of arterial lumina and blood supply to the maternal space and larger portions of infarcted, chorionic villous tree. Extensive parenchymal infarction is associated with a high incidence of fetal hypoxia, growth restriction, and intrauterine demise. Thus, the significance of chorionic villous infarction should be interpreted in the context of a variety of factors. These include the period of gestation and the correlative expected placental weight range; the site, volumetric percentage, and zonal distribution of infarction; the presence of any underlying maternal disease and chorionic villous dysmaturation; the presence of fetal vascular thrombosis that would alter supply of the villous tree (see section on 'Lesions due to disturbances of fetal blood flow'); the type of placentation and cord insertion; and the presence of RH or MH.

'X cell' or 'septal' cysts (or 'chorionic cysts')

Gross These are subchorionic and intratrabecular cysts. They are sometimes referred to as 'chorionic cysts'[3], but they not intrachorionic. They are formed by proliferations of *extra*villous cytotrophoblasts (the term '*extra*villous cytotrophoblast' is shortened to 'X cell') that line the undersurface of the chorionic plate and form the solid, trabecular or anchoring, villi of the placenta that attach to the basal plate of the trophoblast or to the crests of decidual septa. Thus, the anchoring villi span the maternal space from the inferior surface of the chorionic plate to the basal plate, and add stability to the placental structure. Extravillous cytotrophoblastic cellular viability is dependent upon diffusion, and, with X cell proliferation, the central aspects of these aggregates and columns undergo cellular degeneration and liquefaction. They may enlarge to form grossly detectable, 0.3–1.5-cm diameter, ovoid cysts that contain clear to gray, gelatinous fluid (Figure 35a). These so-called 'X cell cysts' and 'septal cysts' can be seen in mature placentas and, most commonly, are located in the subchorionic and parabasal zones.

Incidence They are seen in 11–20% of placentas[3].

Histology The cysts are lined by trophoblastic epithelium[4]. The *extra*villous cytotrophoblasts are distinguished from the chorionic villous trophoblasts because they do not provide surface for exchange and are often embedded in fibrinoid material. These extravillous cytotrophoblasts elaborate a proteinaceous, mucin-like fluid, and central cellular degeneration leads to accumulation of pools of this amorphous, eosinophilic, and weakly periodic acid-Schiff (PAS)-positive fluid (Figure 35b).

X cell cysts have also been referred to as 'septal cysts'[3], due to their basal location. Placental *septa* are the triangular-shaped or folded portions of *decidua*, seen by light microscopy, projecting upwards into the maternal space from the base of the placenta. They lie between the terminal branches of the chorionic villous tree, and their crests include roots of anchoring villi and proliferating and infiltrating cytotrophoblasts. The bases of the septa are largely pyramidal masses of intervening decidua that remained as interstices between the paths of the invading masses of syncytiotrophoblasts and cytotrophoblasts. Their apices contain trophoblastic cells and cytotrophoblastic-derived matrix fibrinoid, and these appear to contribute to the septal configurations as the placenta grows. Since the bases of these pyramids remain in the uterus after delivery of the placenta, retention of the decidual base results in the gross 'defects' that demarcate the borders of the cotyledons on the maternal surface (see also Chapter 3.) Thus, X cell cysts may lie atop, merge with, or become enfolded within the crests of the decidual septal component and may be called 'septal cysts'.

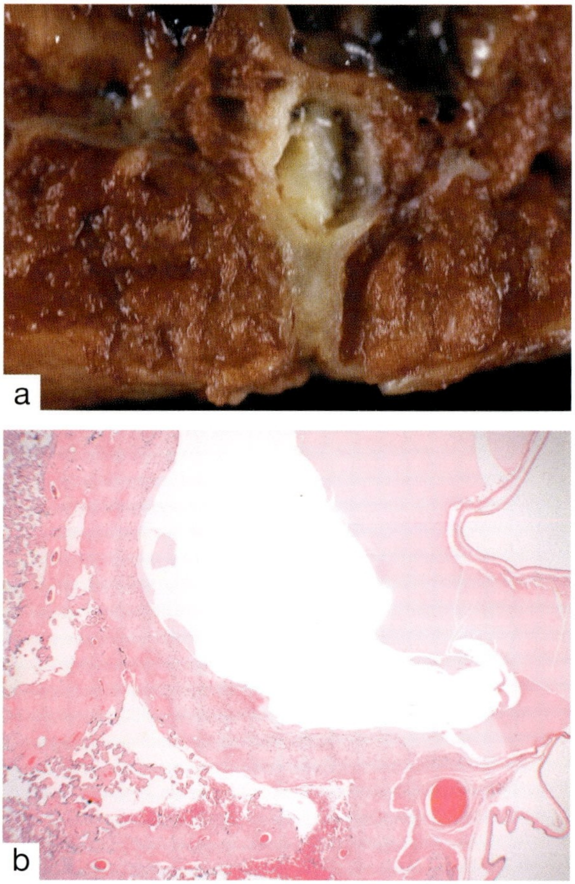

Figure 35 (a) A cystic cavity is present at the crest of this maternal septum. Except for their locations, this cyst and the one seen in Figure 26b have similar gross appearances. Both are lined by extravillous cytotrophoblast cells and contain clear, mucinous material. (b) The typical histology of the X cell cyst is seen in this large subchorionic example

The X cells may also form floating cell islands without core stroma that are suspended from chorionic villous tips. They resemble the structures of primary villi that failed to become infiltrated by mesenchyme[4]. Again, while they may be attached to chorionic villi as free-floating masses or columns, they do not add functional surface area.

Pathogenesis and significance Extravillous cytotrophoblastic proliferation, like chorionic villous cytotrophoblastic proliferation, is stimulated by hypoxia (see section on 'Excessive numbers of cytotrophoblastic cells' in Chapter 9). Thus, X cell cysts are characteristically seen in the subchorial and basal zones, since these are relatively hypoxic zones in even normal placentas. Fox[3] has reported that these may be seen in 19% of term placentas from uncomplicated gestations. They are pathologically increased in placentas from gestations complicated by placental bed underperfusion and maternal diabetes mellitus. In addition, they are characteristic findings in maternal floor infarction and massive perivillous fibrinoid deposition (see section on 'Maternal floor infarction' in Chapter 10). In these pathologic states, the chorionic and non-villous cytotrophoblasts are isolated and effectively distanced from their oxygen supply by their cloaks of fibrinoid. In addition, the progressive fibrinoid deposition forms a meshwork that seems to create baffles and alterations in the blood flow patterns in the maternal space and regions of true placental ischemia. Finally, for unclear reasons, edematous placentas (e.g. Rh isoimmunization) may also show increased numbers of X cell cysts[3].

LESIONS DUE TO DISTURBANCES OF FETAL BLOOD FLOW

Intervillous thrombus

Gross features An acute to recent intervillous thrombus (IVT) is a central, 2–5-cm, oval, soft, dark-red, parenchymal lesion. In the historical literature, *acute* IVTs were referred to as *Kline's hemorrhages*[58] on close gross inspection of placental sections, these can be detected as fresh liquid or semifluid intervillous blood pools. A *chronic* thrombus is firm to hard, whitish, and laminated. Thrombi of intermediate age have soft, cystic-appearing, red-brown centers bordered by a firm laminated periphery. As with the basal intervillous thrombus (see above section on 'Lesions due to disturbances of maternal blood flow'), chorionic villous structures are pushed aside and are not part of the lesion. Chorionic villous infarctions are generally firmer and more granular than IVTs, but parenchymal thrombi are often grossly misidentified as infarctions, so, histologic sampling is advised.

Histology Acute to recent thrombi contain fibrin lamellae admixed with erythrocytes; histologic examination will often reveal the presence of numerous nucleated erythrocytes in early IVTs. Acute to recent thrombi may show bordering macrophages that contain phagocytosed fetal erythrocytes. The erythrocytes gradually degenerate and the laminations may become more compacted. Chorionic villi are not integral components, but may be seen as displaced structures at the borders of an IVT. Chronic IVTs consist largely of persistent fibrin lamellae, and there may be hemosiderin-laden macrophages at the periphery. In subacute and chronic IVTs, peripheral chorionic villi may show features of ischemia, crowding, or infarction, likely reflecting chorionic villous compression and blood flow pattern alterations within the maternal space.

Incidence Reported occurrence ranges from 3 to 50% of full-term uncomplicated pregnancies[3,59]. IVTs are increased in placentas from gestations complicated by ischemic conditions such as pre-eclampsia and ischemia-associated fetal growth restriction[59–61].

Pathogenesis IVTs are an admixture of fetal and maternal blood. Early studies of *Kline's hemorrhages*[58] convincingly showed that their frequency and size correlated positively with the quantity of fetal cells in the maternal circulation, as determined by Kleihauer–Betke (KB) testing[4]. Kaplan and colleagues[9] later confirmed the fetal origin of the nucleated erythrocytes in IVT by immunoperoxidase staining methodology, employing a labeled antibody directed against fetal hemoglobin.

Rolschau, and Batcup and colleagues[60,62], concluded that fetal erythrocytes gain access to the maternal space and initiate the formation of IVT at sites of chorionic villous damage and hemorrhage, and investigations by Soma and co-workers[63] and others[3,4] have supported these conclusions. Loss of chorionic villous integrity may be due to spontaneously occurring breaks and/or villous tree trauma due to fetal movement, and not to ischemia[4]. Whatever the mechanism, fetal red blood cell (RBC) extravasation presumably initiates coagulation in the maternal space via exposure to tissue thromboplastin from damaged vasculosyncytial membranes[62], fetal red cells (erythrocyte stroma is a potent thromboplastin), and/or chorionic villous stroma. Exposure to incompatible fetal ABO blood-group antigens was responsible for only a small percentage of intervillous thrombus formations, in the study by Batcup and colleagues[62]. Rh isoimmunization has been proposed to be linked to IVT formation[64,65], but the connection between IVT and Rh isoimmunization is likely of less significance, today, due to prophylactic administration of Rh immunoglobulin to Rh-negative women.

Fetal blood cells have been found in the maternal circulation in up to 95% of pregnancies[66] and detected during all three trimesters of gestation, but their volumes, as estimated by the Kleihauer–Betke method, are usually minuscule (0.07–0.13 ml)[33]. IVTs probably denote sites of additionally lost fetal RBCs that have been 'entrapped' and localized within the maternal space, and not freed to the circulation to enable detection by KB testing.

Significance Most clinicopathologic studies of IVT have mainly involved evaluations of third-trimester to term gestation placentas. These studies have revealed that IVTs are usually non-specific or incidental findings, and do not result in fetal anemia or other gestational complications[3]. Fox has gone so far as to state that they have no effect on placental function or fetal well-being, and that they merely mark sites of fetal blood leakage. Others have shown that IVTs are frequent co-lesions with those of placental bed ischemia, such as chorionic villous infarction, fibrin plaques, and accelerated chorionic villous maturation[59–61]. Becroft and colleagues[57], in their study of term placentas, concluded that IVTs were not independently, significantly associated with fetal growth restriction or pregnancy-induced hypertension, but noted that IVT, chorionic villous infarction, and intervillous fibrinoid plaques co-occurred in a two- to four-fold incidence over incidences in placentas without the associated lesions. Their observation of the association of IVT with intervillous fibrinoid plaques and chorionic villous infarction led them to postulate that maternal thrombophilia may be a common factor in the pathogenesis and co-occurrence of these lesions. (They noted that fetal hemorrhage into the maternal space is presumably contained by the formation of IVT, but that the ultimate relative composition of the fibrin (fibrinoid) is unknown.) More research is necessary to clarify whether the presence of IVT with the other two lesions should be regarded as a *forme fruste* of underlying maternal thrombophilia, but the association of the three lesions is now well documented.

Other studies indicate that IVT formation can occur earlier than the third trimester, and that this may have important implications. Large IVTs, observed either by serial antenatal ultrasonography and/or on pathologic examination[67,68], have been clinicopathologically linked to mid-gestational unexplained elevations in maternal serum α-fetoprotein levels and a positive KB test. Of note is that there are no studies, to date, comparing the clinicopathologic correlations of IVTs found in second- and early third-trimester placentas with those found in late-gestation deliveries. Since the reserve of the placenta is different earlier in gestation, even small, ongoing, or multifocal losses in chorionic villous integrity and fetal blood may have different clinicopathologic implications for the fetus and the developing chorionic villous tree. Thus, while IVTs are regarded as having little independent clinical significance, careful inspection of serial sections of placentas (especially those from mid-gestational to early third-trimester deliveries and those without an accompanying history of pre-eclampsia) may disclose an unusual extent or multifocality of these lesions and provide clues to otherwise unexplained gestational complications or adverse outcomes.

Fetomaternal hemorrhage (major)

General On the other end of the spectrum from the essentially non-compromising hemorrhages described above are fetomaternal hemorrhages that result in fetal hypovolemia and anemia. Hemodynamically significant fetomaternal hemorrhage (FMH) is primarily a clinical diagnosis and a condition that often warrants emergency cesarean section delivery. Resolution of acute and chronic FMH may also involve intrauterine transfusion and, certainly, immediate postnatal transfusion. The pathologist examining the placenta (and/or the infant) in such cases will render a more meaningful examination if he/she has some understanding of the clinical parameters used to identify FMH and treat the affected infant. A brief clinical overview is presented.

Clinical suspicion of FMH is raised upon maternal report of decreased fetal movement, new onset of ultrasonographic and Doppler flow velocity evidence of fetal distress, including fetal edema or effusions, and/or rhythm irregularities on fetal heart rate monitor tracings; a sinusoidal fetal heart rate tracing is regarded as a particularly ominous sign and a strong indicator of severe fetal anemia. A positive KB test, in the face of negative direct and indirect antibody tests, is used to confirm the clinical suspicion. Gradually developing anemia is usually better tolerated than an acute large loss, since, over a period of time, the fetus can more easily reconstitute blood volume and, eventually, red cell mass. Treatment of the fetal anemia will depend upon the medical means and expertise available and the fetal condition, but possibilities include intrauterine serial intravascular transfusions via the umbilical cord, even in cases of fetal hydrops[69–71]. The live-born infant will be pale, tachycardic, and tachypneic, and may also be hydropic, and transfusion therapy is rapidly instituted[33,72–75]. The stillborn is characteristically hydropic and pale; autopsy examination will reveal an abundance of circulating nucleated fetal erythrocytes in all organs, and may reveal marked effusions and collapse of large vessels[66].

While FMH is recognized as a predominantly clinical diagnosis, it is also important to note that clinical means of intrauterine assessment of fetal well-being do not yet fully forecast gestational outcomes, and that, to date, no reliably predictive risk factors for FMH have been identified[33,76–80]. For example, in a large series, by Dayal and colleagues[80], a normal score for a gestational biophysical profile did not exclude a subsequent FMH in the study of stillbirth occurring within 1 week of a negative maternal examination. Moreover, FMH was found to be the leading cause of stillbirth (ahead of cord accident and abruptio placentae), and generally occurred within 3–4 days of the negative examinations. Thus, the pathologist's examination of the placenta may play a pivotal role in confirming and even detecting the presence of FMH, and identifying its etiology[4,81] and its role in cases of term perinatal demise[82].

Gross From a pathologic standpoint, fetal viability, and thereby the pathology in the placenta, is related to the volume and rapidity of fetal blood loss. Massive, sudden FMH, with fetal exsanguination, usually has no gross placental correlate, and despite concerted efforts, an obvious site of FMH often remains undetectable. Serial sectioning of the placenta, however, may disclose the presence of a hemorrhagic, disrupted chorangioma or reveal a massive, central, fresh IVT that explains an otherwise idiopathic fetal demise. An acute FMH that does not result in the immediate demise will result in fetal anemia and congestive cardiac failure, and the placenta will correspondingly show edema or hydrops and increased weight, a thickened, edematous umbilical cord, and a diffusely pale, edematous, spongy chorionic villous parenchyma. In other cases, one may see a mixture of chorionic villous pallor and acute IVT. In one such rare instance, one author (OF-P) found a diffusely spreading, red to dark-red IVT in the upper to middle parenchymal zones that, on serial section, dissected between and displaced the villous tree, and extended to the deeper mid- and upper basal zones. Grossly, it extended toward one placental margin, but no marginal hematoma was present. The chorionic plate was not elevated. The IVT appeared to dissipate at its mid- to basal aspect, potentially reflecting circulatory patterns in the maternal space. The displaced chorionic villi were alternatively pale or congested and firm, evidence of secondary ischemia (Figure 36). The baby was profoundly anemic and acutely stillborn at term; no other cause after an exhaustive autopsy was identified. In others' studies of FMH, the umbilical vein has been reported as showing thrombosis[66,78,81,83]. In the author's case, a chorionic plate vessel showed acute thrombosis on one section, but no site of chorionic plate vascular disruption or thrombosis was grossly identified. Chronic FMH may also be manifested as placental hydropic change and chorionic villous pallor, but the placenta may be relatively small for the period of gestation. Sections may show acute and/or chronic IVTs.

Histology Acute FMH consists of numerous fetal erythrocytes admixed with the blood of the maternal space. Sections of a massive IVT may show abundant fetal erythrocytes, and minimal peripheral fibrin lamellae. Transmural sections may show decreasing numbers of nucleated fetal red cells in the maternal space as one nears the basal aspect. There may be associated acute chorionic villous ischemia at the periphery of the IVT. A discrete site of hemorrhage is rarely, if ever, identified. The chorionic villi may be congested at the limits of the IVT, but other villi may show capillary collapse or an almost 'bloodless' appearance due to intrauterine fetal cardiac failure and poor chorionic villous perfusion. Sections from hydropic placentas show chorionic villous edema, and fetal vessels contain many nucleated erythrocytes. A left shift to the basophilic normoblast stage may be seen as well, depending upon the severity and duration of the hemorrhage[3,4].

Incidence Hemodynamically significant FMH is uncommon; reported incidences have varied from as few as 1/2800 pregnancies[66] to approximately 1–6 per 1000 gestations[33]. Clinically, large hemorrhages have been defined as ≥ 2% fetal blood cells in the maternal circulation, as determined by KB test[76,84]. FMHs of ≥ 80 ml were found in 1/3893 pregnancies, and losses of ≥ 150 ml in 1/4360 pregnancies in the review by de Almeida and Bowman[85]. When significant loss is defined as ≥ 20 ml, FMH has been found to have an overall prevalence of 4.4% in cases of third-trimester intrauterine fetal death and of 35.7% in cases of fetal death with major fetal anomalies, revealing that gestations of fetuses with malformations may also be complicated by FMH[76]. Redline[82] also found FMH to be an important cause of term stillbirth.

The incidence of FMH may be underappreciated, however, since the diagnosis of FMH (and thereby its reported incidence) is dependent upon the detection of fetal erythrocytes in the maternal circulation, by KB test. While this manual test remains the standard, a variety of more technical methodologies have recently been developed and compared with the standard KB test; some reports cite that the manual KB test underestimates the volume of fetal blood lost. Flow cytometry, using antibody directed at fetal hemoglobin or anti-D to sort cells, or an automated or rosette expanded KB test has replaced the standard manual KB test in some institutions[86–89]. Others have proposed using determination of the cord blood hemoglobin or the initial neonatal hemoglobin[84] as a measure of significant FMH. Dayal and colleagues[80] propose use of the false-negative rate of the biophysical profile to derive its incidence.

Pathogenesis and significance Careful examination of the parenchyma may serendipitously reveal a region of FMH that, by light microscopy, clearly demonstrates numerous fetal erythrocytoses in the maternal space. However, the cause of FMH is often undetermined. Etiologic structural lesions include chorangiomas and, very rarely, hemorrhage due to a primary placental choriocarcinoma (of note is that primary placental choriocarcinomas may be detectable only by microscopic examination; see section on 'Non-trophoblastic tumors of the placenta'). Umbilical vein thrombosis may also cause FMH[66,81,83], and Hoag[81] proposed that the entire umbilical cord should be serially sectioned and inspected, in cases of FMH. Also, intrauterine cordocentesis procedures may be complicated by FMH[4,33]. Placental abruption is not commonly complicated by significant fetal blood loss, but, when due to maternal abdominal trauma (e.g. automobile accident or physical abuse to the mother), the risk for FMH is increased.

As inferred from the preceding paragraphs, FMH, while uncommon, is associated with very high

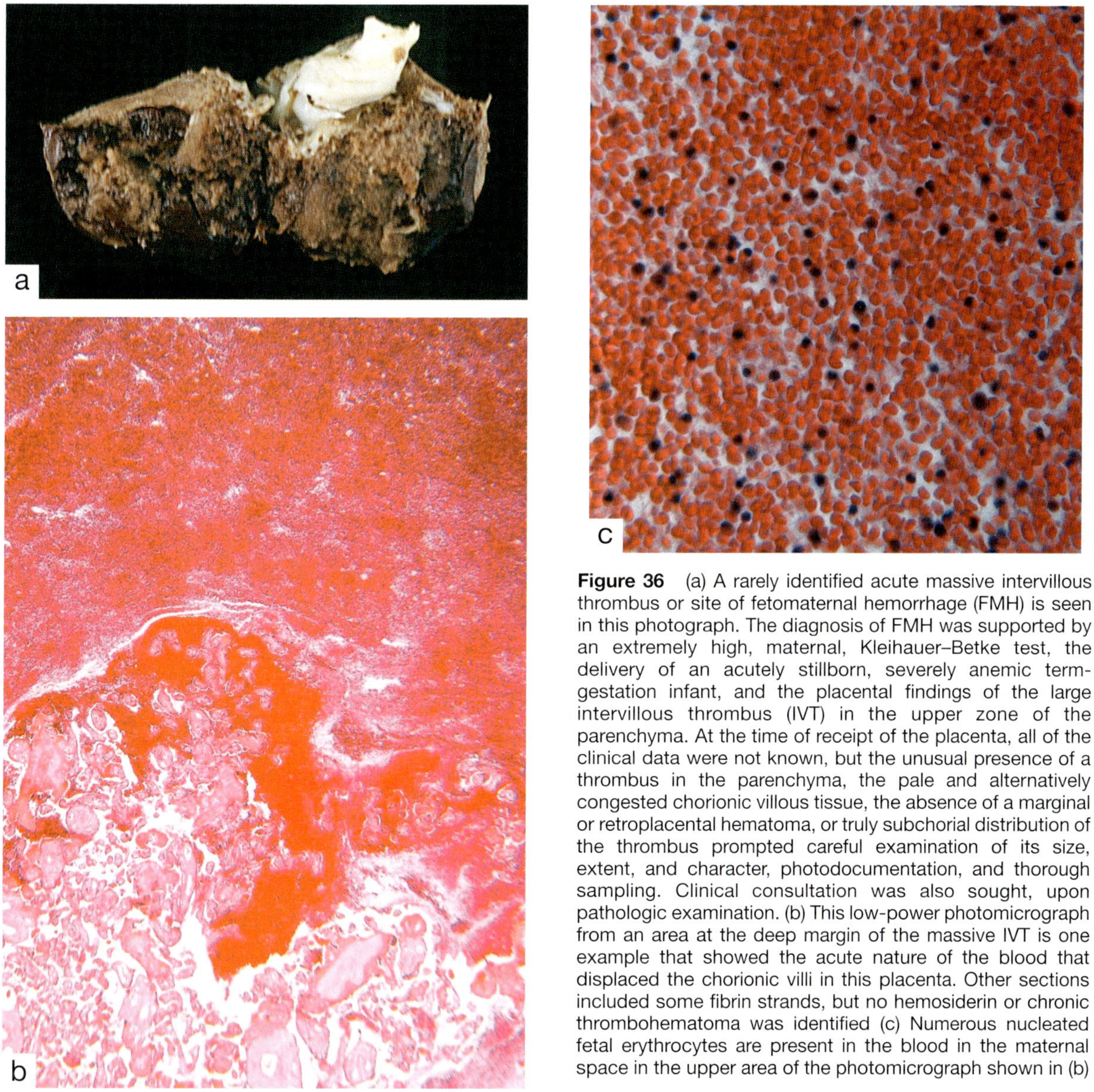

Figure 36 (a) A rarely identified acute massive intervillous thrombus or site of fetomaternal hemorrhage (FMH) is seen in this photograph. The diagnosis of FMH was supported by an extremely high, maternal, Kleihauer–Betke test, the delivery of an acutely stillborn, severely anemic term-gestation infant, and the placental findings of the large intervillous thrombus (IVT) in the upper zone of the parenchyma. At the time of receipt of the placenta, all of the clinical data were not known, but the unusual presence of a thrombus in the parenchyma, the pale and alternatively congested chorionic villous tissue, the absence of a marginal or retroplacental hematoma, or truly subchorial distribution of the thrombus prompted careful examination of its size, extent, and character, photodocumentation, and thorough sampling. Clinical consultation was also sought, upon pathologic examination. (b) This low-power photomicrograph from an area at the deep margin of the massive IVT is one example that showed the acute nature of the blood that displaced the chorionic villi in this placenta. Other sections included some fibrin strands, but no hemosiderin or chronic thrombohematoma was identified (c) Numerous nucleated fetal erythrocytes are present in the blood in the maternal space in the upper area of the photomicrograph shown in (b)

risks of fetal morbidity and perinatal mortality, and a given infant's outcome will be dependent upon the volume and rapidity of the loss, and the time interval from onset of hemorrhage to delivery. For example, a KB of 2% translates to a 70-ml red cell loss for a 3000-g infant, or 140 ml of whole blood; this represents the loss of about a third of the baby's total fetoplacental blood volume, and an acute loss would almost certainly result in fetal death. (Normal fetoplacental blood volume at term is 125 ml/kg and hemoglobin//hematocrit is 17.9 g/dl//50.) Complications of FMH include fetal hypotension, diminished fetoplacental perfusion, intrauterine fetal hypoxia, fetal tachycardia and cardiac rhythm abnormalities, congestive heart failure, hydrops, and intrauterine fetal death; perinatal sequelae include profound anemia of the newborn, cerebral infarction, intraventricular hemorrhage, and cerebral palsy[3,4,33]. Unfortunately, after an acute, very large hemorrhage, obstetrical management may have little effect on the infant's outcome. In the review by de Almeida and Bowman[85], massive FMH of ≥ 80 ml was associated with a 46% rate of adverse outcome; some 83% of the affected infants died in the perinatal period, with all deaths occurring by age 6 months. (The reader is referred to the article by Biankin and colleagues[66] for a full discussion of the autopsy findings in cases of fetal demise due to FMH.) More chronic FMH may permit obstetrical intervention (such as intrauterine transfusions) and timely delivery of a live-born infant who can be successfully treated with transfusions in the neonatal period[69,72,73].

Subamniotic hematoma

This is a collection of fetal blood that lies between the amnion and chorion, on the fetal surface. It is usually small, generally due to disruption of a venous vessel on the fetal surface, near the cord insertion site, and related to cord traction with delivery of the placenta or cord blood sampling (Figure 37). Since it usually occurs after delivery of the infant, it is of no clinical significance. However, very rarely, spontaneous subamniotic hematoma (SH) may develop *in utero*. It may be detected on prenatal ultrasonography and/or associated with an unexplained elevation of maternal serum α-fetoprotein, fetal intrauterine growth restriction, or even intrauterine fetal demise, due to FMH[4,90,91]. Trauma to fetal plate vessels can result in SH and intra-amniotic contamination by fetal blood; iatrogenic subamniotic hematoma may very rarely occur during amniocentesis. Also rare is SH with velamentous cord insertion. Benirschke[92] reported a case that resulted in fetal exsanguination. One of the authors (OF-P, unpublished observations) has seen a case in which rapid intrapartum fetal demise occurred after artificial rupture of membranes had been performed. An acute FMH was clinically suspected, and placental examination revealed extensive velamentous insertion of the cord with a site of vascular disruption and SH formation in the free membranes. The hemorrhage was concluded to be due to iatrogenic laceration of a velamentous vessel in this clinically unsuspected instance of vasa previa. *Chronic* SH was reported by DeSa[93] and found to be associated with fetal growth restriction and chorionic plate venous thrombosis.

Histologically, incidental SH consists of hemorrhage alone, without thrombus formation. Fibrin thrombus formation occurs in antenatal or intrapartum, infant birth-related events; thus, SH occurring in these settings will be manifested by fibrin deposition on both sides of the vascular rupture/laceration site and as true fibrin laminations in the hematoma. Chronic SH is further associated with chorionic hemosiderosis.

Fetal arterial thrombosis

Fetal arterial thrombosis may occur in the fetal plate or stem villous ramifications of the umbilical arteries. Careful inspection and palpation of the fetal surface arteries (which nearly always overlie the veins) may reveal pale, white-tan and firm, to overtly calcified, vascular segments. Obstruction of large branches is generally accompanied by considerable segmental propagation, and, thus, these obstructions are more easily detected. More often, however, medium-sized or smaller branches are affected and multiple vessel sites may be involved. One can more easily detect sites of occlusion on fresh, unfixed placentas by exerting mild pressure on proximal aspects of the arterial tree; luminal blood will not be easily displaced past points of obstruction. (This technique, of course, works poorly on fixed placentas!) Sectioning of occluded vessels may reveal acute, red-brown, laminated, or white chronic thrombi. Transmural placental sections should always be submitted in instances of questionable fetal plate thrombosis.

The pathologic features of this lesion are largely covered in Chapter 9, section on 'Lesions involving fetal stem vessels' since fetal arterial thrombosis is a type of fetal thrombotic vasculopathy. However, to summarize briefly, fetal arterial thrombosis at the chorionic plate, stem, or intermediate villous level results in ischemia and/or sclerosis in the dependent portions of the villous tree, and renders them

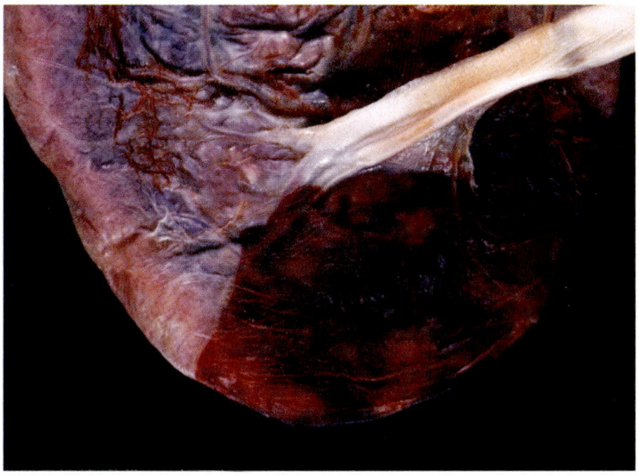

Figure 37 Cord traction to facilitate delivery of the placenta can result in a typical cord-associated distribution of artifactual subamniotic extravasation of fetal blood ('hematoma') that should not be overinterpreted

dysfunctional. In addition, fetal arterial thrombosis is often multifocal or compounded by thromboembolic sequelae. The site, degree, and timing of arterial luminal compromise determine the distal effect on the villous tree. The more complete is the occlusion, the more proximal is its location, the earlier it occurs in the development of the villous tree, and the greater is its distribution within the tree, the greater is the composite loss of chorionic villous surface available for exchange, and the greater is the risk for fetal morbidity and mortality. Moreover, while recanalization may occur, luminal size and integrity are not fully restored, and the compensatory growth and maturation of the villous tree may not be sufficient to prevent chronic hypoxia or fetal growth restriction. Finally, since the placental arterial tree is an extension of the fetal cardiovascular system, the factors that predispose to thrombosis within the placenta may also result in thromboembolic phenomena in the fetus.

9

Histologic lesions of the placenta: villi, fetal stem arteries, intervillous space and maternal arteries in decidua

Histopathologic lesions of the placenta can be categorized by pathogenic mechanism (e.g. placental bed underperfusion) and by type of underlying maternal disorder (e.g. diabetes mellitus, heritable thrombophilias, metabolic diseases). However, pathologists are often faced with the task of evaluating placentas without the benefit of much accompanying clinical history. Therefore, we have chosen to adopt the categorization by site (Table 8) and, secondarily, to list the differential diagnoses of these lesions, in overview. Use of this histologic scheme, however, is predicated on: first, basic knowledge of the normal maturational gross and microscopic changes that occur during gestation (as described in Chapter 2 and amplified below); and second, appreciation of the fact that the gross and microscopic features seen at the time of pathologic examination represent a point of 'arrest' in the continuum of placental development in the given case. Hence, any gross or microscopic assessment of a placental specimen should be made with reference to the features normally expected for the gestational period in question and to maternal and fetal disease processes, abnormalities occurring during labor and delivery, and primary placental abnormalities. Some features, such as syncytiotrophoblastic knots (see below) for example, are normally present at term, but pathologic when present early in gestation or when relatively increased in numbers in late gestation. The structures of normal villous types and highlights of normal villous development are shown in Figure 38.

Table 8 Basic histologic 'lesions'* of the placenta. Adapted from reference 3

Lesions of the villi involving

Trophoblast
- excessive number of syncytiotrophoblastic knots, excessive number of cytotrophoblastic cells, deficiency of vasculosyncytial membrane, fibrinoid necrosis of villi (intravillous fibrinoid)

Trophoblastic basement membrane
- thickening, dystrophic mineralization

Stroma
- stromal fibrosis, villous edema, excessive number of Hofbauer cells

Blood vessels
- hypovascularity, hypervascularity

Generalized villous population
- villous immaturity, accelerated villous maturation

Lesions of fetal (placental) stem arteries

Thrombosis/fetal thrombotic vasculopathy (including 'endarteritis obliterans')

Fibromuscular sclerosis

Hemorrhagic endovasculitis/endovasculosis

Lesions of intervillous space

Lesions of the decidua

Lesions of maternal arteries in decidua

*Many of these 'lesions' can be present in the normal placenta

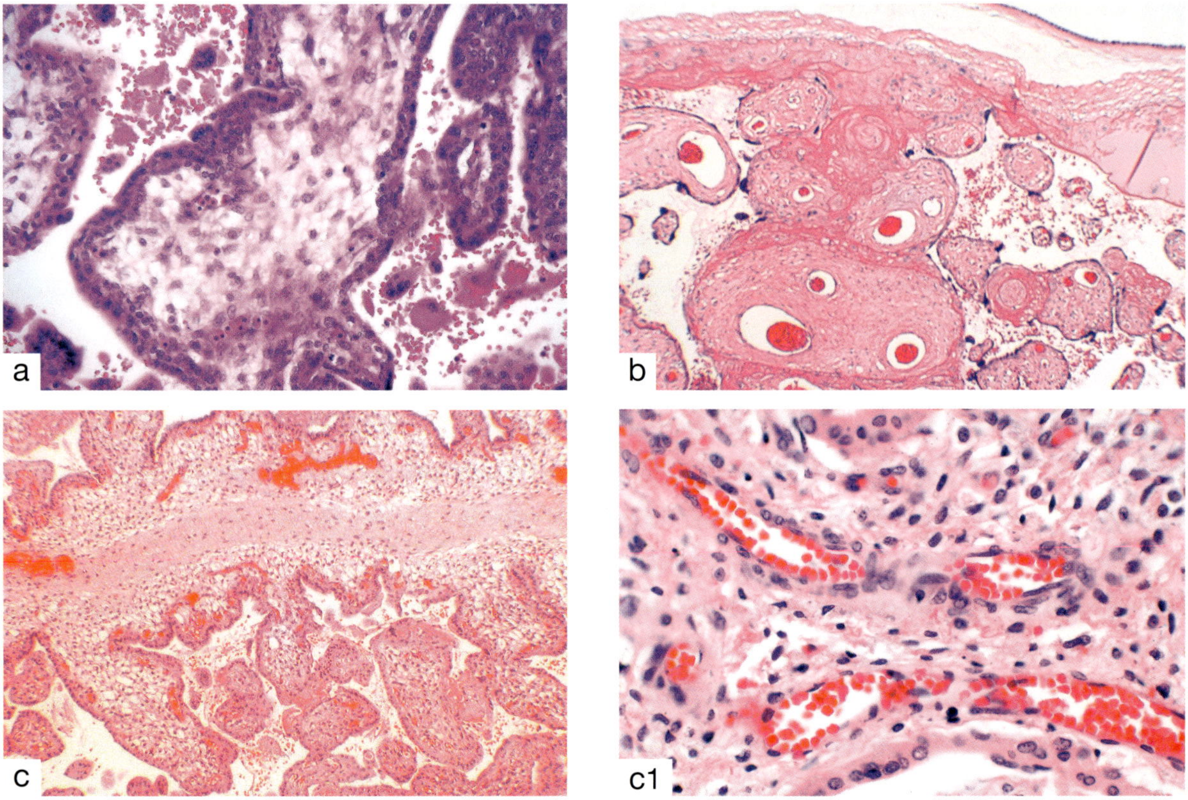

Figure 38 Types of villi and their structure. (a) First-trimester villi are characterized by a double layer of trophoblasts, abundant loose stroma, easily seen Hofbauer cells, and one to only a few, centrally positioned capillaries containing nucleated erythrocytes. These mesenchymal villi are the most primitive villi. (b) Stem villi: these connect the chorionic plate with the villous tree and are composed of condensed fibrous stroma, with one to only a few central arteries and veins, and branches with media or adventitia. They constitute about 20–25% of the villous volume of a term placenta. The mature, large, main stem villi emerge from the floor of the chorionic plate, as shown here, and have a cytotrophoblastic covering with a dense fibrous core with thick-walled arteries and large veins. These branch serially to form four short, thick orders, which then branch further to create some ten suborders of progressively thinning trunks of the deeper tree, 70–80 μm in final diameter (see Figures 6 and 38c). The last generations of these give rise to intermediate villi. Intermediate villi show two basic developmental forms: immature and mature. (c) This field from a second-trimester placenta shows an immature stem villus branching to immature intermediate villi: bulbous, ~ 200 μm in diameter structures with loose, reticular stroma, easily identified Hofbauer cells, and scattered capillaries (c-1). Immature intermediate villi are most numerous in second-trimester placentas and are scattered in low-power fields of sections from third-trimester placentas, especially of placentas from gestations between 25 and 32 weeks. Immature intermediate villi remain detectable in small percentages in term placentas. (d) The immature intermediate villous branchings of the second-trimester placenta lead to smaller-diameter intermediate villi with villous surface and tip extensions, that show a single layer of plump cytotrophoblasts and trophoblastic villous ‘sprouts’ and ‘buds’ (future intermediate villous branch and villous growth points). Many of the buds in this photomicrograph appear to be ‘free-floating’ because their connection to a villus is not caught in the plane of section. The villous stroma is loose, and the capillaries that contain some nucleated fetal erythrocytes are several micrometers away from the trophoblastic epithelial villous surface (see d-1). Note: compare these villi with those in (a) and (f). (e) Mature intermediate villi. The prominent central collagenization of the stroma marks maturational change of the intermediate villus and cessation of its intermediate branching with correlative increase in the development of its terminal villous tree. Note the presence of peripheral collagen in the stroma of these two intermediate villi, which show arterioles and venules, and the complex formations of terminal villi, captured at various levels in this photomicrograph extending from the intermediate villus in the center. (f) Terminal villi. These are grape-like ramifications of mature intermediate villi and appear at about 32 weeks of gestation. One is cut in cross-section and several villus tips surround it. They have a high degree of capillarization and show initiation of the formation of vasculosyncytial membranes (VSM), as seen in the upper right corner of the field in the villus tip with the multinucleated syncytiotrophoblast layer, which increase the efficiency of gas and nutrient exchange. This photomicrograph is from a 33–34 week gestation placenta, so not all the villi have VSM, but the capillaries more closely approximate the villous surface than they do in the second trimester villus (d-1).

Continued

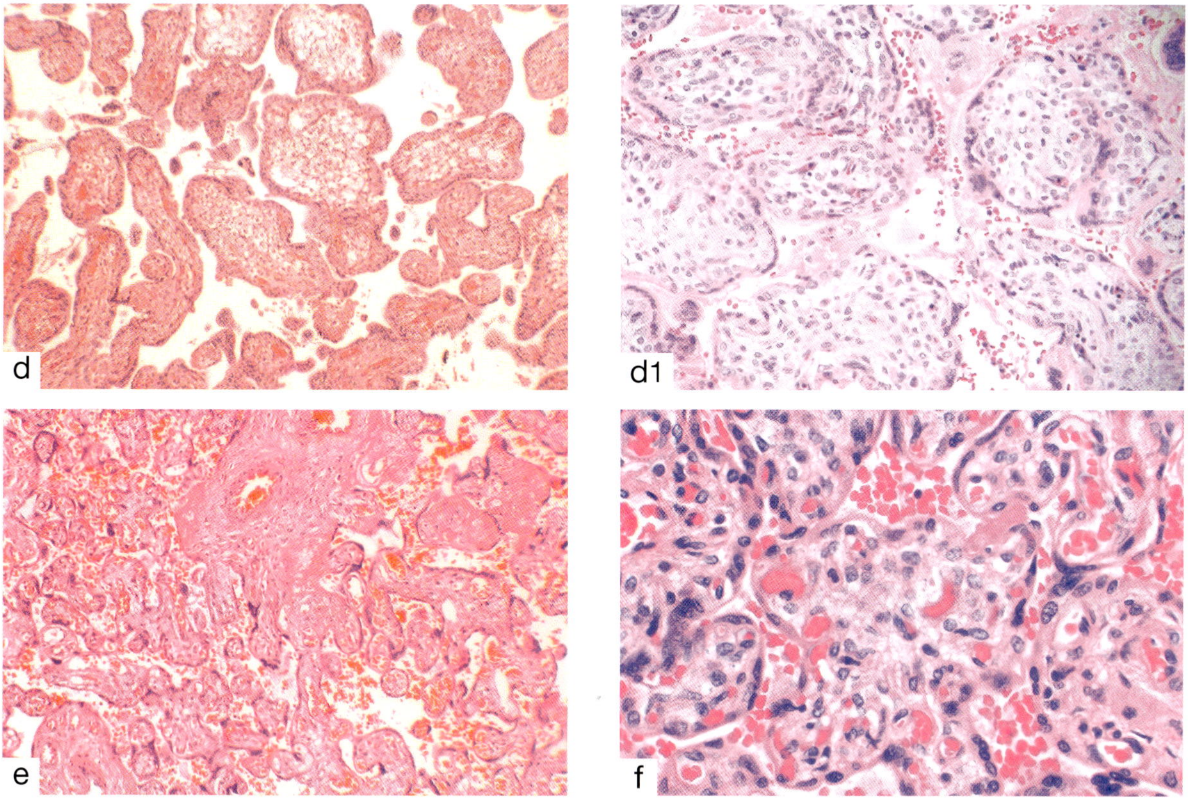

Figure 38 *Continued*
Note that there are no nucleated fetal erythrocytes in this field; nucleated red blood cells are uncommon and generally make up less than 3–5% of circulating red cells seen in the villi in normal gestations. (g) Term villi. At term, the development of vasculosyncytial membranes is maximal (compare with d-1 and f). Syncytial knots, with cytoplasmic thinning and localization of the syncytiotrophoblastic nuclei to a lateral focus in the syncytiotrophoblast, optimize villous transport and function. These nuclei undergo apoptosis and are progressively shed into the maternal space; the viability of the syncytiotrophoblast is dependent upon its replenishment by the underlying cytotrophoblast

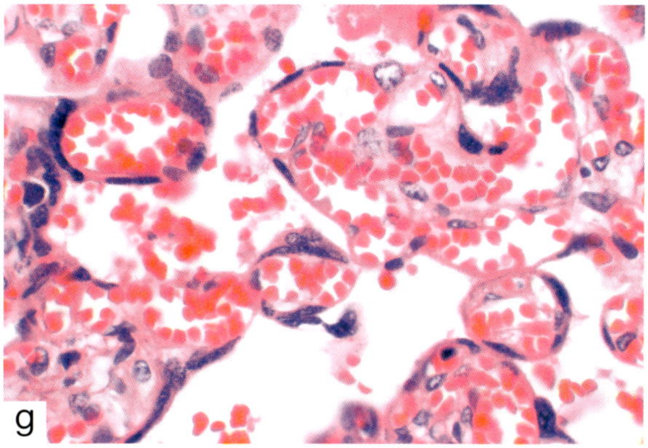

LESIONS OF THE CHORIONIC VILLI INVOLVING THE TROPHOBLAST

Excessive numbers of syncytiotrophoblastic knots

Incidence In order to address their normal occurrence or relative increase during gestation, syncytiotrophoblastic knots must first be distinguished from other types of syncytiotrophoblastic accumulations: syncytiotrophoblastic sprouts and syncytiotrophoblastic bridges. Unfortunately, these terms have been used interchangeably in the literature. In addition, there may be pathologically significant implications for subtyping knots into 'syncytiotrophoblastic' versus 'apoptotic' forms.

In normal gestation, chorionic villous cytotrophoblasts proliferate and subpopulations differentiate, later to fuse with, and become incorporated into, the continuous, external syncytial layer. This process is incompletely understood, but normal growth and development of the chorionic villous tree appear to require a balance of cellular proliferation, differentiation, and senescence, as well as a specialized milieu of maternal hematologic, hormonal, nutritional, and biochemical factors, and locally generated trophoblastic mediators. The number and morphology of the various syncytiotrophoblastic formations are, thereby, temporally and milieu-dependent.

Syncytiotrophoblastic sprouts are large, loose clusters of normochromatic and normally sized syncytiotrophoblastic nuclei that form prominent, bulging protrusions from the chorionic villous surface. In the first half of gestation, they occur in limited numbers and are sites of chorionic villous sprouting, but, in late gestation, true sprouts are rare, and their 'presence' nearly always represents tangential sectioning through villous syncytiotrophoblast. Sprouts are shed into the maternal circulation. Similarly, *syncytiotrophoblastic bridges* are early structures that result from the fusion of intervillous abutments of neighboring syncytiotrophoblastic aggregates. Bridges may impart some structural stability to the chorionic villous tree, but their functional significance, if any, is unclear. Like the 'sprouts' of later gestation, 'bridges' in the third trimester are sectional artifacts through adjacent villous convolutions. '*Syncytiotrophoblastic buds*' are stromal syncytiotrophoblastic inclusions and are mentioned, herein, only to clarify that they are also artifacts created by a plane of section through scalloped or protruding chorionic villous contours. *Syncytiotrophoblastic knots*, in contrast to sprouts, are localized accumulations of syncytiotrophoblastic nuclei that produce focal thickenings in the syncytial surfaces of terminal villi.

Pathogenesis and significance Syncytiotrophoblastic knots are a normal component of terminal villous development, and their numbers/low-power field increase with passing gestational weeks. Terminal villi (exchange villi) are formed as foci of branching and lengthening, capillaries that protrude directly from mature intermediate villi (conduit villi). The proliferative cytotrophoblast, covering the terminal villi, forms and replenishes the overlying syncytial layer, as needed. Progressive attenuation of villous stroma increasingly facilitates oxygen and nutritional transport, across the villus. Moreover, the cytoplasm of the syncytial layer also thins and becomes depopulated of organelles at sites of its direct apposition to bulging capillary loops. These flattened, mirrored profiles of cytoplasm and basal lamina of the endoepithelial interface are called *vasculosyncytial membranes*. The vascular loops impinge upon the overlying epithelium and the syncytiotrophoblastic nuclei are 'displaced' laterally, forming collections called *syncytiotrophoblastic knots* (or *syncytial knots*). The knots are composed of aggregates of small, closely packed, densely staining syncytiotrophoblastic nuclei in various stages of apoptosis, and are sites of sequestration and extrusion of these 'nuclear suicides' into the maternal space[94]. The process of cytotrophoblastic turnover, from fusion to the syncytial layer to aggregate expulsion, is accomplished in 2–4 weeks[95]. Because they are particularly associated with angiogenesis, which begins at about 26 weeks[96], and terminal villous differentiation, syncytial knots are sparsely identifiable before 32 weeks of gestation but detectable on 11–30% of villi by term[3]. Their presence on routine histologic section of term placentas largely reflects sectional thickness and angle through the syncytial layer.

Excessive numbers of syncytiotrophoblastic knots or *syncytial knotting* results from excessive capillary proliferation in the terminal villi, which is stimulated by hypoxia. Irregular, knob-like outgrowths of tortuous and complex capillary configurations create irregularly contoured terminal villi, numerous syncytial–capillary interfaces, and, thereby, increased numbers and shapes of knots seen by flat section. At low power, the terminal villi appear to be clustered together and small, because of their abnormally branched configurations, and their proximity to one another results in elongated 'bridge' and bulbous 'sprout' configurations. The villous clustering and increase in syncytial knot frequency, for a given period of gestation, is called 'Tenney–Parker change', and it results in increased chorionic villous surface area available for exchange.

It is at this juncture that terminology becomes problematic. Histomorphometric investigations suggest that increased *syncytial knottings* result from excessive capillary proliferation and abnormal terminal villous configurations stimulated by hypoxia, and that *apoptotic knots*, which show apoptotic nuclear and cytoplasmic degenerative changes, are knots of normal villous maturation[94]. It appears that apoptosis is a factor essential to the normal processes of chorionic villous proliferation, development, remodeling, and cell turnover throughout gestation[95,97,98]. In addition, trophoblastic cell turnover, which is well regulated and changes during gestation, directly influences placental function[94,99]. Rates of syncytial apoptosis in term placentas (as determined by immunohistochemical terminal deoxynucleotidase end-nick labeling (TUNEL) marker studies) are 0.03–0.05%[100,101]. However, as will subsequently be discussed, hypoxia *also* accelerates cytotrophoblastic cell turnover and apoptosis.

Despite the morphogenetic differences, the pathologic and developmental syncytiotrophoblastic knots show overlapping light microscopic features of nuclear condensation, crowding, and variability of size and shape, and immunohistochemical and ultrastructural features (aging nuclei in various stages of apoptosis)[94,95,101,102]. Therefore, the descriptive term 'syncytiotrophoblastic knot' is used to denote collections of aged, apoptotic syncytial nuclei of *any* morphogenetic derivation. A relative increase in numbers of these multinucleated profiles reflects alterations in the normal course of cytotrophoblastic turnover. Due to the 'relative ischemia' of the subchorial and basal zones of the placenta, chorionic villous morphology and knot number are best assessed in the mid-parenchymal zone of a well-fixed and thinly cut (5 μm) transplacental section. The extent of knotting can be estimated by careful low-power scan, but more thoroughly assessed by counting the number of knots/100 villi. At term, less than a third of villi should exhibit syncytial knots.

Excessive syncytiotrophoblastic knotting (Figure 39) is a histopathologic indicator of excessive chorionic villous capillary proliferation and/or exaggerated senescence (increased cell turnover) induced by hypoxia that may be due to several maternal or fetal pathologic conditions. They include hypoperfusion and/or reduction of oxygen availability of the intervillous space, villous capillary hypoperfusion, and fetal anemia. Conditions that lead to hypoperfusion of the maternal space include maternal chronic hypertension, diabetes, primary thrombophilia and some connective-tissue disorders (e.g. systemic lupus erythematosus[103]), in which there are maternal arterial occlusive changes, and pre-eclampsia, in which there is inadequate physiological transformation of superficial, intramyometrial spiral arteries. Thrombophilic conditions may also be associated with increased perivillous fibrin deposition, further reducing the perfusion of intervillous space[104]. Maternal anemia from any cause (e.g. malaria in tropical countries[105]) and lung disease cause hypoxia due to reduced oxygen availability in the intervillous space. The fetal conditions include fetal anemia due to any cause (e.g. Rh isoimmunization), requiring increased villous surface and fetal artery thrombosis due to primary or secondary hypercoagulability states or vasculitis (e.g. in syphilis[106,107]). Excessive syncytiotrophoblastic knots are also seen in postmaturity[108] and after 2 or more days of intrauterine retention of the fetoplacental unit, following intrauterine

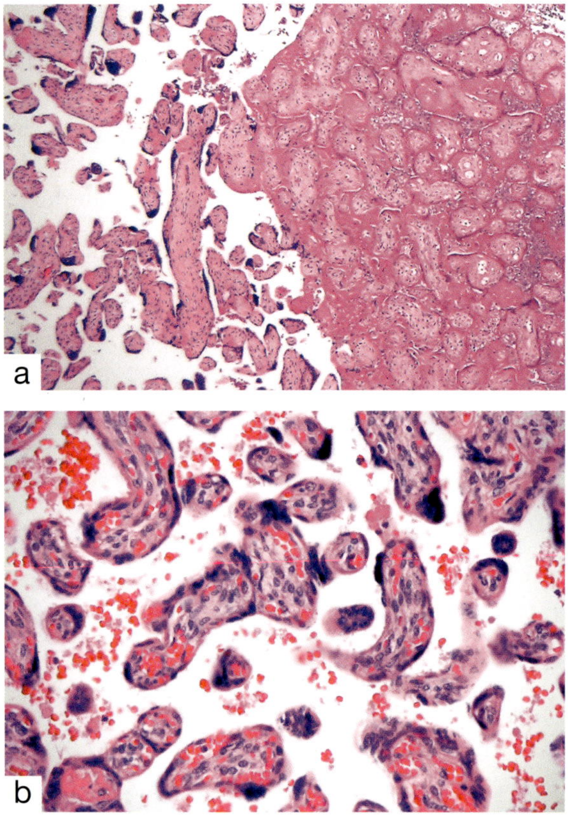

Figure 39 (a) Excessive syncytial knotting. Excessive knotting is seen in the ischemic villi bordering an acute chorionic villous infarct. (b) Additional photomicrograph showing third-trimester chorionic villi not associated with an infarct, but which are closely crowded together and which demonstrate increased numbers of syncytial knots, features suggestive of acute ischemia

fetal demise[109] (see Chapter 15, section on 'Features of intrauterine retention').

Increased knottings for period of gestation are associated with increased risk of fetal intrauterine growth restriction and perinatal morbidity and mortality. In addition, while multinucleated trophoblasts are found in the maternal circulation during gestation[48], and several hundred thousand trophoblasts are normally deported/hour into the maternal uterine vein during labor in the third trimester[110], they are shed in increased numbers into the maternal circulation in pathologic conditions with increased apoptosis and necrosis, such as pre-eclampsia[102,110–112]. This marked increase in deportation of syncytiotrophoblastic aggregates, that is, up to 30 times higher in pre-eclampsia (~ 10^7 trophoblasts/hour)[110], may have important implications for the mother, including contributing to the morbidity of pre-eclampsia[113–116]. These deported cells may potentially even serve as the source of soluble fms-like tyrosine kinase 1 (sFlt1), a plasma factor recently identified to induce several key features of pre-clampsia (hypertension, proteinuria, and glomerular endotheliosis) in rats[117], and noted to be elevated in women with pre-eclampsia. A pathologic increase in the numbers of these circulating cells may also explain the potential predictive value of using sFlt1 elevation, in combination with lowered plasma levels of placental growth factor (PlGF), to identify pregnant women at risk for the development of pre-eclampsia[118,119]. Moreover, sudden death from trophoblastic embolism[120] and with trophoblastic embolism associated with pre-eclampsia has also been reported[121–123].

Excessive numbers of cytotrophoblastic cells

Incidence The villous cytotrophoblastic cells (also known as Langhan's cells) form a complete mantle around immature villi. With advancing gestation and progressive villous maturation, the increase in chorionic villous surface far exceeds the increase in the number of cytotrophoblasts, and the cytotrophoblasts form a discontinous layer. The cytotrophoblastic cells become inconspicuous, giving a spurious impression of their 'near absence' on routine histologic assessment of mature terminal villi. Thus, between 20%[4] and 40%[3] of normal mature villi will show cytotrophoblast, by careful light microscopic examination, depending upon the thickness and orientation of section.

The cytotrophoblastic cell compartment is largely proliferative and undifferentiated, with a few cells showing ultrastructural, immunohistochemical, and enzymatic features similar to syncytiotrophoblasts. These more differentiated cytotrophoblasts regenerate the syncytium by fusing with the overlying syncytiotrophoblast. Fusion is accompanied by progressive dispersion of, and functional changes in, incorporated cytotrophoblast organelles, and apoptotic changes in their nuclei. The stem cytotrophoblastic cells lie external to the chorionic villous basement membrane and can best be distinguished from the syncytial layer by PAS stain; syncytial cytoplasm and the basement membrane are PAS-positive, whereas the undifferentiated cytotrophoblastic cell cytoplasm is not. (Lack of PAS staining is a likely histochemical correlate of the essential absence of enzymes of aerobic and anaerobic glycolysis in the stem cell.) PAS stain will, therefore, bracket the cytotrophoblast (Figure 40) and the presence of cytotrophoblastic hyperplasia. A thin section of plastic embedded material will also reveal the presence of excessive numbers of cytotrophoblasts.

A greater proportion of chorionic villi may show cytotrophoblasts in placentas from pregnancies complicated by maternal diabetes, pre-eclampsia, and/or hypertension; gestation at high altitude; fetal anemia (e.g. immune-mediated hemolysis); prolonged gestation; or recent intrauterine fetal demise after prolonged hypoxia. The conditions that are associated with excessive numbers of cytotrophoblastic cells are similar to those in which there is increased syncytial knotting.

Pathogenesis and significance Excessive numbers of cytotrophoblasts reflect proliferation of precursor cells beyond what is normally required to maintain the growth, survival, and functional integrity of the syncytiotrophoblastic layer. Hypoxia enhances apoptosis in the syncytium, damages the syncytiotrophoblast (see above), and hinders differentiation[4,94,98]. It is also a major stimulus of cytotrophoblastic (stem) cell proliferation, triggering an increase in mitotic rate, shortening of the cell cycle, and changes in the molecular and functional phenotype of the cytotrophoblast. It appears to effect a kind of return to the intermediate cytotrophoblast cell phenotype present in early gestation. A variety of mediators of this process have been identified (e.g. hypoxia inducible factor-1α subunit, HIF-1 heteromeric dimer, transforming growth factor-β_3, focal adhesion kinase)[124], but the process remains

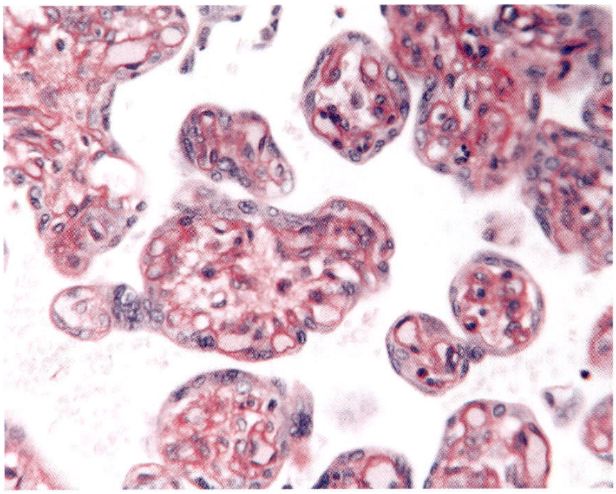

Figure 40 Periodic acid–Schiff (PAS) stain brackets the plump, immature cytotrophoblast cells of these 33-week gestation chorionic villi. The cell cytoplasm of the thin, mature syncytiotrophoblast and its basement membrane, as well as the basement membranes of the capillaries, are PAS-positive, whereas the cytotrophoblastic cell cytoplasm (and aggregates) is not

incompletely understood. Suffice to say, hypoxia results in increased need for syncytial regeneration and repair and increased numbers of cells for the tasks. Cytotrophoblastic hyperplasia appears to be an indicator of ischemia and its degree an indicator of the severity of ischemia.

Deficiency of vasculosyncytial membranes

Incidence A distinct, continuous basement membrane separates the trophoblast from the villous stroma. However, as described in the previous section on chorionic villous morphogenesis, there are sites in the syncytium, adjacent to knots, in which the syncytial cytoplasm is thinned, shows organelle paucity, and is directly apposed to the basement membranes of endothelial cells of the underlying, ectatic capillaries. Studies have revealed that some of these locations show actual fusion of the facing cells' basement membranes. These specialized sites, the *vasculosyncytial membranes* (VSM), when particularly thin, are places of diffusional gas and water and, it appears, facilitated glucose transfer. Thicker VSM, with more organelles and enzymatic activity, are presumed sites of active transport of amino acids[94]. VSM are very uncommon before 32 weeks of gestation, but increase rapidly as branching angiogenesis continues and more terminal villi are formed. They have been identified, with careful fixation and section, to constitute 20–40% of the chorionic villous surface at term[3,125].

Deficiency of VSM (< 5% of villi showing VSM) may be seen in placentas from gestations complicated by maternal diabetes, immune-mediated hemolytic disease of the fetus, chromosomal anomalies of the conceptus, and acute stillbirth.

Pathogenesis and significance VSM are a manifestation of villous maturation. Normal synchronous, maturational progression results in a normal capillary to villus ratio of about 5 : 1 at term[126], and normal numbers of vasculosyncytial membranous formations. Decreased VSM for period of gestation reflect a delayed or defective villous maturational process. In the placenta with a deficiency of VSM, the histopathologic picture is dominated by immature-appearing, larger-diameter (up to 150–250 μm) intermediate villi with cellular stroma, few terminal villous branchings, and true sprouts admixed with more mature-appearing, intermediate villi. Hence, the villous morphology is often reminiscent of that seen in the early third trimester (26–32 weeks)[4], and likely represents the sequelae of a maturational disturbance(s) occurring early in gestation. Maturational disturbances may be synchronous as seen in Rh incompatibility or asynchronous (i.e. mismatch of interrelated processes of capillary and trophoblastic proliferation) as seen in diabetes (Figure 41) (see below, also, section on 'Maternal diabetes' in Chapter 14).

Whatever the etiology, a deficiency of VSM results in increased risks of deficiencies in placental transport, abnormalities of placental volume, fetal intrauterine growth restriction, and perinatal morbidity and mortality.

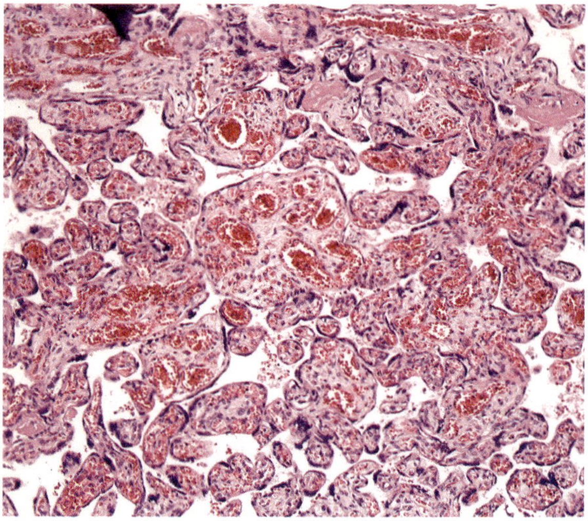

Figure 41 An example of deficiency of vasculosyncytial membranes is present in this section that was widely representative of this 820-g placenta from a 36.5-week gestation complicated by maternal diabetes mellitus. The terminal villi are bulky and dysmature-appearing, with excessive stroma, poor development of vasculosyncytial membranes, and abnormal vascularity. The villi in the center of the field additionally have a chorangiomatous morphology

Fibrinoid necrosis of villi (intravillous fibrinoid)

Incidence Homogeneous fibrinoid material is seen beneath the syncytiotrophoblast and external to the basement membrane in the earliest stage of the lesion. Increasing amounts of the acellular, eosinophilic material eventually form a large fibrinoid nodule bordered by a few attenuated nuclei of syncytiotrophoblast that virtually replaces the villous stroma (Figure 16). This intravillous lesion is distinct from *peri*villous fibrinoid deposition in which fibrinoid material partially or completely envelops the villous *surface*. About 3% of villi in mature placentas show fibrinoid necrosis. Increased deposition is seen in placentas from preterm deliveries, and moderate increases are seen in pre-eclampsia, erythroblastosis fetalis, and diabetes mellitus[3] of both insulin-dependent and gestational types[127]; active and active-chronic malarial infection[28,105]; and postmaturity[126].

Pathogenesis and significance It appears to be due, at least in part, to immunologic factors[3,105,127], and particularly to placental aging[128]. Degeneration from placental aging and/or hypoxic damage to the trophoblast appears to contribute to the process of fibrinoid formation. Excessive amounts of fibrinoid necrosis are likely associated with reduced efficiency of transport across and function within the chorionic villus, thereby further contributing to the fetal pathology of diabetes, pre-eclampsia, and postmaturity.

LESIONS OF THE VILLI INVOLVING THE TROPHOBLASTIC BASEMENT MEMBRANE

Thickening

Incidence Assessment of thickening is based on subjective criteria, but PAS stain and immunohistochemistry for collagen IV or laminin[4] can be used to distinguish between normal and thickened basement membrane. Thickened basement membrane is found in approximately 1% of term placentas, but increased foci of thickening can be seen in postmaturity. Marked, and often generalized, changes in membrane thickness can be seen in pre-eclampsia, essential hypertension, diabetes mellitus, fetal growth restriction with absent end-diastolic umbilical blood flow, immune-mediated fetal anemia, excessive perivillous fibrinoid deposition[3,4], and malarial infection[105,129]. Placentas from cases of macerated stillbirth commonly show basement membranous thickening that is likely due to prolonged hypoxia of the chorionic villi that occurs with retention.

Pathogenesis and significance The basement membrane is produced by the trophoblast. Cytotrophoblastic hyperplasia results in increased elaboration of membrane components, possibly with reduced membrane turnover. Aberrations of cytotrophoblastic proliferation and function are presumed to cause basement membrane thickening[4]. The role of immunoglobulin and immune complex deposition remains undetermined[3].

As discussed above, cytotrophoblastic hyperplasia appears to be an indicator of ischemia and ischemic severity. Thus, conditions that result in chorionic villous ischemia show basement membrane thickening. Thickened membranes presumably impair chorionic villous transport. The occurrence of thickened basement membranes is associated with fetal hypoxia, growth restriction (particularly in cases of active malarial infection[129]), and stillbirth.

Dystrophic mineralization

Incidence Purple-blue-staining, dystrophic mineralizations of the basement membrane (on hematoxylin–eosin stain) have been mostly reported in cases of fetal demise with intrauterine retention of the conceptus[4]. The basement membranous mineralizations are often linearly deposited, especially in instances of prolonged intrauterine retention, but may be discontinuous or accompanied by stromal stippling (Figure 42). The encrustations and dusty deposits stain positively for both calcium and iron (von Kossa and Prussian blue stains, respectively), and involve the subtrophoblastic region of stem, intermediate, and terminal villi. While they are very common in stillbirths, they may also be occasionally seen in mature placentas from live births, and not infrequently observed in anencephaly, fetoplacental chromosomal anomalies, viral non-immune fetal hydrops, and chronic villitis; congenital anomalies, including isolated heart defects; fetal Bartter's syndrome; sclerotic villi in pre-eclampsia, hypertension,

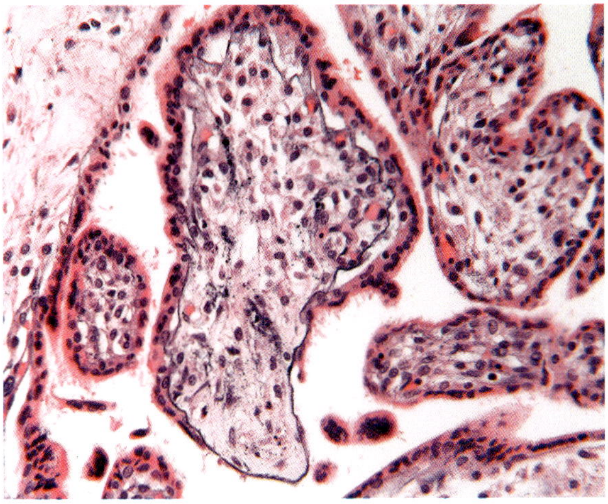

Figure 42 Dystrophic mineralization is seen along villous basement membranes and in stroma in these late second-trimester villi from a placenta from a stillborn delivery

and postmaturity; and devitalized chorionic villi of fetal thrombotic vasculopathy (see below)[130–133].

Pathogenesis and significance The exact nature of the deposits and their pathogenesis are not known, but a crystalline pattern of calcium hydroxyapatite has been identified by electron microscopy diffraction[134]. Presumably, the precipitates represent sites and/or sequelae of defective transport of materials across the trophoblast. In fetal death, the trophoblast continues to transport material for a time, but without fetal circulatory removal and uptake. Similarly, defective fetal cardiac function might also result in circulatory abnormalities in the villi and abnormal clearance of molecules and ions, such as calcium and iron. In villous sclerosis and villous damage, the trophoblast may persist and retain some transport function and/or lose membranous integrity and restrictive permeability. A defective interface with maternal blood might permit villous penetration and dystrophic deposition of calcium and iron on an altered basement membrane 'barrier'. Alternatively, loss of villous vascularity may retard their removal. Defects in fetal renal ion excretion have been proposed to be responsible for the mineralizations in Bartter's syndrome[131] and may contribute to encrustations in other conditions, too. The pathogenic mechanisms are unclear, but the mineralizations are linear tombstones, if not hallmarks, of altered pathways of villous transport and/or clearance functions[133].

LESIONS OF THE VILLI INVOLVING STROMA

Stromal fibrosis

Incidence Fibrosis is a feature of *stem* villous maturation and begins centrally, in large stem villi, at about week 15 of gestation. The process of fibrosis then progressively replaces the loose, reticular stroma of stem and immature intermediate villi, so that, by 30 weeks, collagenized, mature intermediate villi begin to dominate the placental histologic picture. By about 35 weeks, only a scant rim of subtrophoblastic reticular stroma remains to delineate the origins of the intermediate villi, and, by week 38, the stroma is completely fibrosed. However, in contrast to the conducting branches of the villous tree, there is little collagen in the stroma of *terminal* villi. Generally, $\leq 3\%$ of villi of term placentas will show fibrosis. Excessive, if not extensive, intermediate and terminal villous stromal fibrosis is seen in diabetes mellitus; fetal vascular obstruction; non-acute intrauterine fetal demise; fetal intrauterine growth restriction; and prolonged pregnancy, in which up to 33% of villi may be fibrotic[3]. Villous avascularity is often a component in these conditions, and both villous fibrosis and avascularity have been reported to be independent predictors of poor fetal growth in studies of preterm infants born at 32 weeks of gestational age[135]. Chronic villitis of cytomegalovirus (CMV) and rubella infections are characterized by villous scarring, and the chronic stage of villitis of unknown etiology may show patchy fibrosis. Pre-eclampsia has been associated with villous fibrosis, but the villous lesion may reflect coincident fetal malperfusion of the villous capillaries[3,4]. Rh incompatibility is not associated with villous fibrosis.

Pathogenesis and significance The underlying cause(s) of terminal villous fibrosis is unclear. One theory holds that collagen production may be stimulated by increased partial pressures of intravillous oxygen. Diffusion of oxygen from the maternal space into the stroma, in the face of inadequate uptake by fetal capillaries due to poor fetal perfusion of the villous tree, might result in increased oxygen content in the stroma and stimulate collagen synthesis[4]. Such a theory might partially explain the normal process of collagenization of the relatively hypovascular conducting stem and intermediate villi. It might also explain the abnormal collagenization that occurs with cessation of fetal blood flow in fetal demise and decreasing placental function that occurs with postmaturity. However, as stated above, Rh incompatibility is not associated with villous fibrosis. It is, in fact, characterized by delayed villous maturation (i.e. persistence of immature intermediate villi) and edema, the latter likely reflecting compromised fetal cardiac function. The underlying cause of the deficiency of 'normal' fibrosis (and absence of excessive fibrosis) in immune-mediated hydrops is also unclear. Currently available evidence indicates that villous fibrosis may be a marker of reduced fetoplacental perfusion (of a segmental or diffuse distribution), and positively associated with fetal growth restriction.

Villous edema

Incidence Despite the fact that chorionic villi have no lymphatics, villous edema is not normally seen. Immature intermediate villi with loose stroma and stromal channels in preterm placentas may be mistakenly diagnosed as edematous, since their lack of collagen makes their stroma poorly basophilic. In addition, the central aspects of the villous tree in term placentas typically contain a few remaining immature intermediate villi. These presumably represent sites of reserve and potential for proliferative capability. Hence, the presence of villous edema in conditions such as pre-eclampsia may be suspect, especially if the edema is 'patchy' and does not affect the terminal villi. True villous edema may be seen in Rh incompatibility in conjunction with delayed maturation (Figure 43), other major blood group incompatibilities that can elicit an anti-IgG antibody response, such as Kell antigen, many infections (e.g. parvovirus B19, CMV, toxoplasmosis, and syphilis), and diabetes mellitus. In these disorders, stromal channels are markedly distended and contain scattered Hofbauer cells. Villous edema is also seen in degenerated villi in first-trimester abortuses and, of course, in complete and partial molar specimens. Finally, villous edema may be seen in placentas from cesarean section deliveries; its presence probably at least partly reflects fluid shifts associated with clinical administration of maternal intravenous support.

Pathogenesis and significance The pathogenesis and significance of villous edema are unclear. True edema probably represents the sequelae of trophoblastic and cellular dysfunction/damage and osmotic imbalances between the stroma and the maternal space. However, functional insufficiency of the fetal circulation and/or fetal hypoproteinemia may be contributing factors, since not all processes that result in cellular damage are associated with stromal edema. Fetal hypoproteinemia has been suggested as the etiology of the profound villous edema of Finnish type congenital nephrosis[136].

The clinical significance of villous edema is incompletely understood and also controversial. Part of the debate reflects differences among investigators' interpretations of villous edema. Some have stated that villous edema has no discernible, significant deleterious effect. Others have questioned whether the apparent absence of clinical disorder has reflected a histological misinterpretation of the open reticular interstitium, of normal immature intermediate villi, as being manifestations of villous edema[3,4]. Villous edema does increase maternofetal diffusional distances, but whether this results in clinically significant pathology probably depends on its degree, distribution, time of onset, and duration. Whether it compresses villous capillaries and/or results in fetal hypoxia due to decreased fetoplacental blood flow[137–140] is unclear. However, placental villous edema with chorioamnionitis has been reported to be associated with preterm birth and low birth weight[141,142] and fetal hypoxia[141], and, when villous edema is marked, with neurologic impairment in very-low-birth-weight children[143].

Excessive numbers of Hofbauer cells

Hofbauer cells are tissue macrophages derived from villous mesenchyme and, especially in late gestation, from circulating fetal blood monocytes. They are located in the stromal channels of the villi and are most prominent early in gestation. Their numbers appear to decline sharply by the 4–5th gestational month, since they become inconspicuous with advancing gestation. However, they do not decrease in number; their presence is merely masked by the progressive collagenization of villous maturation. They can be seen at term on terminal villi and, of course, within the residual central immature intermediate villi. Excessive numbers of Hofbauer cells then may be an 'artifact' of villous edema or

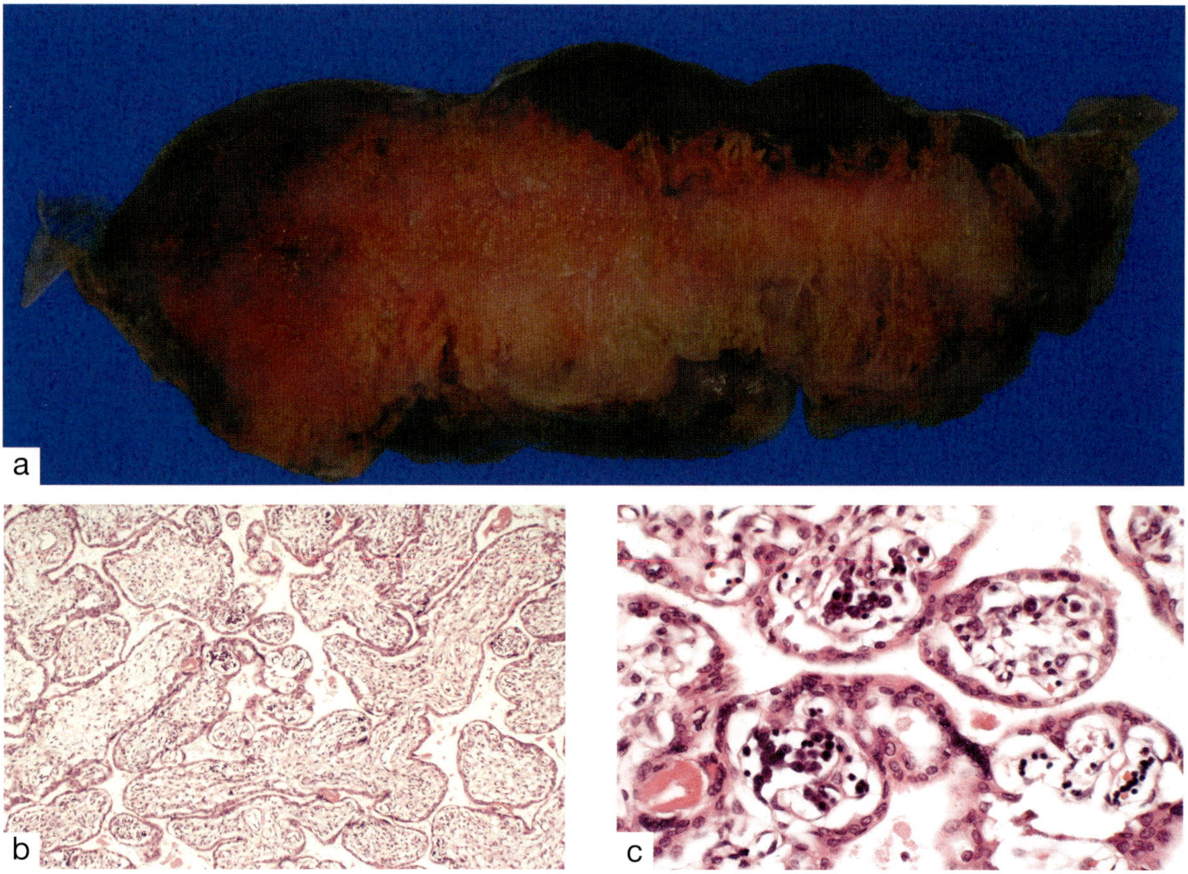

Figure 43 (a) Section from a 745-g, 34-week gestation, hydropic, pale placenta reflecting fetal anemia due to rhesus incompatibility. (b) Diffuse chorionic villous edema and delayed villous maturation are present. (c) Higher-power examination reveals a marked reactive left shift in the circulating fetal erythrocytes, in this case

represent a true proliferative response, as in villitis. Their numbers are also relatively increased in diabetes mellitus and Rh incompatibility, conditions associated with delayed villous maturation.

ABNORMALITIES OF VILLOUS BLOOD VESSELS

Assessment of terminal villous vascularity is complicated by capillary collapse that occurs after delivery, and artifactual changes that occur with storage prior to specimen fixation and fixation in inadequate volumes of fixative. Inadequate volumes of fixative result in villous distortion and/or compressive shifts in blood within the villous tree, which produce variable fields of villous collapse or capillary distension. Conclusions about abnormalities of the villous tree should be made with these factors in mind.

Villous hypovascularity

A lesser degree of capillarization is seen in immature villi, so knowledge of the period of gestation is critical to a valid assessment of villous vascularity. Besides primary reduction of vessel number, the term 'villous hypovascularity' has also been used to imply a relative reduction of vessel caliber. It is seen secondary to fetal arterial thrombosis (see above) or as a consequence of intrauterine fetal death (see below, section on 'Features of intrauterine retention' in Chapter 15) due to cessation of fetal blood flow. In both conditions, loss of vessel caliber is followed by villous atrophy and villous avascularity. Primary reduction of vessel number followed by avascularity is seen in the healing or late stage of villitis of various etiologies (see below, 'Villitis' section in Chapter 10).

Villous hypervascularity

Normal terminal villi contain about five vascular channels. Hypervascularity implies an increased number of vascular channels, not mere congestion or dilatation. It occurs in diabetes mellitus, preeclampsia, and Rh incompatibility.

Chorangiosis

Incidence Altshuler[126] defined quantitative criteria for a special category of hypervascularity that he labeled *chorangiosis*. He found it in 5.5% of placentas from infants who required admission to a newborn intensive care unit. Chorangiosis has been called the 'rule of ten': it is the identification of ten or more vascular channels, in each of ten or more *terminal* villi, in ten or more ×10 (low-power) fields, in three different areas of non-ischemic placental tissue (Figure 44). It is a finding that rarely, if ever, occurs in normal placentas. It is a feature of underperfusion of the placental bed, very-high-altitude gestations, severe maternal anemia, and diabetes mellitus, and is also associated with maternal tobacco use. Judging from its distinctive appearance and distribution, it probably requires several weeks of chronic hypoxia to produce chorangiosis[4]. Placentas with chorangiosis often also exhibit acute or chronic ischemic changes (45%) including Tenney–Parker change and infarction[126].

Pathogenesis and significance Chorangiosis is a manifestation of chronic hypoxia-stimulated angiogenesis, but other causal or potentiating factors include increased villous capillary pressure (e.g. cord occlusions) and inflammatory cytokines, since it may also be seen in conjunction with villitis of unknown etiology (27%)[144]. It is a rare, but ominous condition, associated with a higher incidence of perinatal morbidity, including requisite cesarean section delivery (32%), Apgar scores of 5 or less (22%), and major congenital anomalies (28%). It has a risk of perinatal death of 27% and term infant neonatal death rate of 39%[126,145]. It is also seen in placentas from infants with cerebral palsy and umbilical cord problems[146]. Its etiopathogenesis in diabetes mellitus is likely chronic hypoxia, but there may be other factors. Finally, chorangiotic villi are seen in Beckwith–Wiedemann syndrome (see section on 'Large placenta' in Chapter 10).

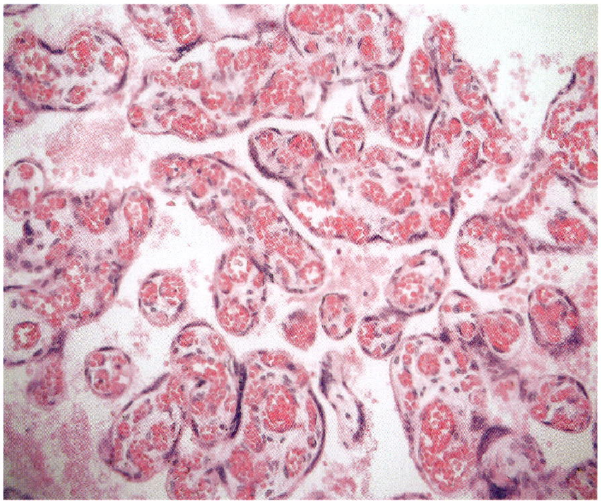

Figure 44 Chorangiosis. Most of the villi in this field show ten or more capillary profiles. Microscopic examination of this placenta satisfied the criteria for chorangiosis. The photomicrograph is purposefully taken with a greater than x10 objective (x100 total magnification) in order to show the numerous discrete capillary loops of this pathologic condition more clearly. See also Figure 41 in which some villi showed ten or more capillaries, but insufficient numbers and fields of villi were seen

GENERALIZED ABNORMALITIES OF THE VILLI

Villous immaturity

The assessment of villous immaturity is difficult in placentas delivered prior to 37 weeks of gestation. At term, the villi are small and have dilated vessels that compress the stroma. Term villi also show syncytial knots (Figure 38g).

As discussed in the sections above covering excessive syncytial knotting and deficiency of VSM, immature villi are larger and have a small caliber, simply configured vessels, a relatively larger amount of stroma, and scant to few syncytial knots. Immature villi remain normally present, at term, in small groups, in the central villous tree; their presence is evidence of continued growth until term and of villous proliferative reserve. This pattern, of a few isolated immature villi in a mature villous background, is seen in 97% of term placentas and is within normal limits. A second type of distribution, characterized by a more generalized population of immature villi, is seen in pathologic villous developmental delay. Delay in villous maturation occurs in diabetes mellitus (Figure 41), Rh incompatibility (Figure 43b), syphilis, and chromosomal anomalies, including Down's syndrome.

Distal villous hypoplasia/terminal villous deficiency ('accelerated villous maturation')

This is characterized by the presence of excessively thin and poorly vascularized villi, which, at low power, mimic the villous morphology of term, but which are morphologically abnormal and also may be seen in early- to mid-third-trimester placentas (Figure 45). The long, slender, filiform villi of distal villous hypoplasia[149] show sparse numbers of vascular channels and are compatible with villous maldevelopment marked by a predominance of non-branching angiogenesis. (Normal villous development is first a predominance of branching angiogenesis that is followed by a carefully controlled switch to non-branching angiogenesis in the intermediate villi and later the terminal villi, in which the capillaries lengthen and bulge into the overlying trophoblast[4].) This pathologic histomorphology has been referred to by a number of descriptive terms, including 'terminal villous deficiency' and 'accelerated villous maturation'[4,147]. However, since it affects the distal villous tree, which includes the distal stem villi, and it is not 'acceleration' to a normal stage of villous development, the designation 'distal villous hypoplasia' may be more accurate[147]. It is seen in placentas from gestations complicated by pre-eclampsia, maternal hypertension, and other conditions associated with underperfusion of the placental bed (such as thrombotic maternal vascular disease or reduced cardiac output) and maternal hypoxia (lung disease, smoking, anemia). It may also be seen in placentas from preterm births, fetoplacental aneuploidy, and confined placental mosaicism (CPM). Moreover, it is characteristically seen in cases of marked fetal intrauterine growth restriction (IUGR) that clinically may be associated with the absence of end-diastolic

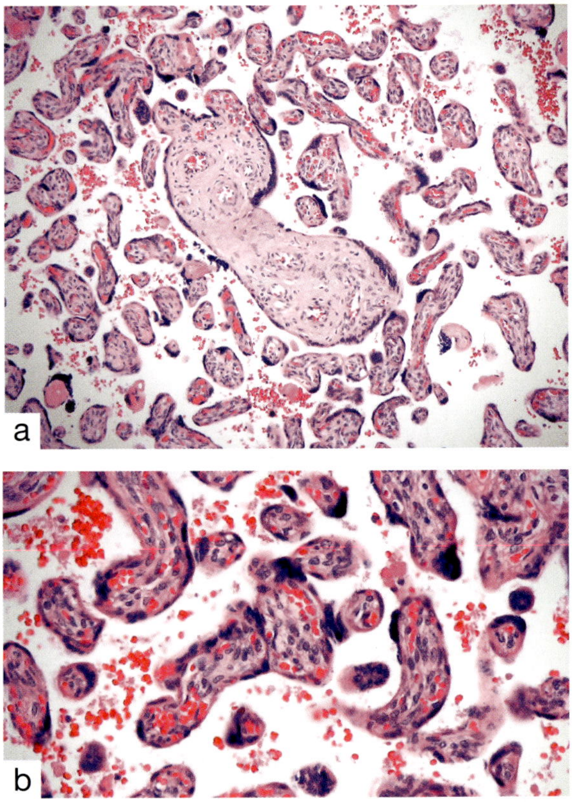

Figure 45 Histopathology of distal villous hypoplasia (DVH). (a) A distal branching stem villus is surrounded by abnormally configured, hypoplastic, slender, poorly vascularized villi with frequently seen syncytial knots. Some knots are likely isolated from their villi, by the plane of section, as single clumps of nuclei; others present may be shed, apoptotic aggregates of nuclear debris. (b) High-power photomicrograph of DVH

blood flow in the umbilical arteries. In this condition, there is high resistance to blood flow in the (fetal) placental vasculature, and perfusion of the chorionic villous tree is suboptimal (potentially due to fetal thrombotic vasculopathy (see below), or to some structural placental problem associated with chorionic villous tree maldevelopment). Of note is that the oxygen concentration in the maternal space itself in IUGR with absent end-diastolic umbilical artery blood flow is typically normal or may even be elevated. Fetal growth restriction may, thereby, become progressively severe and there is a high risk of fetal asphyxia[4].

LESIONS INVOLVING FETAL STEM VESSELS

A spectrum of lesions can be seen in the vascular segments of the chorionic plate and stem and distal villous tree, and different investigators have applied a variety of terms to describe these histopathologic lesions. Assessment of stem vessel pathology is also complicated by the fact that the pathogenesis and significance of some entities, such as hemorrhagic endovasculitis, are not uniformly agreed upon. Finally, some findings represent degenerative changes of intrauterine retention of the placenta and can be used to estimate the period of retention (Chapter 15, section on 'Features of intrauterine retention'). Because of the recent re-examination of these processes and the increased interest and research in thrombophilias, cytokines, and the placental pathologic correlates of poor perinatal outcome, we have chosen to group the lesions into categories that reflect antemortem pathology, those that are associated with postmortem retention of the placenta, and those for which the pathogenesis is unclear. In practice, however, the distinction between antemortem and postmortem changes may be difficult to make, particularly since both primary and secondary types of lesions can be seen with stillbirth. Further complicating the issue of diagnosis of fetal stem villous lesions is the fact that placentas from *live*-born infants may exhibit chronic, obstructing thrombi with downstream histopathologic sequelae that demonstrate considerable histomorphologic overlap with postmortem changes. However, distinguishing between true thromboembolic phenomena and sequelae of postmortem change is critical, because thrombi are due to antemortem, coagulopathic conditions affecting a *viable* fetus. Thrombi are associated with significant perinatal morbidity and mortality, and, if genetically based, with increased risks of recurrence in subsequent gestations. Thus, careful assessment of a stillborn's placenta is necessary to disclose whether the fetal vasculopathy identified represents primary pathology, and/or whether there is (superimposed) postmortem retention change. The following sections are primarily focused on the pathologies of stem and distal villous ramifications, but, as will become evident, vasculopathic changes in these segments often occur as complications of cord and chorionic plate vessel lesions. Our separation of the fetal cord and fetal plate vessels from the branch vascular 'compartments' is, to some extent, artificial, since the fetal vascular tree is continuous.

Thrombosis/fetal thrombotic vasculopathy and related terms

Incidence As discussed in the above chapter on gross pathology (Chapter 7), careful examination of the umbilical cord and fetal plate (and membranes, in the case of velamentous vascular segments) may reveal the presence of an acute or chronic thrombus. Histologically, however, distinguishing arteries from veins in the chorionic plate may be virtually impossible, unless the section fortuitously includes both types of vessels in vertical alignment, with the artery overlying the vein. A thorough re-examination of the gross specimen is advised when prominent thrombi are noted microscopically. Stem villous thrombi are usually very difficult to detect, grossly, but are most commonly present in veins.

Chorionic villous tree thrombi (Figure 21) are not uncommon, and mural, acute thrombi are far more frequently identified than sites of luminal obliteration. Acute, laminated thrombi, when optimally sectioned, show early attachment to the endothelial surfaces of arteries or veins. Acute thrombi in the fetal plate have been correlated with cord complications and stasis with knots, complex entanglements, prolapse, and excessive twisting. Chronic thrombotic changes may be evidenced by peripheral fibrointimal proliferation and ingrowth into the thrombus, cushion formation, and dystrophic mineralization. Old thrombi may undergo '*cushion*' transformation, which produces sites of organization and thickenings in the vessel wall[148]. (Note that branch points of larger vessels, especially of the chorionic plate, may be sectioned tangentially and resemble 'cushions'; cautious interpretation is advised when mural thickenings are encountered in the absence of other fetal vasculopathy.) Recanalization may be seen in arteries.

The presence of single arterial thrombus has been noted in 4.5% of term placentas, and fetal arterial thrombi are seen in 10% of placentas from diabetic gestations[3]. Arterial thrombi may show stem villous propagation and/or thromboembolic organization and occlusions in the villous ramifications, and secondary villous atrophy and fibrosis. Luminal obliterations often calcify if chronic. The term *fetal thrombotic vasculopathy* (FTV)[149] has been applied to describe collectively fetal branch vessel thrombemboli with associated clustered villous atrophy and fibrosis; chronic non-infectious villitis may also be seen[150,151]. FTV has an incidence of 3–10/1000 placentas[146]. It may include villous venous pathology but it is primarily an arterial process.

'*Endarteritis obliterans*' is another term that has been used to designate lesions of the stem and villous vessels in which there is near to complete occlusion of the lumen. Endarteritis obliterans is a misnomer, in that it is a non-inflammatory lesion, but it does result in luminal stenosis and/or occlusion with mural thickening and reduplication of the basal lamina of the vessel. It was focally seen in 10% of term normal placentas, but seen more frequently and extensively in pre-eclampsia/toxemia, essential hypertension, heavy maternal tobacco use, and diabetes mellitus, in studies by Fox[3]. It is believed to result most often from a proximal thrombus, and is one of the terms incorporated under the umbrella of FTV. It is also a lesion of infection with syphilis, CMV, and rubella.

One of the authors (OF-P) has seen a case in which there was velamentous insertion and extensive intramembranous branching of the umbilical cord vasculature (Figure 46a and a-1). This case showed the gamut of FTV, with arterial chorionic plate chronic (Figure 46b) and acute propagating thrombosis and stem villous thombosis with associated chorionic villous sclerosis (Figure 46c). Acute umbilical arterial branch thrombi were seen (Figure 46d). Chronic and propagating acute thrombi were also seen in many veins (Figure 46e and e-1), but chronic lesions were not detected in sampled velamentous vessels. The widespread intramembranous distribution of the vessels likely contributed to fetal vascular damage, compromise, and alteration of flow dynamics in the placental bed and potentially within the fetus. The infant, while a term, live-born with Apgar scores of 8 and 9 at 1 and 5 min, respectively, was intrauterine growth-restricted. Because of the placental pathology and its associated risks, the newborn's pediatrician was immediately contacted. The newborn, other than being small, was normal, but a computed tomography (CT) scan of the baby's head, performed at age 5 weeks, revealed severe, bilateral, periventricular leukomalacia. The findings were consistent with bilateral cerebral infarctions in the distribution of the middle cerebral arteries, due to intrauterine thromboembolic phenomena. Figure 47 shows another placenta with extensive chronic, chorionic plate, venous thrombotic vasculopathy.

Pathogenesis and significance The etiology of FTV is likely multifactorial. Fetal plate and stem villous thrombi are seen in association with overly long umbilical cords[146]; stasis and vascular injury with coiled cords, cord knots, and velamentous cord insertions[4,151,152]; fetal trisomy; maternal hypertension/ toxemia[4]; Rh incompatibility[148]; and maternal hemolytic uremic syndrome[153]. Fetal thrombophilias of both heritable (i.e. factor V Leiden mutation, protein C or S deficiencies) and secondary types have also been reported to be associated with FTV[4,154]. However, there are conflicting data as to whether maternal heritable thrombophilia or fetal thrombophilia due to a single mutation are sufficient to result in FTV, or whether cofactors, such as hypoxia or infection (see later), are additionally necessary. In the discordant, diamniotic dichorionic, twin gestation reported by Khong and Hague[154], in which only one twin's placenta was affected, the fetal vasculopathy represented the inheritance of two (biparental) mutations in the affected twin. Ariel and colleagues[155] found that fetal thrombophilia (due to factor V Leiden, prothrombin II, or methyltetrahydrofolate reductase (MTHFR) mutation) was not associated with increased incidence of FTV, even when present in conjunction with maternal thrombophilia and/or maternal conditions associated with underperfusion of the placental bed. They concluded that fetal thrombophilia might, however, be an underlying risk factor for the formation of vascular lesions initiated by other pathologic processes.

In contrast to the role of fetal thrombophilia, there is ample evidence that fetal coagulopathic states are associated with infections by vasotropic, vasculopathic organisms (e.g. cytomegalovirus, treponemal pathogens; bacterial infections by group B streptococcal and *Pseudomonas* species) and cytokine release in severe chorioamnionitis[4,143,152]. Cytomegalovirus is particularly associated with luminal calcifications of the fetal plate and stem villous vessels (see section on 'Villitis' in Chapter 10). Non-infectious disorders such as diabetes mellitus may be associated with reactive erythrocythemia, excessive thromboxane production, and vascularization abnormalities that predispose to FTV[156–158]. Fox[3] found that 10% of diabetic placentas showed a single arterial stem vessel occlusion (versus 4.5% of term placentas from uncomplicated gestations). Hypoxia due to hypertension or maternal smoking during pregnancy may also be an important, contributing factor.

Whatever their pathogeneses, thrombi are associated with serious consequences. Venous thrombi are more common and may embolize, via the umbilical vein, and through the fetal foramen ovale or ductus arteriosus, to the preferentially perfused fetal brain and upper extremities, and to the fetal viscera. Arterial thrombosis and FTV may result in atrophy of a significant amount of the villous tree and/or impedence to blood flow within the placenta, fetal growth restriction, and fetal demise. Kraus and Acheen[151] found that extensive vasculopathic lesions (affecting 35–50% of the placental parenchyma) were strongly associated with, and seemed singularly sufficient to cause, fetal death, probably through sudden or progressive loss of placental reserve. Neonatal hemolytic anemia, thrombocytopenia, and hypofibrinogenemia due to consumptive coagulopathy have also been documented. Somatic thromboemboli have been seen in 37.5% of stillborns or neonates with FTV, and may result in fetal brain damage that becomes manifested as infarction, cerebral palsy, and other neurologic deficits in childhood[151,159], visceral infarctions, including thromboembolic perinatal liver disease[160], and limb reductions[151]. Thus, long-term follow-up of infants born with placentas showing FTV may reveal the presence of neuropathology or renal disease clinically unrecognized in the neonatal period.

In summary, it may become useful to separate FTV into groups by etiologies that are caused by primary thrombophilias, versus infectious pathogens, and non-infectious etiologies. However, because of its significant sequelae, the presence, pattern of distribution (fetal plate and/or stem villous vessels), and extent of villous atrophy and fibrosis should be noted in the final, placental diagnosis. Moreover, the presence of thrombi and FTV, especially in the absence of chorioamnionitis or infectious placentitis, may denote the existence of an unrecognized parental thrombophilic mutation(s) and an increased risk of fetal morbidity and mortality in subsequent pregnancies.

Fibromuscular sclerosis

Incidence In fibromuscular sclerosis, the intimal and medial layers of stem vessels are markedly thickened and there is luminal obliteration. Arteries are most commonly affected. The lesional process is most often localized, and seen in an artery supplying a portion of the villous tree that shows ischemic infarction (villous infarction is due to interruption of

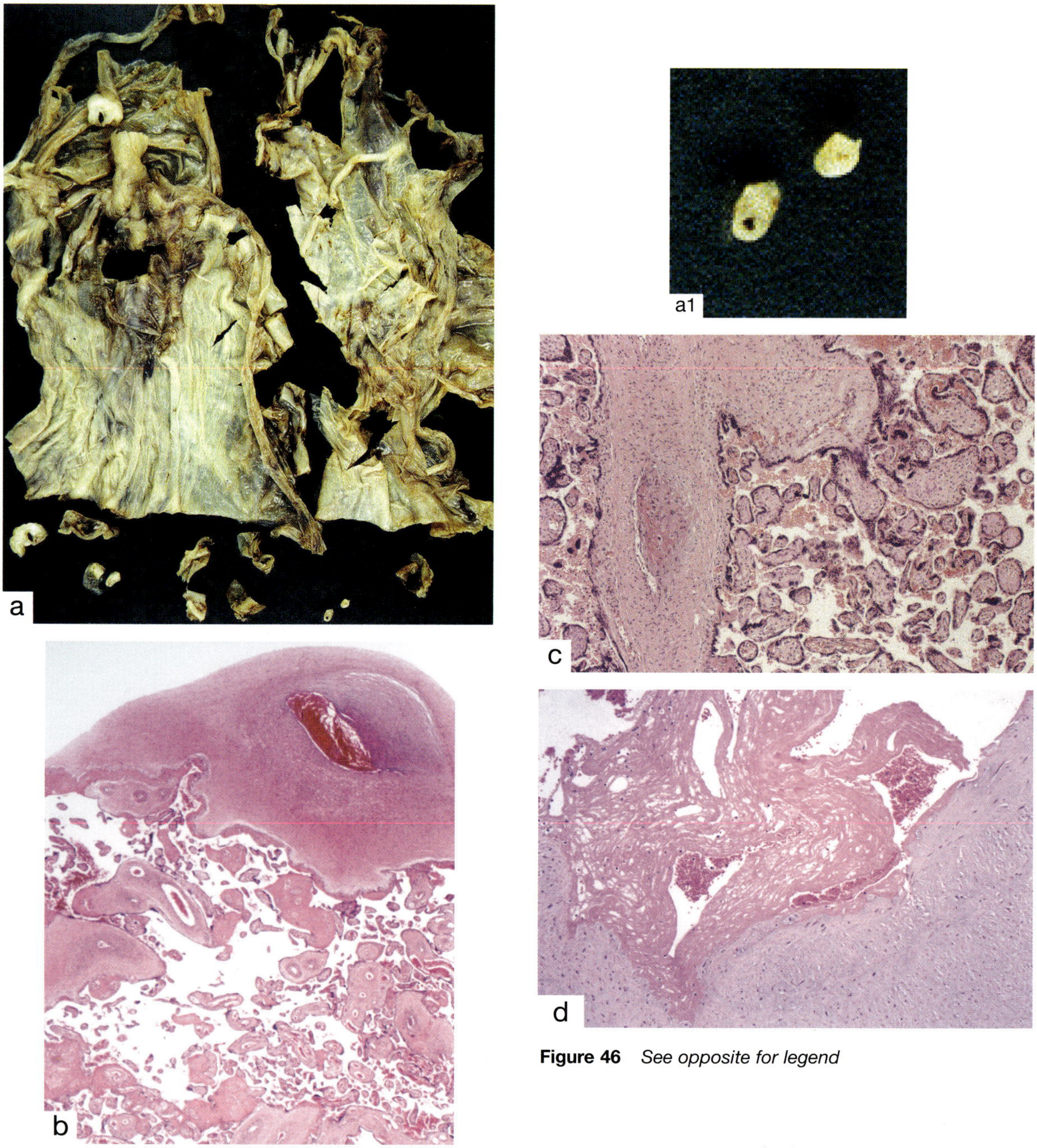

Figure 46 *See opposite for legend*

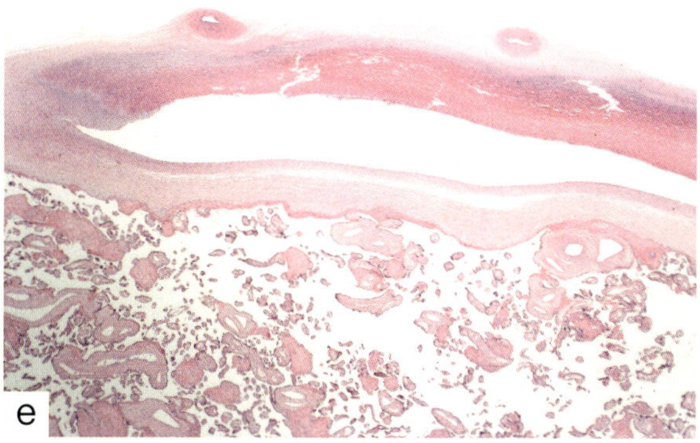

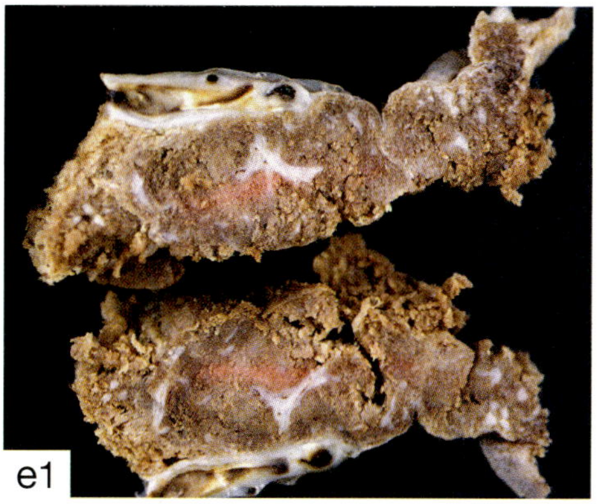

Figure 46 (a and a-1) This umbilical cord from a term-gestation placenta showed extensive velamentous insertion and intramembranous branching. A few umbilical arterial branches contained acute, subtotally occlusive thrombi. (b) Example of chronic chorionic plate arterial thrombus found. Foci with mural calcification were also seen. (c) Fetal thrombotic vasculopathy with chronic stem villous arterial thrombus. Many of the villi in the field are sclerotic, and are likely downstream of this or similarly affected stem villi. (d) Acute thrombus in umbilical arterial branch; microscopic examination of the fetal plate arteries and veins and stem villous vessels showed chronic and propagating acute thrombi. (e) Section demonstrating a hemisected chronic thrombus in a large, chorionic plate vein, near the site of velamentous insertion of the vessels at the placental margin. Note the thin rim of adjacent and basal ischemic and infarcted parenchyma included in this sampled section. (e-1) Corresponding photomicrograph of the thrombus in (e) (note two arteries overlying the vein)

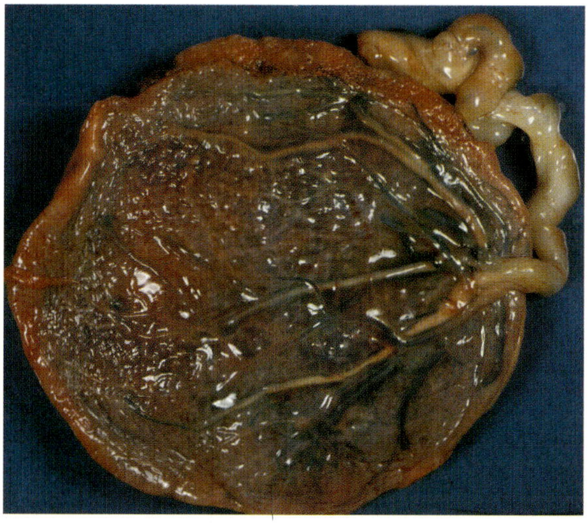

Figure 47 Placenta demonstrating extensive chronic thrombosis of large chorionic plate vein and branch point confluence with adjoining surface vein. (Arteries overlie veins on the chorionic plate)

maternal blood supply), or that is embedded in fibrinoid material, and in arteries distal to an occlusion. Generalized fetal plate and stem villous vascular sclerosis is characteristically seen in cases of intrauterine fetal death, and its extent is directly related to the duration of retention[3,109] (see section on 'Features of intrauterine retention', Chapter 15).

Pathogenesis and significance Both localized and generalized distribution of fibromuscular sclerosis is regarded as a secondary phenomenon. Fox[3] proposes that it represents true fibrous proliferation, and his conclusions are supported by the observations of postmortem chorionic villous change with intrauterine retention by Genest[109]. Others, however, submit that the histopathologic picture of mural thickening and luminal obliteration probably represents sequelae of vascular collapse and condensation of mural components[4]. The etiology of the process is unclear; it may reflect a combination of both condensation and fibroblastic proliferation, especially when seen in association with the birth of a viable infant. Widespread arterial fibromuscular sclerosis in placentas from live-born infants is very uncommon, and is associated with the absence or reversal of end-diastolic umbilical arterial blood flow by Doppler study and, often, severe fetal growth restriction[4]. The chorionic villous arterial tree presumably develops high resistance to blood flow in these instances.

Hemorrhagic endovasculitis/ endovasculosis

Incidence Hemorrhagic endovasculitis (HEV) is a vaso-occlusive lesion that involves vessels of all sizes from fetal stem and branch arteries to the villous capillaries. It has a variably reported incidence from 0.67% (serially examined placentas from normal-weight, > 20-week gestational age live-borns[161]) to 8.8–22% of placentas from live births[162,163]. However, it has a well-accepted increased frequency among placentas from stillbirths; rates of 32–52% have been reported[162,163]. In HEV, the arteries show recent or old thrombi, endothelial and medial hyperplasia, mural diapedesis of erythrocytes and red cell fragmentation, fetal normoblastemia, and occasional hemosiderin deposition in the villous stroma[163–165] (Figure 48). Coexistent chronic villitis of unknown etiology is very common; 75% of cases in the study by Stevens and Sander[163] showed villitis, and subsequent studies have also noted the association[161,165–168]. It has been further divided into active (Figure 48c; mural red cell diapedesis, marked fragmentation with vasodestruction/vaso-occlusion and luminal/mural nucleocytoplasmic debris or non-exudative necrosis), bland (Figure 46b and d; mural hemorrhage, minimal mural disruption and red cell fragmentation, luminal septation and bridging by endothelial or myointimal cells), and healed forms (Figure 46b and d; villous stromal fibrosis, evidence of residual wall disruption, hemosiderin deposition). The occurrence of clustered capillary, destructive lesions, and intravillous hemorrhage of HEV is considered a severe and terminal villous expression of the active stage. The active stage has been reported as being associated with an increased risk of perinatal pathology[165].

In addition to stillbirth, HEV has been associated with growth restriction of viable term infants (15–16%)[166,167], and with fetal intrauterine growth restriction and reversed end-diastolic umbilical arterial blood flow[167], meconium passage, umbilical cord complications, postmaturity[161,163], non-immune hydrops[169], and abnormal heart rate tracings[167]. It is more common with maternal pre-eclampsia[163], toxemia, and preterm birth[170], and it has been reported to have a 28.9% recurrence risk, especially as related to recurrent stillbirth (64.3%)[168].

Pathogenesis and significance HEV is a lesion of some controversy, since it has been replicated in explants of chorionic villous tissue culture that were allowed to degenerate passively as organ cultures in media with progressively decreasing oxygen content, following their procurement from term live-born infants' placentas[171]. Others have found that it was not associated with low birth weight or maternal disease, and that its occurrence was distinctly related to the duration of intrauterine retention[162]. The histologic features of the degenerative placental changes of intrauterine retention[109] have also shown overlap with septation of the healed form of HEV (see section on 'Features of intrauterine retention' in Chapter 15). However, while there is histopathologic overlap with the features of changes associated with short-term organ culture and those of retention, there are instances of arterial fetal plate and stem vessel thrombosis that clearly demonstrate the vaso-occlusive pathology of HEV. The association with cord complications and HEV have led some to conclude that interference with umbilical blood flow or regional compromise of villous perfusion and hypoxia with vascular smooth muscle contraction may explain both naturally occurring and culture-induced lesions[161,171].

There has been no conclusive light microscopic or electron microscopic evidence that HEV is an infectious process, although viral and a mycoplasma-like pathogens were postulated to be etiologic agents[4,172], and some have preferred the term 'endovasculosis' over 'endovasculitis'. The lesional complex is thought to represent a microangiopathic process since it can be seen in placentas from live births and fresh stillbirths.

HISTOPATHOLOGY OF MATERNAL UTEROPLACENTAL ARTERIES

Adequate perfusion of the placental bed is dependent upon a variety of factors (e.g. normal maternal cardiac

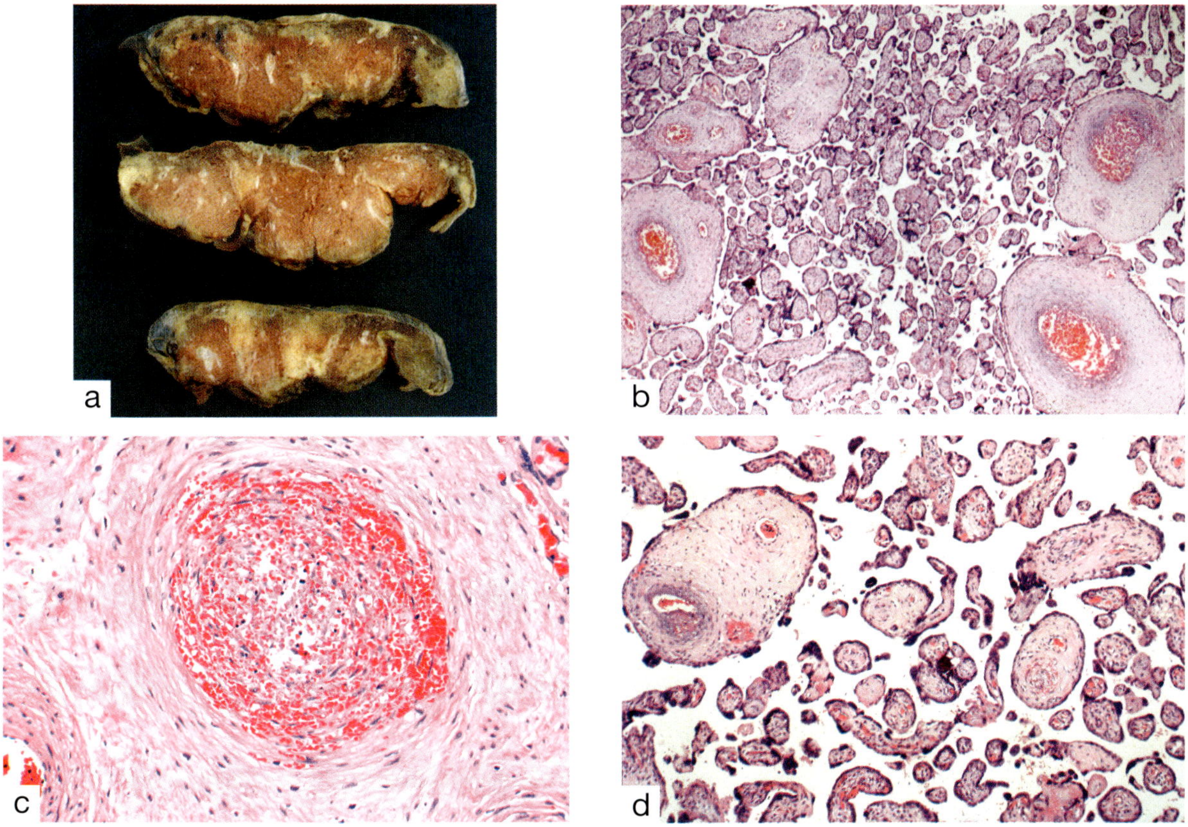

Figure 48 (a) Serial sections of a 315-g, small (372–542-g expected) placenta for 36.5 weeks of gestation with hemorrhagic endovasculitis/endovasculosis (HEV) show numerous subchorionic triangular areas of pale firm chorionic villous parenchyma with focal extension into the basal regions. Their distribution is compatible with stem villous and branch villous vasocclusive lesions, with loss of perfusion to respective dependent portions of the villous tree. While some are basal and marginal, and comparable to those seen in ischemic chorionic villous infarction (see Figure 33), the distribution of these HEV-associated lesions is different from that of infarctions due to placental bed underperfusion associated with maternal vascular disease. (b) A spectrum of lesions of HEV is present in this photomicrograph from the placenta in (a). Large stem villi show arteries with partial occlusion, mural hemorrhage, and septation, and some diapedesis of red cells. A smaller stem villus (upper center left) shows nearly complete replacement of its vascular lumen by fibroblast overgrowth, with scattered red blood cells in the stroma. (c) 'Active' lesion of HEV with mural disruption, red cell fragmentation, and loss of luminal patency. (d) Higher-power view of several villi also from the placenta in (a) showing bland lesions (stem villus on left) and healed forms (smaller stem and intermediate villi on right) of HEV. Note that distal villous hypoplasia is also present and that the placenta was small. The infant was also intrauterine growth-restricted

output, blood pressure regulation, hemostasis, and dietary intake; normoxemia; the absence of maternal vascular disease). However, the most important factor is the early-gestational 'physiological conversion'[173] of the spiral arteries of the decidua and superficial myometrium (Figure 49). Physiological conversion is a cytotrophoblastic cell-dependent process in which extravillous cytotrophoblastic cells invade and/or plug decidual arterioles, infiltrate the arterial wall, and, through events that are incompletely understood, destroy both the elastin and myocytes of the tunica media, invade the endothelium[174–176], and change to express an endothelial phenotype[111,177–179]. The normally thick-walled, high-resistance, muscularized, spiral arteries of the decidua and subjacent myometrium are remodeled into thin-walled, dilated, low-pressure conduits (Figure 8), having ostia of up to 2000 μm in diameter, and poor response to regional or systemic vasoactive substances. This cytotrophoblast-dependent vascular transformation is a two-stage process. The first phase is completed by the end of the first trimester and accomplishes remodeling of the intradecidual segments of the vessels, i.e. it is delimited at the deciduo-myometrial junction. The second phase effects remodeling of the intramyometrial portions of the vessels and occurs sometime between the 14th and 16th weeks of gestation. Its exact duration is unknown, but it appears to be mostly completed within a few weeks, at most, but recent evidence suggests that it may continue throughout gestation. A number of cellular and extracellular factors (growth factors, cell adhesion molecules, extracellular matrix molecules, and metalloproteinases, and their receptors); nitric oxide; cytokines and immunologic factors; plasminogen activators and inhibitors; maternal plasma prostacyclin/thromboxane ratios; maternal hormones[4,176,178,180–185]; and maternal dietary factors (vitamins C and E, calcium, zinc, n-3 essential fatty acids)[186–189] all play roles in this complex process. Work by Starzyk and colleagues[190] has also suggested that an underlying adequate number and distribution of maternal endometrial/decidual arteries are likely required.

The notable features of the dual-phase trophoblastic-dependent process of conversion are:

(1) This change in the spiral arteries/arterioles is localized to the decidua basalis (i.e. the placental bed) and does not occur in the basal arteries of the decidua vera or capsularis[3].

(2) The second wave, the critical step for full conversion, is begun and largely completed well before the third trimester of gestation, when the typical clinicopathologic features of pre-eclampsia and intrauterine fetal growth restriction become manifested.

(3) Abnormalities of decidual arteries/arterioles are primarily due to failure of the cytotrophoblast, but aberrations of the other factors likely contribute to, or result in, decidual arteriopathy.

(4) Physiological conversion results in replacement of the arterial musculoelastic wall by a mixture of fibrinoid and fibrous and amorphous tissue

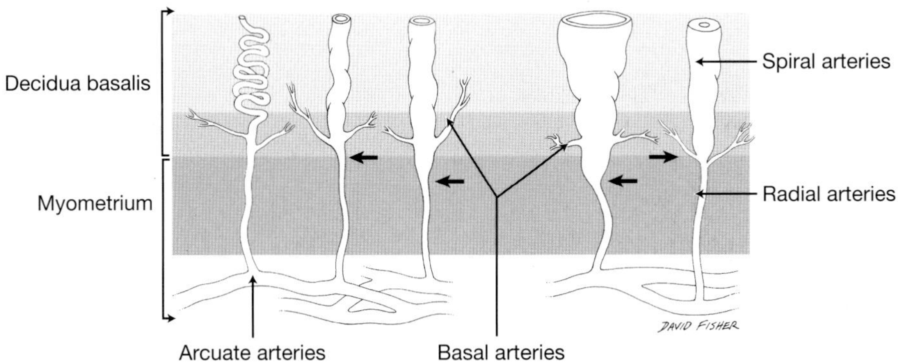

Figure 49 Normal physiological conversion of maternal spiral arteries versus vasculopathy of pre-eclampsia. This illustration depicts, from left to right: an unmodified spiral artery of the superficial myometrium and endometrium (future decidua); the first stage of physiological conversion of the spiral arteries of the placental bed with arterial dilatation limited to the decidua basalis and excluding the basal arteries achieved by the end of the first trimester; the second stage of physiological arterial conversion with extension of process into the superficial intramyometrial segments of the vessels, and begun within gestational weeks 14–16 and completed some time before mid-gestation; late third-trimester spiral artery: the low-resistance, high-capacitance artery is maximally dilated to ensure optimal perfusion of the maternal space; and far right, a representation of a thick-walled, spiral artery of pre-eclampsia, with a small lumen, that lacks the intramyometrial component of physiological conversion, and, therefore, is functionally compromised

in which modified myointimal cells and degenerate trophoblasts and smooth muscle cells are embedded. Mild fibrinoid change/necrosis is, therefore, a normal finding (see below), and is not, in itself, a feature of arterial pathology in this setting.

(5) Physiologic conversion is not a uniform process in decidua basalis or within a given vessel.

Atherosis

Incidence Atherosis is a lesion of unconverted arteries/arterioles. Therefore, it is seen in the decidua basalis, with failure of physiologic conversion in the intramyometrial segments of these vessels, and in arterioles of the decidua parietalis, which normally do not undergo physiologic change. The term 'acute atherosis' was introduced by Zeek and Assali[191]; it is used to describe the pathologic presence of foamy, lipid-laden macrophages and smooth muscle cells lying within thickened, hyalinized, decidual arterial walls (Figure 50) (see also section on 'Decidual vasculopathy' in Chapter 13). 'Acute atherosis' must be distinguished from simple intimal vacuolation, which is common to placental bed and non-placental bed arteries, increases with gestational age, and is considered a non-specific feature[175]. Atherosis is often accompanied by mural 'fibrinoid necrosis' and luminal stenosis and/or thrombosis. The lipid accumulations may be due to abnormal imbibition, by endothelial cells, of plasma constituents[4], and/or to pinocytosis, by macrophages and intramural myocytes, of degenerated membranous components of endothelial cells. The fibrinoid is partly derived from trophoblastic secretions of proteinaceous substances or degeneration and necrosis of the trophoblast itself[192], and, as stated above, is not necessarily pathologic.

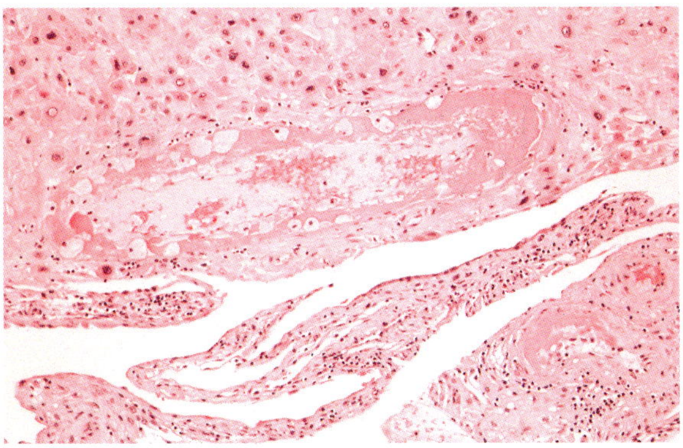

Figure 50 Atherosis, with foamy macrophages and lipid-laden smooth muscle cells lying in thickened hyalinized wall, is present in an artery in decidua basalis. Two smaller arterioles are also present in the portion of decidua basalis in the lower right corner. One shows focal atherosis, the other, a lack of physiological conversion as evidenced by mural thickening and a constricted lumen. The central fragmented portions of tissue show dilated venous channels. (see also section on 'Decidual vasculopathy' and Figure 98

Since the process of physiologic conversion is non-uniform, trophoblastic cell-dependent, and multifactorially influenced, atherosis is non-uniformly distributed among arteries and within a given vessel. Moreover, the affected portions of the vessels lie largely within the superficial myometrium. Therefore, detection of atherosis is sample-dependent; a decidual layer shave, taken parallel to the maternal surface, increases the likelihood of sampling an abnormal vessel, and is easier and more cost-effective than submitting several transmural, placental sections. In addition, rolled free-membrane sections with the attached decidua parietalis provide considerable decidual tissue for examination and may also include affected vessels.

Atherosis, together with thrombosis and fibrinoid change, villous infarctions of varying age, and chorionic villous Tenney–Parker changes with syncytial knot formation, is characteristic of pre-eclampsia. Atherosis with features of superficial implantation (aggregates of immature intermediate trophoblasts and increased numbers of giant cells) may also be seen, especially in cases of preterm delivery with fetal growth restriction[147].

Pathogenesis and significance Pre-eclampsia is a *clinical* syndrome of unknown etiology, and of such challenge that it has been called the 'disease of theories'[119]. It affects 5% of pregnancies and is typified by second-trimester onset of hypertension and proteinuria, and, frequently, peripheral edema. Pre-eclampsia may progress to glomerular dysfunction, hepatopathy, thrombocytopenia, and seizure[118,119,180,193]. It is a leading cause of maternal mortality in developed countries, associated with preterm delivery with fetal intrauterine growth restriction, and necessitates approximately 15% of preterm deliveries; associated with a five-fold increase in perinatal mortality; and seen in term gestations complicated by maternal diabetes, hypertension, and obesity[194]. Core features of pre-eclampsia are abnormal placentation and placental vascular insufficiency, believed to be due to 'failure of the extravillous cytotrophoblast'. The 'failure' presumably leads to inadequate infiltration or survival within the arterial wall and failure of physiologic transformation of the spiral arteries of the placental bed decidua and superficial myometrium[195], secondary hypoperfusion of intervillous space, and hypoxia. However, since normal arterial transformation is a complex process, as outlined above, the roles of maternal endothelial cellular, hematologic, and decidual interstitial factors have also become the foci of much recent research. Research supports the hypothesis that such 'cytotrophoblast failure' could represent a primary or a secondary defect of this cell line, or a combination of a primary and a secondary defect. This failure might then lead to direct or indirect damage to maternal endothelial cells, as discussed below. In pre-eclampsia, the cytotrophoblasts show abnormal differentiation and widespread apoptosis. Primary failures of cellular function could result in insufficient replication of requisite cell numbers, inadequate elaboration of trophoblastic cell receptors and adhesion molecules, or incomplete trophoblastic phenotypic adaptation of endothelial cell markers that enable them to penetrate and remain within maternal vessels[111,178,195,196]. However, malinvasion could also reflect imbalances in requisite local decidual or systemic factors, or in maternal factors that adversely affect the necessary interactions between trophoblasts, endothelial cells, and blood components (platelets, leukocytes, and coagulation factors), as described below.

Pre-eclampsia develops in association with a variety of clinical disorders that include maternal immune-mediated connective-tissue disorders (e.g. systemic lupus erythematosus), thrombophilias (e.g. factor V Leiden, prothrombin, and MTHFR mutations)[39,44,197,198], antiphospholipid/anticardiolipin antibody syndromes[41,199–201], and hypertension, hyperlipidemia, diabetes, and obesity[118,180,202]. Investigations of the mechanisms involved in these numerous conditions led[180] to the hypothesis that maternal endothelial cell damage and/or dysfunction plays a pivotal role in a final common pathway that leads to the clinical manifestations of pre-eclampsia. Evidence supporting their hypothesis has included observations that: first, women with pre-eclampsia may have increased levels of endothelial-related factors (e.g. factor VIII-related antigen, fibronectin, thrombomodulin, endothelin-1, and abnormalities of tissue plasminogen activator/plasminogen activator inhibitor ratios)[118,119,180,194]; and second, other genetic factors involved in cytokine[118,178,203–206] and nitric oxide and reactive oxygen species production[188,207–209] and in type 2 diabetes, hypertension[210,211], and hyperlipidemia[212,213] also appear to affect a woman's risk for developing pre-eclampsia, the severity of her disease, and her risk of passing the predisposition to her offspring[180,193,211,214,215]. A recently proposed mechanism in the pathogenesis of pre-eclampsia and maternal endothelial damage involves a trophoblast-produced molecule, fms-like tyrosine kinase 1 (sFlt1). Increased sFlt1 levels have been found in the circulations of pre-eclamptic women, and the molecule has induced hypertension, proteinuria, and glomerular endotheliosis (the classic lesion of pre-eclampsia) when injected into rats[117]. Presumably, excessive amounts of sFlt1 bind to soluble vascular endothelial growth factor receptor (VEGF) and placental growth factor (PGF) in the maternal circulation, reduce the amount of circulating free VEGF and PGF (vascular 'survival' and functional maintenance signals), and cause endothelial dysfunction in multiple organs and the brain, and the signs of the clinical syndrome. Moreover, hypoxia is a stimulus for increased sFlt1 production[216], and placental bed hypoxia is a critical component of pre-eclampsia. Thus, worsening hypoxia of the placental bed could result in more sFlt1 production, progressive maternal clinical disease and, in turn, more placental dysfunction, and increased risks of fetal and maternal morbidity and mortality. However, there may be other key molecules (e.g. inflammatory mediators) and processes involved[118]; of particular note have been the recent observations that the lesion of 'acute atherosis' in the pre-eclamptic placental bed shares many pathogenetic mechanisms with *atherogenesis* associated with cardiovascular diseases[217]. These observations will also likely lead to new understanding of, and preventive measures for, the clinical pathology of the disorder.

In summary, while the etiology of pre-eclampsia remains unclear, studies indicate that failure of, or damage to, the cytotrophoblast and endothelial cell dysfunction/damage have primary, if not synergistic, roles in development of the clinical condition. Multiple sites exist at which aberrations could impair cytotrophoblastic or endothelial function, and these sites of potential error may help to explain the non-specificity of the histopathology of pre-eclampsia and its variable clinical spectrum and gestational stages of onset, discussed by Sibai[218]. Placental histopathology, indistinguishable from that of pre-eclampsia (including, in some cases, atherosis), may be seen in placentas delivered of women without clinically detected pre-eclampsia, but who have a history of diabetes, hypertension, thrombophilia, or an immune-mediated disorder[219–222]. Recently, Redline and colleagues[147] reported that atherosis and muscularization of basal plate arteries are more specific predictors for clinical correlation with pre-eclampsia (82%) than the several other histopathologic parameters of placental bed underperfusion that they evaluated. However, their series was relatively small (20 cases), the maternal histories of their cases were not specified, sampling limitations may have been operative in their analysis, and placentas from gestations complicated by other maternal disorders, but not pre-eclampsia, were not specifically analyzed for comparison. Therefore, it appears that atherosis, while characteristic of pre-eclampsia, does not identify its underlying etiology, but instead represents a histopathologic 'endpoint' of a process potentially triggered by many factors.

Hypertensive arteriopathy (essential and diabetic)

In essential hypertension, the maternal arteries in the decidua show thickening of the muscle coat with intimal hyperplasia and narrowing of the lumen. The basal arteries, spiral arteries of the placental bed, and myometrial segments of the spiral arteries of the placental bed are affected by these changes. The intradecidual portions of the spiral arteries of the placental bed do not show these alterations since these arteries have already undergone the changes associated with implantation and placental development described above. If pre-eclampsia occurs in a patient with pre-existing hypertension, acute atherosis is superimposed on the arteriosclerotic changes described above. In addition, decidual arteriopathic mural thickening can be seen in placentas from women with diabetes and superimposed pre-eclampsia[147]. Also, as noted above, the blood vessels showing the lesions associated with hypertension and pre-eclampsia are present in the decidua basalis attached to the maternal surface and to the decidua parietalis.

10

Lesions of the placenta as a whole or of the placental disk

PLACENTAL WEIGHT

Placental weight, as a clinicopathologic determinant of intrauterine placental functional adequacy, is not a fully reliable measurement since it is affected by several factors. Placental blood volume in the fetal villous tree and the maternal space varies among normal placentas delivered at similar gestational periods. Alterations also occur with fixation or storage of fresh specimens. For example, placental weight increases, on average, about 10% with fixation. Storage of fresh specimens, of 2–3 h, results in loss of weight due to drainage of most blood within the maternal space. Edematous placentas can lose significant amounts of fluid when stored for a day[4]. At this time, assessment of whether placental growth and function have been adequate, in a given pregnancy, is best made by calculating the fetal : placental weight ratio (Table 9)[223]. (For example, an increased fetal : placental weight ratio of 1.5 or more above the value expected for that period of gestation is highly suggestive of intrauterine growth restriction.) However, such calculation is often precluded by the fact that the corresponding fetal or newborn weight is rarely provided in the clinical history accompanying the placental specimen. Nevertheless, obtaining the weight of the trimmed, fresh (refrigerated) specimen and correlating it with the expected range for the period of gestation (Table 10)[224] can be very informative. The need for sophisticated analysis and the shortcomings of isolated

Table 9 Placental weight at different gestations[223]

Gestational week	*Weight of placenta (g)*		*Ratio of fetal to placental weight*
	Mean	*1 SD*	
24	225	70	2.9
25	235	70	3.1
26	245	70	3.3
27	260	65	3.5
28	270	70	4.9
29	290	70	5.1
30	310	70	5.3
31	335	70	5.4
32	360	70	5.6
33	380	75	5.8
34	400	75	6.0
35	420	75	6.2
36	435	80	6.4
37	450	85	6.5
38	465	85	6.6
39	480	85	6.7
40	490	90	6.8
41	500	90	7.0
42	505	95	7.1

SD, standard deviation

Table 10 Mean weights and centiles for singleton placentas. Adapted from reference 224

Gestational week	*10th–90th centile*	*Cases (n)*
21	114–172	3
22	122–191	6
23	133–211	7
24	145–233	9
25	159–256	19
26	175–280	14
27	192–305	9
28	210–331	16
29	229–357	11
30	249–384	12
31	269–411	14
32	290–438	24
33	311–464	30
34	331–491	32
35	352–516	44
36	372–542	36
37	391–566	32
38	409–589	62
39	426–611	103
40	442–632	193
41	456–651	87

weight measurement can be largely circumvented if weight is determined in conjunction with a thoughtful gross and microscopic evaluation that includes an estimation of the parenchymal volume affected by pathology.

LARGE PLACENTA

A term placenta weighing > 750 g is considered significantly large. Increased weight may or may not be associated with increased fetal surface dimensions or irregularities, but mural thickness will commonly be increased (parenchymal mural thickness at term is usually 2.0–2.5 cm). Cut-off points for large placentas at other periods of gestation are not specified, but Table 10[224] provides very useful guidelines. Increased placental weight can reflect the added mass of a retroplacental hematoma (Figures 27–29), effects of maternal fluid administration during cesarean section, a large intervillous thrombus, or a fetomaternal hemorrhage. Placentomegaly can be seen in conditions of maternal diabetes mellitus, fetal hydrops, Rh incompatibility or hemoglobinopathy, chronic infections (e.g. cytomegalovirus, syphilis, toxoplasmosis), acute placental congestion or edema with acute chorioamnionitis, maternal anemia, and overgrowth syndromes that affect the fetus and placenta, such as Beckwith–Wiedemann syndrome (Figure 51). The color of the placenta is largely due to the presence of fetal hemoglobin, so a large pale placenta is highly suggestive of fetal anemia (Figure 43a).

SMALL PLACENTA

A placental weight less than the lower limit of normal for the gestational period generally reflects true undergrowth of the placenta. Low placental weight may reflect maternal conditions of underperfusion of the placental bed, such as maternal hypertension, pre-eclampsia, or diabetic vasculopathy, and be accompanied by chorionic villous infarction. While small placentas can result in the low birth weight of the infant in these conditions, every instance of the delivery of a small-for-dates baby and a small placenta does not reflect placental insufficiency due to maternal vascular insufficiency. Chronic villitis of unknown etiology and confined placental mosaicism (a condition in which the villus trophoblast or stroma, or both, have populations of cells which are aneuploid, but the fetus is euploid[225–227]) can also result in a small placenta. Cases in which the baby and the placenta are small may reflect conditions in which both the baby and the placenta are 'simultaneously' affected by an abnormality. These conditions include some prolonged intrauterine infections with chronic villitis, fetoplacental chromosomal anomaly (e.g. trisomies), and fetal malformations.

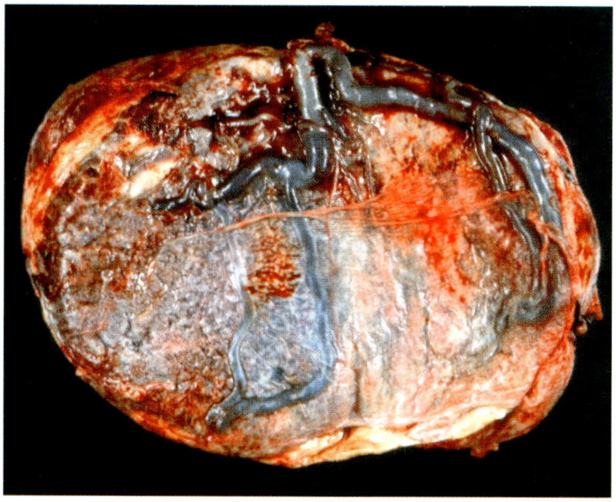

Figure 51 A 1090-g, placenta which had a 140-cm umbilical cord affected with Beckwith–Wiedemann syndrome (BWS) (large-for-gestational-age infant born with an omphalocele, macroglossia, and ear lobe creases, and later conclusively diagnosed with BWS). Placentas with BWS characteristically have excessively long umbilical cords with numerous false knots. In the authors' experience, the BWS placenta also has unusually ectatic, but sparsely distributed, chorionic plate vessels (especially veins) with large intervening areas of net-like chorionic vascular patterns, as seen here

EXTRACHORIAL PLACENTA

In normal placentas, the transition from villous to membranous chorion occurs at the edge of the placenta. Grossly, the zone is a roughly 1-cm wide ring of mild opacification and represents the site where terminal, small branches of chorionic vessels turn downward to supply the marginal chorionic villous tree. Microscopically, it is manifested by reactive cytotrophoblastic proliferation and collagen deposition[4]. In extrachorial placentas, the chorionic plate is *smaller* than the basal plate. Thus, the fetal membranes do not arise at the placental perimeter, but from a site some distance in from its circumference. As a result, a rim of chorionic villous tissue projects beyond the limits of the chorionic plate. This extrachorial rim may involve all or only part of the placental circumference and may range from one to several centimeters in width. Fox[3] has noted that between 18 and 30% of placentas exhibit some feature of extrachorialis.

There are two forms of extrachorialis, circum-marginate and circumvallate (Figures 52–54), and they may occur together. Circum-margination is typified by a thin ridge of fibrinoid at the site of anomalous reflection of the membranes from the fetal surface. This, and the fact that the membrane reflection includes chorionic matrix, distinguishes it from artifactual amniotic detachment due to specimen manipulation. Circumvallation is characterized by a folded redundancy of the membranes at the abbreviated limits of the chorionic plate. Traction of the membranes near their line of attachment can enhance gross detection of membrane plication and appreciation of the extent of its circumferential involvement. Examination of this overfolded edge may reveal associated, chronic marginal hematoma and a yellowish tinge to the membranes, due to hemosiderosis (see section on 'Marginal hematoma' in Chapter 8). The parenchyma of the circumvallate placenta is characteristically thick. Microscopically, well-oriented histologic sections of plica and associated marginal tissue reveal a 'doubled-back' overfold of the marginal chorioamnion, with abundant fibrinoid, degenerated cytotrophoblast, and/or senescent villi and decidua, seen interposed at its lateral aspects (Figure 52). Chorionic hemosiderosis may be present. Interposed and adjacent decidua often show necrosis, evidence of chronic hemorrhage and hematoma formation, and, in some cases of acute antepartum bleeding, superimposed acute hemorrhage. Fibrinoid may also extend inwards to the subchorion of the fetal plate with thrombohematoma formation.

There are no recognized pathologic sequelae with circum-margination, and some degree of circum-margination is commonly identified in placentas submitted to pathologic examination. Circumvallation, of partial or complete extent, occurs in up to 6.9% of placentas[3], and multiparity and early amniorrhea are risks for its occurrence. The exposed chorionic villi are underperfused or completely avascular and sclerosed[4]. Circumvallation may be associated with normal obstetrical outcome, but such instances likely reflect limited placental involvement by the abnormality. Many investigators have found

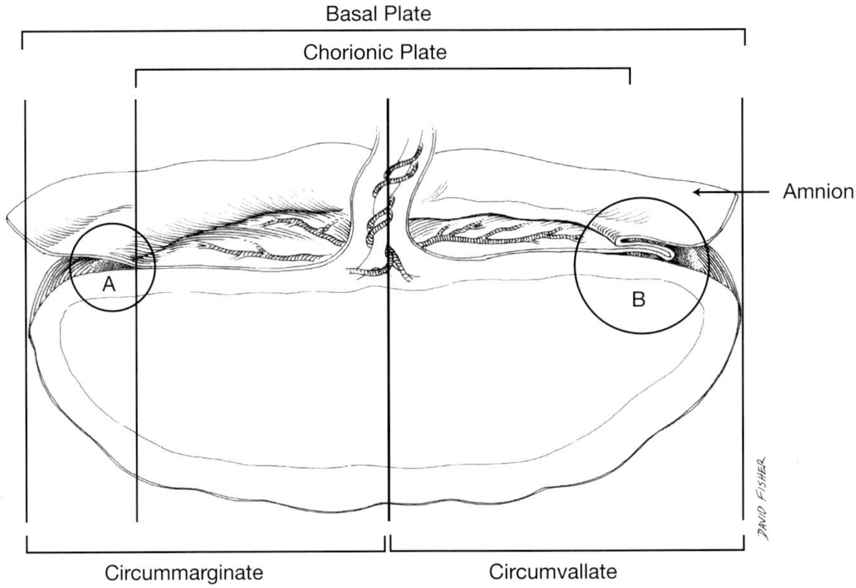

Figure 52 As described in the text, in the circum-marginate placenta, a thin rim of fibrin is deposited at the extrachorial line (A). In the circumvallate extrachorial placenta, fibrin and necrotic decidua are interposed between over-folded layers of chorioamnion, the plica marking a site consistent with damage and repair (B).

prominent or complete circumvallation to be associated with increased risks of preterm delivery, antepartum bleeding, placental abruption, stillbirth, fetal intrauterine growth restriction, and single umbilical artery and other congenital malformations[3,4,228]. In extensive or complete circumvallation, the chorionic plate, and, thereby, the size of the amniotic cavity, can be substantially reduced; restriction of fetal movement may result in fetal joint contractures/or a short umbilical cord[4].

The pathogenesis of extrachorial placentation is unclear. Suggested mechanisms have included unusually deep implantation of the blastocyst; lack of coordination between placental and uterine growth; deficiency in amniotic fluid pressure needed for appropriate growth and lateral extension of the membranes to the placental edge; and hemorrhage around the placental edge. The most favored mechanism for circumvallation implicates marginal decidual hemorrhage. The hemorrhage presumably leads to premature separation of the placenta, medial hemorrhage into the chorionic villous parenchyma, uplifting of the chorioamnion, and compromise of its vascular branches to the villous tree. Marginal tissue repair could be accompanied by organization and/or potential resorption of the thrombohematoma, a re-annealing and subsequent layered plication of the damaged, uplifted free membranes at their medial edge of remaining attachment, and a subsequent loss of chorionic villous integrity and function in the rim of extrachorial tissue[3,4,8]. Recurrent bleeding at the site of the marginal hematoma might explain maternal episodes of vaginal bleeding and the association of circumvallation with placental abruption.

PLACENTA MEMBRANACEA

In this rare type of placentation, the placenta has the appearance of being a large, bag-like cast of the uterine cavity. Its configuration is reminiscent of its early development, when chorionic villi fully cover the outer aspect of the gestational sac (Figure 55). As

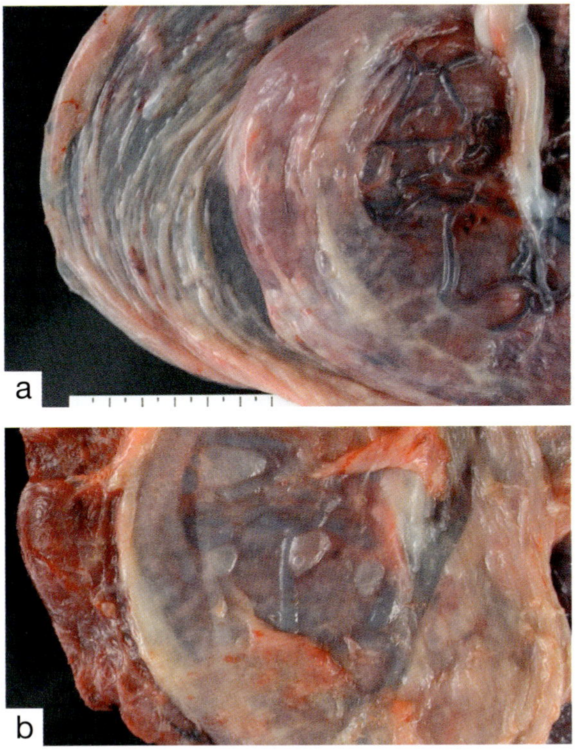

Figure 53 (a) A rim of circum-margination is seen as a paramarginal, crescentic deposition of fibrinoid of variable width on this placenta. Note that the amnion rises smoothly as it passes over the deposition, and that there is no discoloration of the membranes or plication at the edge of the fibrinoid rim. (b) The amnion is now retracted to the right to reveal the extrachorial component of the placenta, which extends beyond the rim of fibrinoid circum-margination. The rim incorporates chorion, but there is no thrombohematoma or hemosiderosis

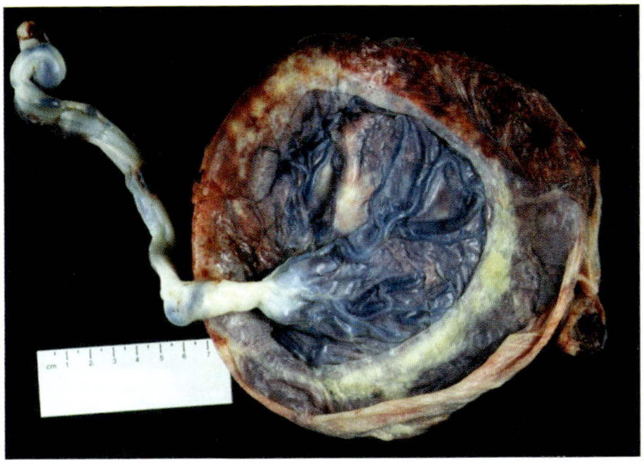

Figure 54 Circumvallate placenta. In contrast to Figure 53, this placenta shows a definitive plication of the membranes that is nearly circumferential

alluded to in Chapter 2, normal configuration of the chorion frondosum is achieved through selective involution of chorionic villi that do not lie opposite the ventral surface of the fetus. The pathogenesis of placenta membranacea (also called 'placenta diffusa') represents complete failure of this normal process of atrophy. While some separate the so-called '*ring placenta*' or '*band placenta*' from membranacea (Figure 56), we agree with Fox[3] that this more cylindrical form is a variant of placenta membranacea. The underlying cause of the failure of chorionic regression is unknown. Theories have included shallow implantation; abnormal trophoblastic function; abnormal excessive vascularization of the endometrium that permits more generalized survival of the chorionic villi; and/or failure of development of an appropriate decidua basalis. As the name implies, the placental parenchyma is generally extremely thin and diffuse, but patchy areas of normal parenchymal thickness may be seen. The chorionic villi are generally ischemic-appearing and/or infarcted. In many instances, fully formed villi are not seen, but instead a layer of trophoblasts that appears to invade the membranes is present[229]. Because of the diffuse attachment of the 'membranous' placenta to the uterine cavity, there may be sites of accretion (especially within the lower uterine segment). This, together with the fact that the placenta often overlies the cervical os, commonly results in recurrent hemorrhage and maternal vaginal bleeding. Labor and delivery are also problematic; retention of placental tissue is a frequent complication. Fetuses are usually intrauterine growth-restricted and stillbirth is common[3,8]. Some cases of membranacea may require a hysterectomy to control maternal bleeding[33].

BILOBATE PLACENTA

A bilobate (or 'bipartite') placenta is one composed of two equally sized lobes with insertion on the umbilical cord *between* the two lobes. The insertion is usually velamentous but it may be into a bridge of

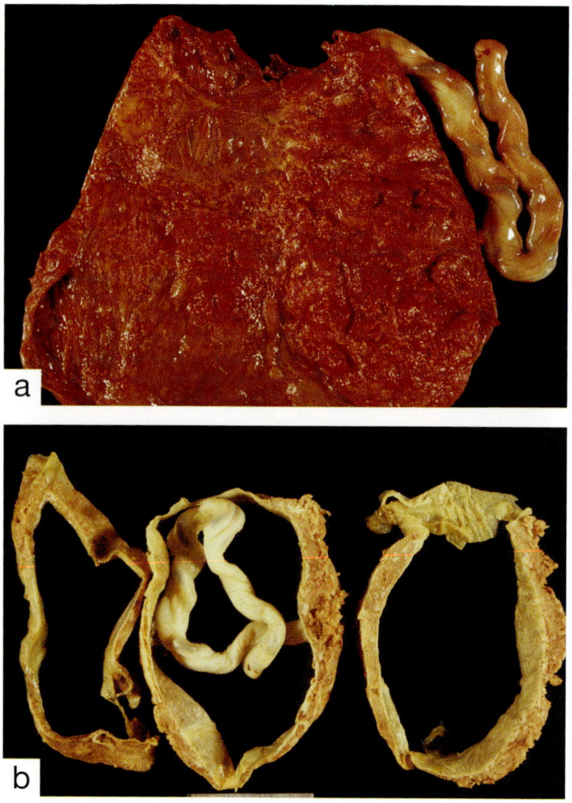

Figure 55 (a) Placenta membranacea. This placenta was a virtual cast of the uterine cavity, with only a small patch of 'free membrane' present, seen at the base of the membranous bag of placental tissue in the photograph. Its parenchyma was very thin and abnormally attached to the inner uterine surface with foci of placenta accreta (see subsequent section) in many histologic sections. A hysterectomy was subsequently performed for continued maternal postpartum hemorrhage. (b) Representative serial sections show the circumferential loops of pale, infarcted, thin, friable, placenta membranacea pictured in (a). The size of the umbilical cord appears in stark contrast to the attenuated mural dimension of the placental parenchyma

chorionic tissue. When defined in this manner, Fox[3] favored an incidence of 0.3%. Bilobation is associated with first-trimester bleeding and adherent placenta, but it is not significantly associated with preterm labor or perinatal morbidity or mortality. Its etiology is unclear but it may represent implantation in a uterine sulcus. *Multilobate* placentas are extremely rare. These show a central velamentous cord insertion with branch vessels forming a radiating distribution that supplies several, separate lobes.

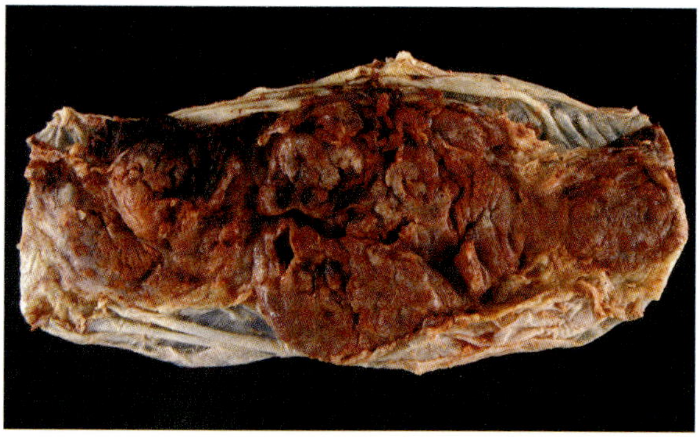

Figure 56 The 'band placenta' is a variant of placenta membranacea

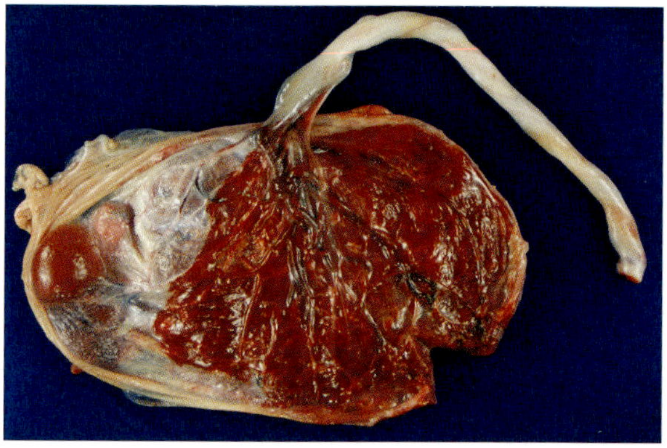

Figure 57 Placenta with accessory lobes

ACCESSORY OR SUCCENTURIATE LOBE

In contrast to the bilobate or multilobate placenta, a placenta with an accessory lobe shows a main lobe evidenced by its larger size and umbilical cord insertion with a smaller dependent lobe some distance from the main disk. The accessory lobe is connected to the main placenta by a vascular bridge, within velamentous or thin chorionic tissue (Figure 57). Accessory lobes are seen in about 3% of placentas and more than one accessory lobe may be present. The finding may represent a very mild expression of abnormal chorionic villous regression or of asymmetric placental development on both the anterior and posterior aspect of the uterine cavity.

The finding has no clinical significance except in rare instances of:

(1) Retention of the accessory lobe following delivery of the main placental disk;

(2) A position over or near the cervical os (see section below on 'Placenta previa');

(3) Disruption of its intramembranous vascular supply and fetal hemorrhage[3,4].

Lobar retention should be suspected when there is a defect or tear in the membranes and intramembranous vascular branches extend to the limits of the tear[33].

PLACENTA PREVIA

Placenta previa is a clinical condition in which the placental implantation site is in the lower uterine segment and diagnosed when the marginal limits of the placenta extend up to or within a few centimeters of the cervical os, or when placental tissue partially or completely covers this opening. Thus defined, it is detected in 0.26–0.55% of pregnancies, and predisposing risk factors include advanced maternal age, multiparity, prior cesarean section delivery, and smoking. Episodic and painless vaginal bleeding is characteristic with previa, and perinatal morbidity and mortality are largely related to its associated increased risk for preterm birth. Surprisingly, clear association with fetal intrauterine growth restriction has not been demonstrated, but an associated 2.5-fold risk for fetal anomalies has been found[33].

The challenges for the pathologist's assessment and meaningful interpretation of a placenta from a gestation with previa relate to the challenges faced by the obstetrician. First, the type of previa in a given gestation may change with progression of pregnancy and, also, with cervical dilatation, during labor. For example, a marginal previa may become partial, as the placenta is uncovered, and a complete previa may change to a partial form, as the edge of the os dilates beyond the presenting placental margin. Second, with intrapartum retraction of the uterine wall, the overlying portion of the placenta becomes detached from its connection to the uterus and severe maternal hemorrhage, which can be difficult to control, may result. Finally, since presentation of the placenta precedes that of the fetus, there are high risks of hemorrhage with vaginal delivery, and almost all cases of previa necessitate a cesarean section delivery. Pathologic correlation of findings in a placenta with history of previa will, thereby, be affected by the clinical course and method of delivery. In a placenta from a cesarean section, pathologic examination may reveal a circular patch of old retroplacental hematoma and chorionic villous infarction that may correspond to the previa site. In a placenta from a vaginal delivery, an irregular hemorrhagic margin or a more central transmural defect in thinned, hemorrhagic and/or infarcted parenchyma may represent the original site of cervical overlay. Membrane rupture and hemorrhage close to the placental margin may indicate a marginal previa. Finally, because nearly 7% of cases of placenta previa are clinically complicated by accreta[33] (see below), and because accreta can be associated with placenta previa in 33%[3] to 88% of cases[230], pathologic evaluation should include careful search for this abnormality. The coexistence of accreta in previa may well be higher than has been previously clinically appreciated. Documentation of the presence of accreta in cases of previa may have implications for the immediate follow-up of the patient, as well as for increased risks of complications in subsequent pregnancies (e.g. spontaneous uterine rupture, during labor).

PLACENTA ACCRETA

Accreta is abnormal adherence of the placenta to the uterine wall, after delivery of the infant. It may affect a portion or the entirety of the placental maternal surface. Its pathologic basis is partial or complete deficiency of the decidua basalis and Nitabuch's membrane of fibrinoid, such that chorionic villi are abnormally contiguous with, or actually extend into, the basal myometrium. Usually, the decidua parietalis is also deficient[3,16]. Three gradations of placenta accreta are recognized:

(1) Placenta accreta vera, in which chorionic villi are attached to, but do not penetrate, the myometrium;

(2) Placenta increta, in which villi show infiltration within the superficial or even deeper myometrium;

(3) Placenta percreta, in which the entire myometrium to or including the uterine serosa is penetrated by chorionic villous tissue (Figure 58).

In placenta percreta, there may be extension to neighboring organs such as the urinary bladder and bowel. Marked thinning of the decidua basalis may be evidenced by the presence of only scattered, small groups of decidual cells in loose connective tissue, and the attenuation may be focal[3]. Since the term 'accreta' is applied to describe any clinical condition of an abnormally firm placental attachment, the pathologist should specify which of the three forms he/she has histopathologically documented, when issuing a final surgical pathology report. A pathologic diagnosis of placenta percreta cannot be made in the absence of the hysterectomy specimen[3,4].

Clinically, accreta is evidenced by partial or complete lack of placental separation, and very frequently there is persistent, maternal bleeding. About 53% of patients with placenta accreta present at term[231], with some 65% of cases of intractable postpartum hemorrhage caused by abnormal adherence of the placenta[33]. Hysterectomy was required in 91% of cases in the review of clinical accreta by Armstrong and colleagues[230], and Dildy[231] has noted that 57% of all hysterectomies are performed for placenta accreta (referring to all forms). Accreta currently clinically complicates 1/2500 deliveries in the United States[232]. Its incidence has increased ten-fold over 50 years, and this has been largely attributed to the increase in rate of cesarean section deliveries[230,232]. Risk factors for all forms of accreta include:

(1) History of uterine trauma including prior cesarean section (the most frequent association, especially if there is a history of two or more such delivery procedures, in which case the risk is 50%), uterine surgery (e.g. dilatation and curettage), manual placental extraction, or myomectomy;

(2) Abnormal location of the placenta (e.g. placenta previa, cornual implantation);

(3) Uterine leiomyomas and malformations (e.g. uterine septum or diverticulum);

(4) Advanced maternal age, multiparity, or postpartum uterine infection and sepsis[33,233–236].

The occurrence of accreta in an unscarred uterus is extremely rare[232,235].

Clinically, placenta percreta is the most rare form of accreta, but also the most ominous. Its incidence ranges from 1/79 000[237] to 1/93 000[233,234] to 1/140 000 deliveries[232], but it has been seen in up to 1/540 deliveries in Thailand and Far Eastern countries; this markedly different occurrence rate is presumably related to the increased rates of molar pregnancies in these nations[238]. While all forms of accreta are associated with both maternal and fetal morbidity and mortality, complications of percreta include severe maternal bleeding that can be life-threatening; percreta is associated with a 7% maternal mortality rate[231] and a 9.6% rate of fetal death[3]. Percreta nearly always necessitates an emergency hysterectomy, but recently conservative management techniques have been successfully employed for a limited number of patients[236].

For the pathologist, it is important to stress that clinical accreta may be placenta accreta or placenta increta histopathologically, and mild accreta in particular may be focal[16,239]. Frequently, pathologic examination is made difficult by the limitations of disrupted tissue, retained tissue, and histologic orientation. With simple accreta and some instances of increta, manual removal, followed by uterine curettage, is successful in many cases. In accreta, the maternal surface is often disrupted, and, especially in cases of manual removal, it may even be fragmented. In cases of clinically diagnosed accreta, defects on the maternal surface may correspond to areas of accreta,

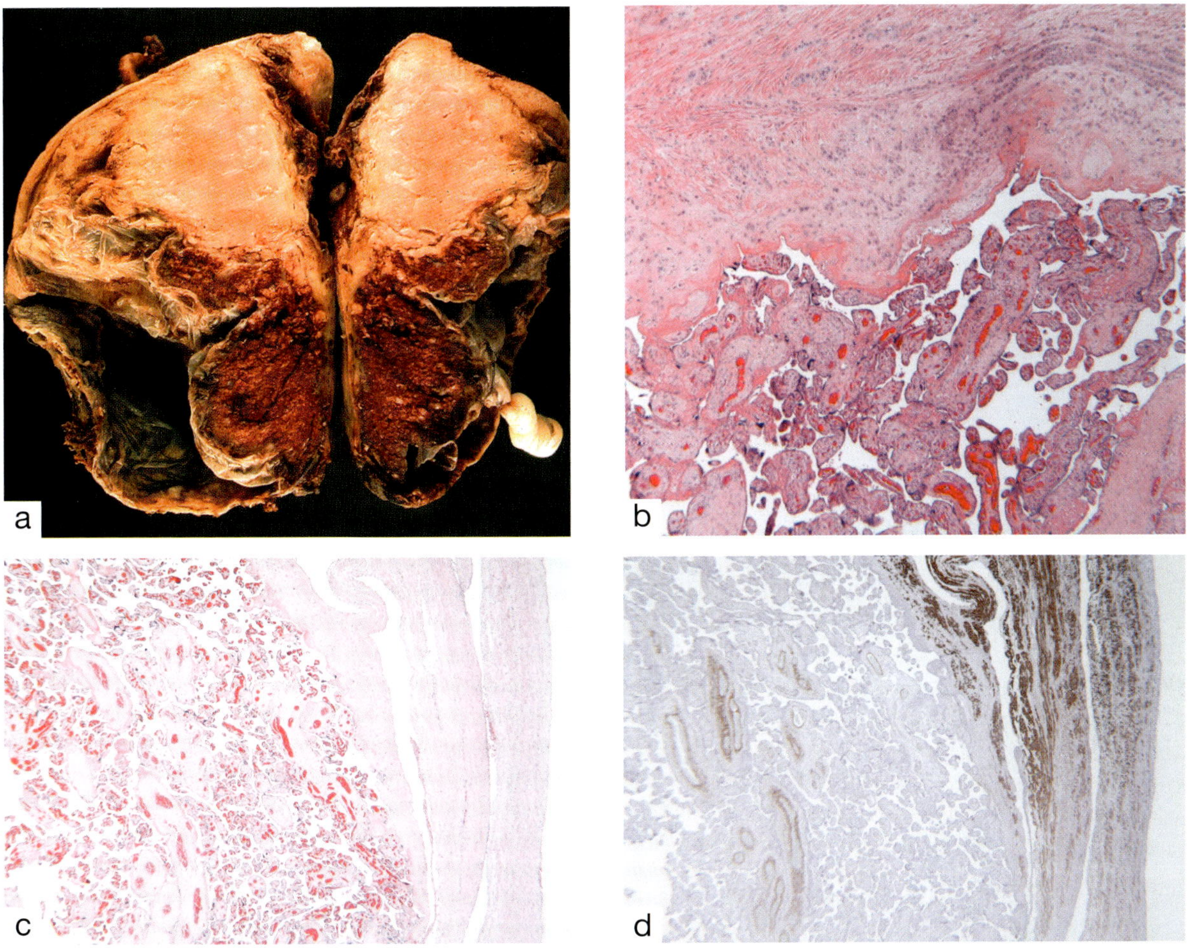

Figure 58 (a) Hemisected hysterectomy specimen of placenta previa with placenta percreta is shown. The uterine fundus shows placentation, but the majority of the placenta involves the lower uterine segment and extends to the cervical os, seen as mirror-image, angled clefts in the bulging inferior masses at the bottom of the photograph. (The serosal surfaces lie in parallel, down the center of the specimen.) On each half, deeply congested, chorionic villous tissue first extends to the limits of the decidua, then into the myometrium, and then deeply to the serosal surface, along the lower uterine segment. Near the cervix, it is present on the serosa itself (placenta percreta). In addition, chorion frondosum is present on a markedly attenuated portion of the opposite uterine wall, seen as a sac-like component with tufts of chorionic villi extending from its cut surface (another region of placenta percreta). Clinically, uterine rupture did occur in this case, at the lower uterine segment. There was also a second rent site at the top of the uterine fundus, where another site of mural attenuation was present; this site is partially shown in the upper left half of the hemisected uterus Microscopically, the spectrum of placenta accreta to percreta was seen in this placenta. (b) Deficiency of decidua basalis is apparent in this section, since fibers of myometrial smooth muscle are readily detectable less than one villus width from the decidual surface. Deeper levels of the block from such sections will often reveal frank infiltration of villi within the underlying myometrium (placenta accreta). (c and d) Hematoxylin–eosin stained and immunoperoxidase stained sections respectively, for smooth muscle actin. Sections are taken from the markedly attenuated region of uterine wall, in (a), near the rupture site. They demonstrate chorionic villi closely approximating the serosal surface, as they confirm the presence of myometrial fibers and also distinguish the smooth muscle of the villous stromal vessels. Other sections showed distuption of the myometrium, necrosis, and hemorrhage and the presence of chorionic villi on the inner and outer aspects of the serosa

but obtaining well-oriented, informative sections can be problematic. Attempts should be made to obtain as well-oriented sections as possible, but, since the tissue in question may no longer be attached to the maternal surface (especially in areas of defect), careful gross examination and sampling of suspicious-appearing foci and tissue adjacent to a defect are recommended. *En face* block, superficially shaved sections of the maternal surface may be of great yield, since a single such 2-cm square samples some 4000 times the amount of decidual surface as that of the standard 5-μm histologic section[16]. Further problems can include documentation of decidual deficiency underlying the accreta; again, such identification may be precluded if the diagnostic tissue has been retained. Associated uterine curettings may provide the evidence necessary to diagnose decidual deficiency, but even with these specimens, section orientation may be suboptimal[3,4]. Use of immunoperoxidase stains for smooth muscle actin[16,239–241] may prove helpful in identifying basal plate myometrial cells in some instances of accreta. However, caution is advised regarding interpretation of the actin staining pattern and position. Superficial skimming of decidual vascular wall tissue in a histologic section and 'edge artifact' are potential confounding factors in the interpretation of these stains. Finally, the rendering of a diagnosis of decidual deficiency, in the absence of chorionic villous contact with the myometrium, is fraught with difficulties. Most important among these is the risk of tangential section and artifactual diminution of decidual tissue. A diagnosis of placenta *increta* or *percreta* rests on the respective demonstration of partial or complete penetration of the myometrium by chorionic villi. A diagnosis of either of these more advanced forms can only be made on hysterectomy specimens, unless a portion of the myometrium is present along the maternal surface of the manually removed specimen[4].

In summary, the pathogenesis of accreta is related to an absence or deficiency of endometrial tissue or its insufficient decidual transformation. Smoking has been considered a risk factor, but this has not been uniformly observed[16]. Whatever its underlying cause, decidual deficiency results in trophoblastic extension of the placental bed beyond normal depth. (Excessive invasiveness of the chorionic villi does not seem to be a factor in the pathogenesis of accreta.) Finally, the extensive sampling performed by Khong and Werger[16], as well as the study by Jacques and colleagues[239], indicates that the presence of mild accreta is more common than clinical manifestations would indicate. The implications of finding mild accreta upon placental examination are unclear, but since it may be a harbinger for impending complications in the woman's postpartum course or for future pregnancies, it seems prudent to include a comment about these potential risks in the pathology report.

RETROPLACENTAL HEMATOMA AND ABRUPTIO PLACENTAE

These have already been described in Chapter 8. It is important to bear in mind the distinction between RH and AP. The former is a pathologic diagnosis, the latter is a clinical syndrome. Although RH is a pathologic hallmark of AP, each can be present without demonstrable presence of the other.

MATERNAL FLOOR INFARCTION/ MASSIVE PERIVILLOUS FIBRINOID DEPOSITION

Definition The term 'maternal floor infarction' (MFI), an entity first described by Benirschke and Driscoll in the 1960s[4], is a misnomer. The pathology of MFI does not represent infarction, but instead is a dense, mesh-like parenchymal network of perivillous fibrin/fibrinoid deposition. In the 'classic' pattern, the deposition is largely basal, but it is frequently more diffuse and can even be transmural. The more extensive type of deposition has been referred to as 'massive diffuse perivillous fibrinoid deposition' (MPFD). Of note is that some investigators have separated MFI from MPFD histopathologically, but such division can be problematic[242]. The entities appear to represent spectral manifestations of closely related, if not highly overlapping, pathogenic processes. For simplicity, we use the acronym MFI to cover the basal and more diffuse patterns.

Incidence MFI is rare; its incidence has been reported to be from as low as 0.028%[243] to 0.09%[244] to 0.5%[245].

Gross features The placenta is characteristically small for the period of gestation, and dense. The maternal surface is diffusely firm, with a pale, yellow-white, thickened, 'corrugated' appearance (Figure 59a and b). Serial placental sections typically reveal a band-like distribution or 'rind' of basal, whitish fibrin/fibrinoid* in 'classic' cases. Often, however, thick, vertically oriented trabeculae of granular fibrin/fibrinoid, extending from the basal tissue into the mid- and subchorionic intervillous space, and irregular lattice-like depositions of intervillous material are present (Figure 59a-1, a-2, b and c). These encase chorionic villi and denote the presence of a more diffuse process, and contribute to the characteristic friable, dry, dense texture and chorionic villous sclerosis of MFI. The deposits of perivillous material alter blood flow patterns in the maternal space and are probably responsible for other commonly seen features of MFI. These include patchy septal and subchorionic 'X cell' cysts (see Chapter 8), and intervillous thrombi. Patchy sites of reddish, spongy parenchyma represent regions of relatively preserved intervillous flow. The gross appearance of MFI is compared with the distribution of pale regions of firm parenchyma of chronic chorionic villous infarction due to ischemia in Figure 59d.

Histologic features MFI is primarily a histopathologic diagnosis and is characterized by a marked, diffuse increase in fibrinoid deposition along the decidua basalis and the perivillous space of basal chorionic villi[4,246–248]. The hallmark feature of MFI is the 'Gitter infarct', the deposition of perivillous fibrinoid in amorphous eosinophilic aggregates that encase regional basal villi and variably extend into the overlying parenchyma. Fibrinoid deposition appears to start on the villous surface, as there is loss of the syncytiotrophoblast; chorionic villi, and especially their tips, become cloaked and matted together in interdigitating accumulations of fibrinoid. Chorionic villi show loss of vascularity and atrophy. Neighboring chorionic villi are not collapsed upon one another (as in ischemia), but rather maintain relatively normal spacing, as individuated and encased units (Figure 60). However, true foci of chorionic villous ischemia and infarction can be seen in transmural sections, as well as intervillous thrombi and basal and subchorial X-cell cysts (See Chapter 8). These findings are compatible with sequelae of altered blood flow patterns and the creation of relatively ischemic or sluggish regions in the maternal space, due to perivillous fibrin/fibrinoid deposition (see below). Inflammation, if present, is a minor component in MFI. Occasionally, lymphocytic or lymphohistiocytic intervillositis within the perivillous fibrinoid and, rarely, chronic villitis (intravillous chronic inflammation) are found. Plasma cells, however, are not part of the inflammatory infiltrate. Decidual arteriolopathy (atherosis, vasculitis, thrombosis) is characteristically *absent* in MFI[4,247–249], except in cases associated with maternal thrombophilia, in which fibrinoid necrosis may be prominent[220]. The relative paucity and scattered distribution of chorionic villous ischemia/ infarction, the essential absence of decidual arteriopathy, and the prevalence of individuated atrophic villi are useful criteria for distinguishing MFI from the pathology of placental bed underperfusion. Ischemic features include Tenney–Parker changes; syncytiotrophoblastic death and necrosis of the villi; and dystrophic mineralization; and, grossly, an ischemic infarct has a triangular shape with its base along the maternal surface. Finally, the intervillous material in placental bed underperfusion is also more characteristically deposited around stem villi and in the subchorionic zone. In MFI, the accumulations are typically around basal terminal villi[246].

Significance MFI is an unusual, but important, cause of perinatal morbidity and mortality[250]. It is associated with high rates of preterm birth (26–60%), intrauterine fetal growth restriction (IUGR) (24–100%), and stillbirth (13–50%)[243–245,248,251,252]. There is also new evidence of its association with long-term adverse neurologic sequelae[253]. Early reports stressed the importance of antenatal ultrasonographic features associated with MFI, and some authors proposed that the antenatal diagnosis of MFI should be seriously considered if prenatal ultrasonograms revealed oligohydramnios; a dense, hyperechoic, small

*The nature of the fibrin/fibrinoid is compatible with a mixture of typical fibrin polymeric formations, of probable maternal and some fetal serologic origin, with trophoblastic cellular matrix material (fibronectin)[5,246]. It is usually referred to as 'fibrinoid', but 'fibrin/fibrinoid' has also been used. Its exact composition is unclear and it may vary among cases.

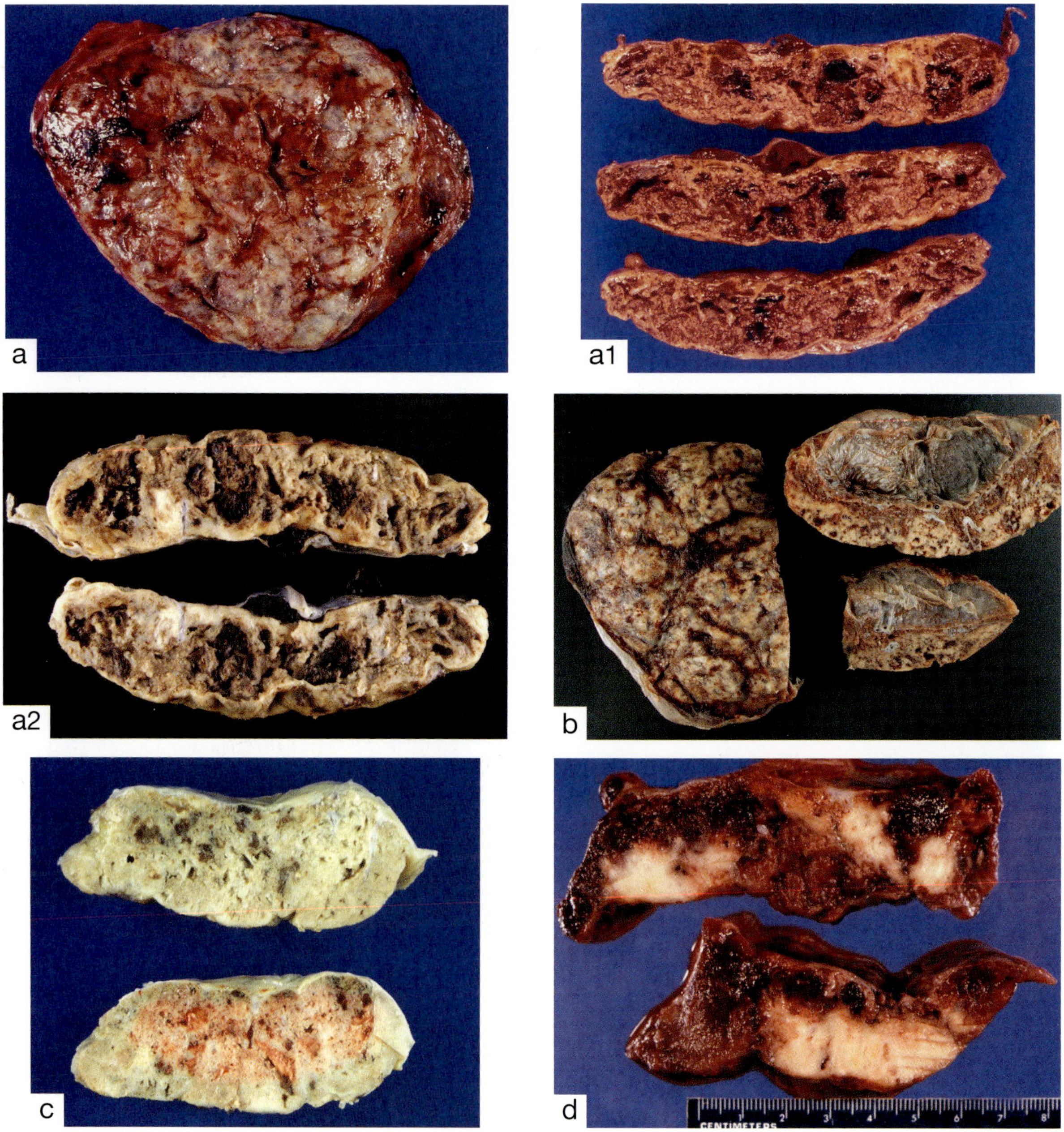

Figure 59 Maternal floor infarction/diffuse perivillous fibrinoid deposition. The characteristic firm, yellow-white, corrugated appearance of the maternal surface of maternal floor infarction (MFI) is seen in two, small but dense, affected placentas in (a) and (b). The fresh, cut surface of (a), seen in (a-1), shows diffuse, fine trabeculae of fibrinoid deposition that extend from the maternal surface in a lattice-like, variably dense pattern up toward the fetal plate. Patchy foci of basal and intervillous thrombi are seen. Fixation brings out the fibrinoid deposition in this case (a-2) and others (b and c). The pattern of fibrinoid deposition in MFI in these cases or in the 'classic' rind-like, basal pattern of MFI is different from that of the pale firm areas of chorionic villous infarction in (d), due to chorionic villous ischemia

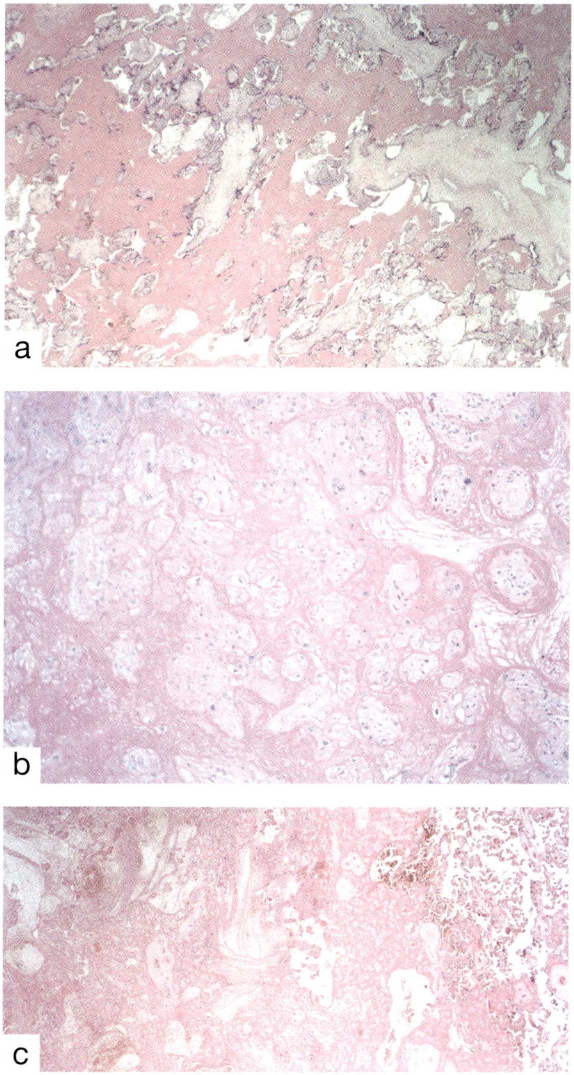

Figure 60 Histopathology of maternal floor infarction. (a) Matted masses of chorionic villi are cloaked in, and often widely separated by, accumulations of perivillous fibrinoid. (b) Entrapped chorionic villi are atrophic. (c) Deposition of fibrinoid changes blood flow patterns creating baffles, and foci of stasis and altered coagulation; intervillous thrombi are formed as seen here

placental mass; and fetal IUGR[254]. Such findings were particularly predictive if the fetal growth lag was early-onset and severe[248].

Color Doppler studies have revealed that MFI is associated with reduced and/or abnormal blood flow within the placenta. The clinically detected flow abnormalities likely reflect the concentrated basal fibrinoid distribution seen in MFI, and altered flow patterns, irregular baffles, and channels created by the intervillous fibrinoid deposition. Thus, massive perivillous fibrinoid deposition seems to have at least two effects: first, impairment of chorionic villous function by deposition of a physical blockade to blood flow and villous exchange; and second, alteration of blood flow patterns in the maternal space, which could compound the placental insufficiency related to MFI by additionally compromising nutritional and oxygen supply to any remaining 'spared' villi. Villous damage could result in the pathogenesis of small fetomaternal hemorrhages at the chorionic villous level (intervillous thrombi), with leakage of fetal α-fetoprotein into the maternal space. MFI is included in the differential diagnosis of unexplained elevation of maternal serum α-fetoprotein (MSAFP)[255–257]. Of interest, however, is that MFI has not been found to be associated with placental abruption[4]. Finally, discordant involvement by MFI may explain relatively rapid development of fetal growth restriction isolated to one twin of a dizygotic gestation[246].

In addition to associations of adverse sequelae for an index gestation, MFI has significant risks for recurrence and potential risks of earlier initiation of and more severe pathology in the subsequent pregnancy. An approximate 50% recurrence rate was found after analysis of Naeye's data[245], but rates of 12%[244] to 78%[252] have been reported. Clewell and Manchester[254] noted that their patient's subsequent pregnancy was characterized by an earlier onset and alarmingly rapid progression of placental fibrinoid deposition, on serial ultrasonography studies. The findings prompted these authors to recommend serial ultrasonographic monitoring during subsequent pregnancies of women with a history of MFI, to aid in clinical assessment for the need and timing of induction of labor or cesarean section delivery.

Because MFI has significant risks for perinatal morbidity and mortality, long-term morbidity, and recurrence, recognition of the gross and histopathologic features of this rare entity is important. Unfortunately, however, its diagnosis is made more difficult by the fact that adequate clinical information is usually not provided to, or recoverable by, the diagnosing pathologist. In other cases, the submitted history may even be misleading; placental hyperechoic regions may be clinically misinterpreted as representing sites of multiple placental chorangiomas[248]. In addition, its histopathology is challenging[242,258]. In their study of the rates of discrepant diagnoses of placental lesions made by practicing pathologists, Sun and colleagues[258] found that when their series' histopathologies were reviewed by placental pathologists, MFI was missed in 66.7% of cases. True, ischemic infarction was the most commonly rendered, erroneous diagnosis. However, such oversights should be minimized if the above-listed criteria are applied.

Pathogenesis The etiopathogenesis of MFI is unknown. Infectious or post-infectious etiologies have been queried, but none has been proved[4,245]. The fibrinoid deposition pattern of MFI likely represents the outcome of a final common pathway potentially triggered by a variety of conditions that disturb the normal and inducible factors of the mechanisms that maintain the integrity of the syncytiotrophoblast and the fluidity of blood in the maternal space. (Trophoblast-generated molecules and elements of the maternal blood contribute to a normal villous surface and maintenance of a fluid maternal space.) The triggers are likely potent and/or in high concentrations since they seem irreversibly to commit the perivillous space to a process of marked fibrinoid deposition and accumulation. A discussion of all of the factors and mechanisms that could initiate MFI is beyond the scope of this manual (the reader is referred to the original articles for details), but potential sites of aberration include trophoblastic factors[18,19,259–262], maternal coagulation factors (including the deleterious effects of circulating, abnormal antibodies)[24,219,263–265], decidual factors[22], and fetal metabolic derangements[266]. Since fibrinoid production and perivillous deposition are normal components of villous repair and normal features of the term placenta[6], the *rarity* of MFI suggests that there are many sites of duplication within the normal protective and reparative systems that prevent pathologic amounts of fibrinoid from being laid down and diffusely distributed.

Potential etiologic aberrations in MFI include:

(1) Aberrant control of plasminogen activation or its inactivation at the trophoblast surface;

(2) Excessive and/or abnormally early reduction of the normal, third-trimester decline in trophoblast urokinase plasminogen receptor expression that leads to a pathologic shift toward perivillous fibrinoid deposition;

(3) Abnormality of maternal hemostasis (gestational or primary) that results in a hypercoagulable state in the unique milieu of maternal space;

(4) Abnormalities of plasma or metabolic factors that are not directly part of the coagulant family, but that interfere with normal coagulant activity;

(5) Auto- or alloimmune antibodies to trophoblast molecules that alter their molecular function or concentrations in perivillous space. The rarity of MFI and research into the effects of rare circulating, abnormal antibodies render these molecules as likely etiologic candidates for at least some of the cases of MFI:

    (a) An antibody specifically capable of binding and inactivating trophoblastic type urokinase-type plasminogen activator and/or urokinase receptors (versus tissue-type plasminogen activators) could lead to intervillous deposition of an unusual, fibrin-like material[24];

    (b) Abnormal antibodies could explain a thrombosis that was localized to the placenta and occurred only during pregnancy[24,219,264,265];

    (c) The perivillous material could contain complexes of molecules unique to the placental trophoblast, molecular remnants of the standard coagulation factors not normally formed, and/or a previously unrecognized variant of fibrin;

(d) The gestational growth of the villous tree would increase the immunologic surface area available for initiation of a para-coagulopathy, and account for the rapidly progressive clinical picture of MFI noted on prenatal ultrasonograms;

(e) The primarily basal distribution of fibrinoid in MFI could represent the effects of the trophoblasts' proximity to the source of the maternal blood flow and/or decidual cells;

(f) Depending upon its density and rapidity of formation, basal deposition might also relatively restrict the passage of maternal blood into the middle and upper zones of the maternal space and further compound the basal concentration of fibrinoid in MFI.

VILLITIS

Overview of the placental barrier and pathogenesis of infectious villitis

It is beyond the scope of this manual to address fully the pathogenic processes that result in villitis, but some recent and pertinent observations regarding the placental barrier and mechanisms of villous infection are presented in overview. The physical and functional barrier of the hemochorial placenta (placenta in which a single layer of fetally derived trophoblasts separates maternal from fetal circulation) impedes hematogenous (vertical) transmission of infection, from mother to fetus. It is an active, rather than passive, barrier composed of the placental trophoblast and its basement membrane, the chorionic villous stroma with its Hofbauer cells, and the villous capillary endothelium with its basement membrane[267]. In humans, the most important part of the barrier to the vertical transmission of many infectious agents, and especially of viruses, appears to be the syncytiotrophoblast[268–271]. In addition to providing a physical barrier, the syncytiotrophoblast has high levels of nitric oxide synthetase and microvillous-associated glycosaminoglycans, and does not express class I or class II major histocompatibility complex antigens, CD4 receptors, or intercellular adhesion molecule-1 (ICAM-1). Functional implications may include production of nitric oxide intermediates that have antimicrobial activity; prevention of adherence of maternal leukocytes to syncytiotrophoblast due to presence of glycosaminoglycans, class I and II antigens, and ICAM-1; and prevention of HIV viral attachment by the absence of CD4 receptors[267]. There is also evidence that the barrier includes an additional immunohumoral component that is of both fetal and maternal origin, and dependent on optimal interactions among all its cellular and chemical constituents[272–277]. For example, the trophoblast secretes interferons that may prevent vertical transmission of herpes and other viruses[267]. The role of the Hofbauer cell in feto-placental defense is partially determined by the specific pathogen. The role of the endothelial cell is very poorly understood[278], except in instances in which it is itself infected, such as in cytomegalovirus placentitis.

Whatever its functional composition, the placental barrier is not completely efficient and/or becomes damaged, since a large number of organisms can cross it to produce placental and subsequent fetal infection. The mechanisms of infection are incompletely understood, but recent studies suggest that damage to the syncytiotrophoblast is a key event and that the presence of receptors for viruses, bacteria, and protozoa on placental cells enable attachment and entry of pathogens into the placental cells and, thereby, into the fetal circulation. Mechanisms of damage include: injury to the syncytiotrophoblast by the pathogens themselves, their toxins, or host reactive inflammatory and immunochemical responses (e.g. tumor necrosis factor-α (TNF-α))[268,273]; and injury resulting in increased apoptosis and reduced capacity for cell renewal of syncytiotrophoblast (e.g. CMV and parvovirus B19 infections)[268,279]. In addition, pathogenicity may involve infection-induced trophoblastic elaboration of cytokines that stimulate viral genome transcription (e.g. HIV infection)[276]. Finally, there is evidence that the immature and extravillous cytotrophoblast is not as resistant as the syncytiotrophoblast to infection, at least with respect to viral pathogens. Immature extravilllous cytotrophoblast has been found to have relatively increased susceptibility to the infectivity of herpes and adenoviruses, in the presence of activated decidual lymphocytes. The immature cytotrophoblast has also been found to show greater numbers of herpes and adenoviral receptors[269]. A relatively greater susceptibility of the immature cytotrophoblast may help to explain the greater morbidity and mortality of viral infections occurring early in pregnancy; immature cells are present in large numbers in the second and early third trimesters of gestation. Moreover, as was discussed in Chapter 9 (section on 'Generalized abnormalities of the villi'), ischemia and vascular insufficiency also result in breaks in the placental barrier. Thus, ischemia, when present, may possibly augment the susceptibility to infectious organisms.

Villitis

Villitis can be acute or chronic. It may be focally or diffusely distributed and vary in severity from mild to marked. In developed countries, the major causes of infectious villitis are viral, whereas in developing countries, bacterial, protozoal, and parasitic villitides predominate, particularly as causes of stillbirth[280]. Acute villitis primarily reflects hematogenous spread of organisms from the maternal blood to the chorionic villi, but spread of organisms from the adjacent basal endometrium may also occur. In very rare instances, organisms may infect the chorionic villi via the fetal circulation, presumed due to complications of fetal septicemia, following intrauterine infection from aspiration or ingestion of infected amniotic fluid[3]. This may be a primary route in cases of intrauterine *Listeria monocytogenes* infection.

Classification of hematogenously transmitted chorionic villitis

A classification of villitis adapted from Altshuler and Russell[281], is listed below. However, the various types may coexist, consistent with histopathologic capture of a point in the progression of a given infectious placentitis.

(1) *Proliferative villitis*: characterized by varying populations of stromal chronic inflammatory infiltrates of lymphocytes, histiocytes, and plasma cells. This type of villitis is seen in CMV, rubella, and treponemal infections. The placentas with these infections are generally grossly bulky and pale, and pathogens can be demonstrated, by routine or special stains.

(2) *Necrotizing villitis:* characterized by chorionic villous necrosis and acute inflammatory infiltrate. This type of villitis is seen as a result of hematogenous spread of bacteria in the maternal space to the chorionic villous tree and chorionic plate. *L. monocytogenes* is the most common cause of this histopathologic finding, but viral and treponemal infections may also be responsible.

(3) *Granulomatous villitis*: characterized by formation of granulomas (histiocytic clusters, lymphohistiocytic infiltrate, and multinucleated giant cells, with or without central necrosis). Placentitis due to toxoplasmosis, treponemal infection, or myobacterial and fungal infection may show this pathology. The term 'granulomatous villitis' has been applied to the florid inflammation that can be seen in cases of *Listeria*, but this organism does not truly elicit a granulomatous response with multinucleated giant cells or clusters of histiocytes.

(4) *Reparative villitis*: characterized by proliferation of granulation tissue and fibroblasts and early sclerosis. This histopathology typifies later-stage villitis and is particularly characteristic of CMV and syphilitic infection.

(5) *Stromal fibrosis and sclerosis*: characterized by fibrosis and hypovascularity with occasional inflammatory cells. This form represents end-stage villous morphology in chronic villitis. It may be focal, patchy, or diffuse.

Bacterial villitis

Enteric and other gram-negative organisms, staphylococci, and group B streptococci can conceivably cause necrotizing villitis as a consequence of maternal septicemia. However, the occurrence of maternal septicemia during pregnancy is very unusual. Ascending infection from the maternal genital tract is the far more common route of transmission of these and other bacterial pathogens, with acute chorioamnionitis as evidence of their presence in the amniotic sac (see section on 'Acute chorioamnionitis', in Chapter 12). Bacterial overgrowth within the chorionic plate and chorionic villi may be seen in severe cases of intrauterine infection caused by bacterial infection, but an inflammatory villitis, with some very notable exceptions, is rarely identified in cases of ascending transmission of bacterial organisms.

Listeria monocytogenes

This appears to be one important exception to the rule that intrauterine bacterial infection results predominantly from an ascending path of transmission. *L. monocytogenes* is a ubiquitous, gram-positive, unencapsulated, motile, bacillary, and facultative anaerobe and a highly important opportunistic, food-borne pathogen. It may be found in a variety of environmental sites including soil and decomposing plant matter, water, and sewage. The incidence of intrauterine infection due to *L. monocytogenes* in live births is 12.7–24/100 000, but outbreaks of food contamination elevate its incidence[282,283]. Unfortunately, *L. monocytogenes* does not reliably respect socioeconomic boundaries; human exposure via food is frequent and recurrent, and likely results in a low-grade chronic T-cell stimulation that confers intercurrent immunity among healthy individuals. *L. monocytogenes* may contaminate milk, cheeses, vegetables, meats, and fish, and especially refrigerated, ready-to-eat products. It is amazingly hardy, and can withstand high salt concentrations and low pHs, and multiply at temperatures of refrigeration. Its special abilities to survive many modern food-processing technologies render it a significant threat to immunocompromised individuals, including pregnant women (pregnancy results in a relatively immunodepressed state), fetuses, and neonates. Maternal infection may be asymptomatic, or accompanied by a flu-like syndrome with gastroenteritis. Rates of intrauterine fetal demise with maternal infection are very high, but may even approach uniformity, since lack of culture documentation due to the absence or only brief periods of maternal symptoms and low rates of bacterial culture of abortuses may compromise detection of *Listeria* in cases of fetal death. *Listeria* should be viewed as an opportunistic, but highly lethal organism[271,282,283].

The pathogenesis of *L. monocytogenes* is related to its rather unique property of being able to cross gastrointestinal mucosal, blood–brain, and placental barriers (especially in cases in which the host is immunocompromised). Its ability to cause severe fetoplacental infection appears to be related to:

(1) The presence of the specific receptor, E-cadherin, to the *L. monocytogenes* bacterial surface antigen, internalin A, on the (maternal) intestinal mucosal cell and the placental syncytiotrophoblast and extracellular cytotrophoblast[271,283];

(2) The fact that *Listeria* confers the property of phagocytosis on cells that ordinarily do not have this ability, including endothelial cells and hepatocytes, so that cell-to-cell transmission also occurs;

(3) Apparent colonization of the trophoblast and translocation of bacteria across the endothelial barrier into the fetal bloodstream and thence to the fetal liver where replication takes place;

(4) A variety of virulence factors, pathways, and interactions (e.g. the inflammatory modulating effects of estriol on the trophoblast and

maternal T-cell and macrophage functions) that effect its infectivity and replication.

Vasquez-Boland and colleagues[283] provide a comprehensive review of the factors involved in the infectivity and severity of disease produced by *L. monocytogenes*. However, it should be stated that not all investigators concur that internalin A is the key factor in the pathogenesis of cellular entry by *Listeria*[284].

It has been difficult to establish whether intrauterine infection with *Listeria* reflects an ascending or a hematogenous route of transmission, since acute chorioamnionitis and striking placentitis with acute necrotizing villitis are generally seen together. The recent work by Lecuit and colleagues[271] on studies of internalin A (see above) suggests that fetoplacental infection is largely due to hematogenous transmission with secondary involvement of the chorioamnion. Goldenberg and Thompson[280] also report that hematogenous transmission largely predominates. However, complementary studies, to determine whether there is passage of *Listeria* through free membranes and/or the presence of internalin A receptor and ligand formation in chorioamniotic epithelial infection, have not been conducted.

The pathology of listeriosis is striking. Grossly, the placenta is enlarged for dates, and sections show diffusely scattered, tiny, yellowish, parenchymal foci of soft necrosis (Figure 61a). Histologically, these foci are villous microabscesses, composed of granuloma-like aggregates of neutrophils (Figure 61b and c). The neutrophilic nature of the infiltrate distinguishes these 'granulomatous' foci of inflammation from the classic granulomatous villitis of acid-fast bacteria (including *Nocardia* species) and fungal organisms, such as *Coccidioides immitis*. Brown–Hopps bacterial stains are useful in revealing gram-positive rods in the villous inflammation, and Warthin–Starry stains may also show bacilli. However, Parkash and colleagues[282] reported that the use of commercially available immunohistochemical stains for the presence of *Listeria* antigen increased sensitivity of detection of this organism over that of routine bacterial stains; in addition, staining was present in extracellular locations and intracellularly, within macrophages and amniotic epithelium. (Since dissemination is generally widespread in the fetus in cases of intrauterine infection with *L. monocytogenes*, with necrotic and abscess foci seen in lungs, liver, adrenals, spleen, bone marrow, and meninges, use of tissue Gram stains on sections of these tissues may also be helpful.)

Treponema pallidum

Treponema pallidum is a vertically transmitted, dangerous pathogen. Untreated, intrauterine infection is associated with a 40–50% stillbirth rate and an estimated 30–40% rate of congenital infection. Despite the decline in the incidence of syphilis in developed countries (for example primary and secondary *T. pallidum* infection in adults in the USA has decreased from 14.3 cases per 100 000 adults in 1990 to 2.5 cases per 100 000 in 1999), the low rates of congenital syphilis (13.4 per 100 000 live-born infants in the USA), and very low rates of stillbirth specifically due to syphilis, syphilis remains a serious global health problem. The overall incidence of syphilis in developing countries is between 5 and 10% and is up to 20% in some populations of African pregnant women. Stillbirth rates with syphilis range from 25 to 50%; syphilis is one of the most important, if not leading, causes of intrauterine fetal demise in some populations[280,284]. As noted by Sheffield and colleagues[107]: the diagnostic guidelines presented by the Centers for Disease Control[285] for congenital syphilis are comprehensive, but do not specifically include examination of the placenta; and detection of congenital syphilis in the asymptomatic infant and macerated stillborn is difficult. For these reasons, as well as the fact that transplacental transmission from asymptomatic mothers may occur, we concur with these investigators that placental examination is an important adjunct to recognition of the presence of intrauterine syphilitic infection. In the series by Sheffield and colleagues, the addition of a placental examination increased the detection of congenital syphilis by 22% in live-born infants and about 6% in stillborns.

The placenta in *T. pallidum* infection tends to be large for the period of gestation and pale, and may

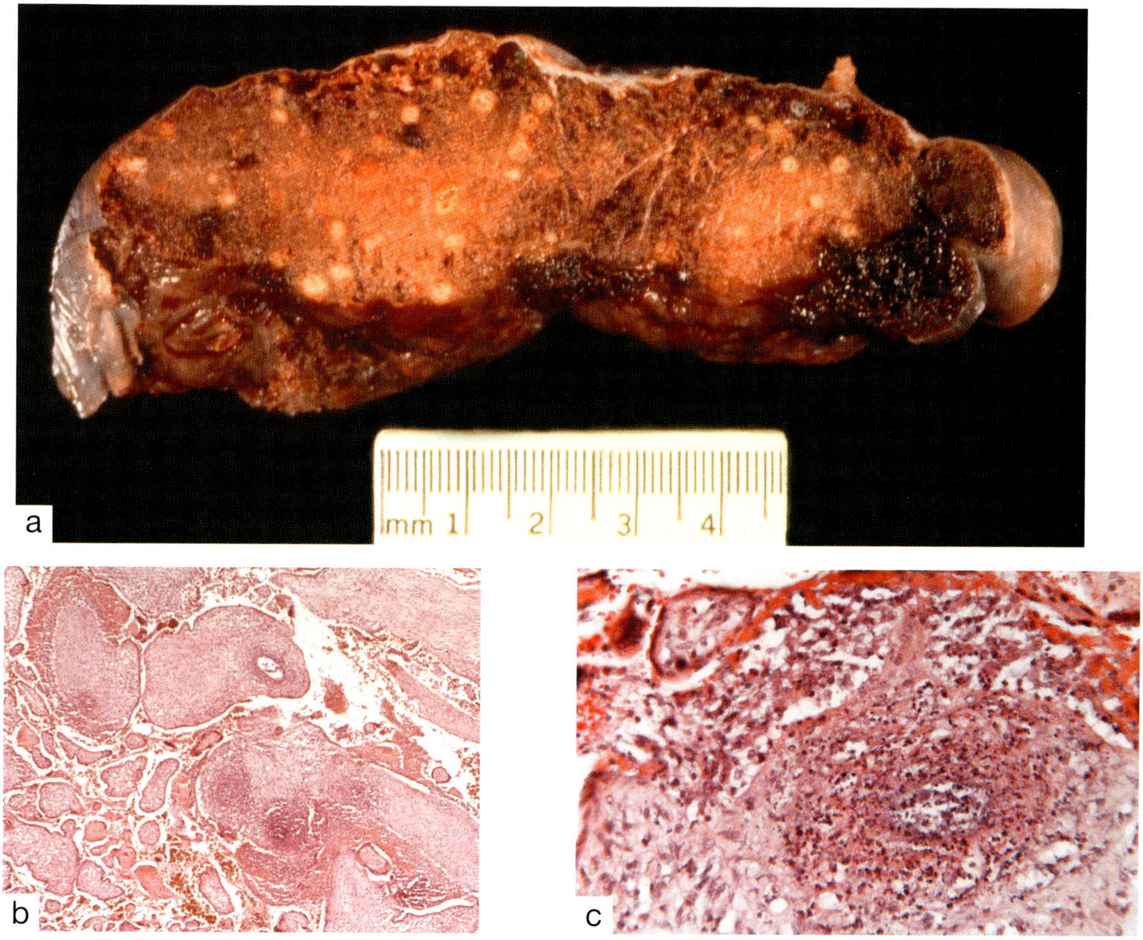

Figure 61 (a) Placenta with gross, yellow, 2–3-mm, parenchymal foci of necrosis due to infection with *Listeria monocytogenes* (case generously contributed by Faisal Qureshi, MD, Hutzel Hospital, Detroit, MI). (b) Acute necrotizing villitis and intervillositis characterisitic of *L. monocytogenes* placentitis. (c) High-power view reveals dense neutrophilic infiltrate and villous necrosis

have yellowish membranes (Figure 62a and b). Histologically, no pattern is specific, but a triad of hypercellular, bulky, immature villi (Figure 62c and d); proliferative fetal vascular changes; and acute (Figure 62e) or chronic villitis is highly suggestive *of T. pallidum* infection[106,107]. Grossly, acute villitis may be manifested as tiny, yellow-white abscesses (much like *Listeria*, as discussed above, or herpes virus placentitis). Acute villitis is indicative of fetal infection and may be admixed with chronic villitis in placentas from both stillborn and live-born infants. For reasons described below, acute syphilitic infection may also be characterized primarily by villous edema. Chronic villitis may be manifested by a lymphoplasmacytic infiltrate, but, contrary to what has often been published, plasma cell infiltrate in the villous stroma is not characteristic of, nor specific for, syphilis[106]. A lymphocytic and especially lymphoplasmacytic deciduitis[4] that may be largely limited to the choriodecidual interface is, however, common and likely reflects maternal disease, since it can be seen without fetal infection. Necrotizing funisitis, with its characteristic perivascular, arc-like deposits of pathogen and inflammatory debris (see below), is an important clue to the presence of *T. pallidum*, but the finding is not specific for syphilis.

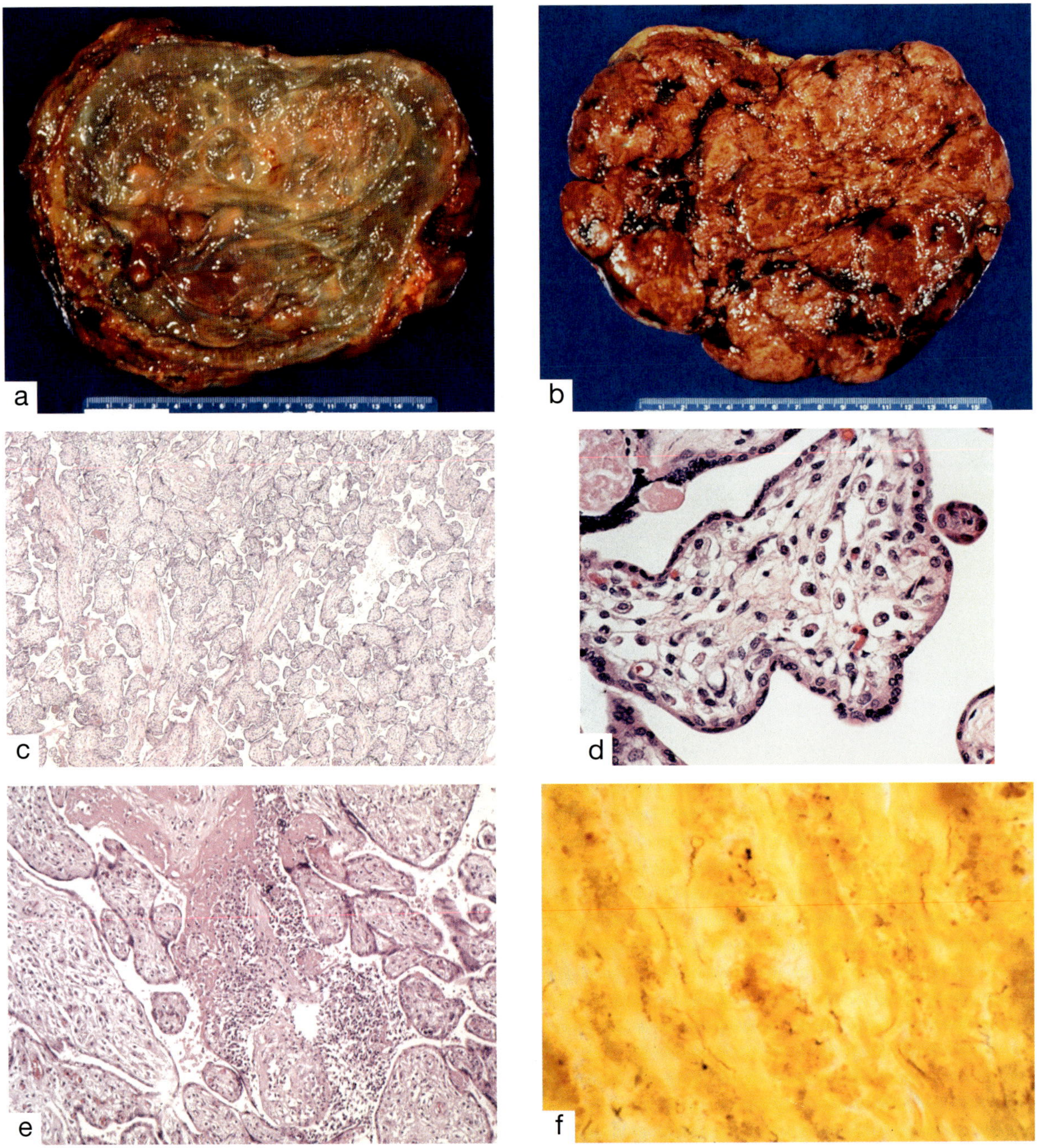

Figure 62 *Treponema pallidum* placentitis. (a) Gross image of syphilitic placenta with meconium and yellowish-stained membranes. (b) Maternal surface shows pale, hydropic cotyledons. (c) Photomicrograph of acute *T. pallidum* placentitis; villi are bulky, immature-appearing and edematous (photomicrograph contributed by Robert Bendon, MD, Kosair Children's Hospital, Louisville, KY). (d) High-power photomicrograph of edematous villus and (e) acute villitis and intervillositis in syphilitic placentitis (contributed by Faisal Qureshi, MD, Hutzel Hospital, Detroit, MI). (f) Positive Warthin–Starry staining of spirochetes in the umbilical vein and Wharton's jelly of the cord

The pathophysiologic mechanisms of *T. pallidum* infection are incompletely understood. However, it is a vasotropic organism, and it attaches to and invades or crosses endothelial cells and activates them[286], initiates an inflammatory cascade that results in edema and neutrophilic perivasculitis, subsequent lymphohistiocytic vasculitis, and thrombotic sequelae, and, eventually, a marked lymphoplasmacytic perivasculitis[107,287,288]. Thrombi can be seen in the umbilical, chorionic plate and stem villous vessels. Their occurrence likely contributes to the intrauterine fetal growth restriction and newborn anemia often associated with congenital syphilis. Notably, Sheffield and colleagues[107] found that placental erythroblastosis was almost exclusively restricted to their cases of stillbirth, and proposed that their findings and similar ones by Young and Crocker[289] suggested that fetal anemia (and/or chronic hypoxia) was an important factor in causing fetal demise in syphilitic infection. The confirmatory detection of spirochetes by Warthin–Starry or Steiner silver stains in placentas exhibiting the triad or two-thirds of the triad listed above can most easily be accomplished on sections of umbilical cord, because of the relative hypocellularity of Wharton's jelly (Figure 62f)[290]. Use of the more sensitive methodology of polymerase chain reaction (PCR) for *T. pallidum*[291] has been limited largely by its cost and low availability.

Mycobacterial infection

Placentitis due to *Mycobacterium tuberculosis* is rare in developed countries, and review of the past dozen years of the English literature on the subject revealed only two instances of perinatal tuberculosis[292] and no cases of stillbirth, despite the significant (30%) neonatal mortality associated with perinatal tuberculosis. Moreover, prenatal detection of tuberculosis in the mother is aggressively treated, reducing the chance of transplacental transmission to the fetoplacental unit[293]. However, hematogenous spread of organisms in *M. tuberculosis* has been well documented, and is found to result in scattered miliary tubercles in the placenta. Classic descriptions and illustrations of past decades have included the finding of granulomatous foci with central and sometimes confluent necrosis and granulomatous or non-specific chronic deciduitis[3]. Nevertheless, intensive search may be required before a necrotizing granuloma is found in chorionic villous or in decidual tissues or acid-fast organisms identified within intervillous fibrinoid. (Benirschke and Kaufmann[4] report that some 2000 sections were required to document placental infection, in one study in their literature review, of congenital tuberculosis!) Therefore, given the potential rarity of granulomatous lesions in intrauterine tuberculous infection, it is possible that some cases of perinatal tuberculosis in infants with a negative placental examination and no known postnatal conditions of exposure have actually been undocumented cases of intrauterine infection; the negative placental examination may have simply reflected practical considerations in placental sampling, histologic levels, and staining for acid-fast bacteria. However, Machin and colleagues[292] postulated that their two cases of perinatal tuberculosis may have resulted from an ascending infection from maternal genital tubercles.

There is a single documentation of chorionic villous granuloma formation with *M. leprae*, or Hansen's disease, in the literature[4]. A careful light and electron microscopic study of 81 placentas delivered of women with Hansen's disease during gestation revealed no granulomas; although a few placental homogenates from women with active leprosy did contain organisms, there was no placental histopathology. The placentas, particularly those delivered of women with lepromatous leprosy, were small, as were the infants[294].

Mycoplasma and Chlamydia

Mycoplasma hominis and *Ureplasma urealyticum* are primarily associated with ascending infection and acute chorioamnionitis. Horne and colleagues[295] described a granulomatous endometritis and chronic villitis, with a pattern similar to what is now referred to as 'villitis of unknown etiology' (VUE) (see below), with *Mycoplasma* infection. Dische and associates[296] described two cases of acute villitis with focal loss of trophoblast, with *Mycoplasma* infection, but, in retrospect, it is unclear whether these may have represented sequelae of co-infection with another organism, since the observation has not again been reported and studies of potential causes of VUE have not demonstrated a link with *Mycoplasma* infection. *M. hominis, U. urealyticum* and *Chlamydia trachomatis* are fastidious organisms and pathogens in bacterial vaginosis, a condition in which the normal vaginal flora of lactobacilli is replaced by other bacteria and associated with increased risk of preterm birth and intrauterine infection (see Chapter 12, section on 'Acute chorioamnionitis'). *C. trachomatis*, the pathogen in neonatal conjunctivitis, is likely implicated in some cases of acute chorioamnionitis, but has not been identified with chorionic villitis. In contrast, *C. psittaci*, although rarely a pathogen of human intrauterine infection and abortion, may cause marked acute villitis and necrosis, with organisms seen within syncytiotrophs. The organism is associated with spontaneous abortion in domestic livestock, and infections occur in pregnant women who become exposed to the pathogen while assisting in the deliveries of infected animals such as sheep, pigs, and other large animals[4].

Viral villitis

Cytomegalovirus

This is the most common viral etiology of perinatal infection and villitis; congenital infection affects 0.5–2% of neonates and reflects vertical maternofetal transmission. In a primary maternal infection during gestation, maternal humoral immunity is produced, but it is not effective in preventing viral shedding, and cell-mediated immunity is required for recovery. The normal state of reduced cell-mediated immune surveillance of the fetoplacental unit is thought to explain its susceptibility to, and the sequelae of, CMV infection; about 40 000 infected infants are born annually in the USA. CMV is a ubiquitous virus most often spread by respiratory droplet transmission, and, primarily because of aerosolization and close contact with other infected individuals, most people become infected by toddlerhood. Rates of serologic evidence of prior infection vary with socioeconomic background; about 45% of pregnant women from higher-income groups and 15% of pregnant women from lower-income groups are susceptible. Horizontal spread from child to parent or between adults can occur during pregnancy and is the basis of primary infection; 1–4% of pregnant women seroconvert during gestation. The risk of vertical transmission in primary infection is 40%. As a result, about 10–15% of newborns with congenital CMV have mild to severe disease that is further linked to a 90% risk of development of sequelae. Sequelae include significant mental retardation and hearing deficits, particularly if the infants are born prematurely. The remaining 85–90% of asymptomatic, but infected newborns have a 5–15% risk of developing sequelae, which are primarily neurological. Of special importance to pathologists is the fact that, in CMV, prior infection does not confer absolute immunity, and that, overall, most cases of congenital CMV are due to recurrent maternal infection that is both asymptomatic in the mother and in the newborn. Maternal immunity is associated with a 0.15–1% risk of vertical transmission of CMV; infected infants, while asymptomatic, have a 1% risk for developing sensorineural hearing loss[33]. Thus, because: recurrent CMV is more common than primary CMV infection during gestation; recurrent CMV is usually asymptomatic in the mother; infants born to mothers with recurrent infection are asymptomatic at birth; and congenital CMV is an important cause of unexplained sensorineural hearing deficits in children, examination of the placenta emerges as a critical means of detection of congenital CMV infection.

CMV placentitis usually results in a boggy, pale, hydropic-appearing placenta, and delivery may be complicated by placental abruption (Figure 63a). However, chronic infections, and those with associated stillbirth, may result in a normal-weight to shrunken, firm, pale, and/or fibrotic mass. Histologically, a spectrum of proliferative and reparative villitis can be seen in CMV placentitis, as well as mononuclear intervillositis. Most cases exhibit chronic villitis and some features of reparative villitis (Figure 63b–d). CMV villitis is characterized by lymphohistiocytic and especially lympho*plasma*cytic inflammation. Plasma cell infiltrate, while not specific for CMV, is highly suggestive of it, even if viral inclusions are inapparent. The authors regard it useful to consider lymphoplasmacytic villitis as due to CMV, until proven otherwise, especially if plasma cells are seen in terminal villi that are not in contiguity with the basal plate. CMV inclusions are usually easily identified in deliveries of infants with clinically apparent disease. The typical eosinophilic and cytoplasmic inclusions are seen in endothelial and Hofbauer cells of the chorionic villi (Figure 63d and e). Other very helpful features that distinguish CMV villitis include bulky dysmature-appearing villi with stromal hemosiderin deposition and fibrosis (Figure 63f), thrombosis, and dystrophic mineralization. CMV infection of endothelial cells likely explains the presence of hemosiderin and thrombosis. Chronic infections may show relatively greater amounts of hemosiderosis. With chronic intrauterine infections, however, inclusions can be *very* difficult to find owing to their reduced numbers or obscuration by intravillous calcifications. The calcifications may represent mineralized 'tombstones' of infected cells and damage in infected villi (Figure 63f). Careful review of multiple sections may be required to identify the presence of CMV inclusions. In such instances, the use of CMV immunoperoxidase stains (Figure 63g) is especially recommended to identify or confirm the presence of CMV in cases with suspicious-appearing histopathology[4,297–299]. The use of PCR for CMV early and late gene antigen gp 64 has been reported[300]. (CMV cultures are usually precluded, as placental specimens are often received in formalin.)

Parvovirus B19

Parvovirus B19 (PVB19) infection of the fetus is an important cause of non-immune hydrops fetalis (NIHF). The incidence of maternal infection during pregnancy, as determined by IgM seroconversion, is 1–5%[301]. Maternal infection may be asymptomatic, but it is usually manifested by skin rash, arthralgia, upper respiratory symptoms, and malaise, and the risk of vertical transmission of PVB19 with primary infection in an IgG-seronegative woman is between 20 and 33%[302,303]. Fortunately, most women of child-bearing age are immune (50–70%)[304]. The severity of resultant fetal infection varies from mild progression to full-blown hydrops (5–10% of cases). However, it is usually self-limited, and even hydrops can spontaneously resolve in up to 33% of cases[33,302]. Fetal susceptibility to infection ranges from high, during the first trimester, to minimal after 20 weeks of gestation; the secondary appearance of hydrops is most common between 20 and 28 weeks, as is the corresponding risk of fetal death[302,303]. In the series reported by Rogers and colleagues[303], PVB19 accounted for 17% of their autopsy cases of NIHF. However, weekly sonographic monitoring with conservative management and/or a single intrauterine transfusion can result in the resolution of fetal hydrops[33,305]. Placental examination is of crucial importance for the diagnosis of fetal infection (see below).

PVB19 infects cells with the P blood group antigen globoside. Many cells express this molecule, but most important among these, for the fetoplacental unit, are erythrocytes, megakaryocytes, cardiac myocytes, and villous trophoblasts. First-trimester villous trophoblasts exhibit strong and abundant expression, whereas diminished to minimal expression is seen in the second- and third-trimester placenta, respectively[306]. The loss of expression with villous maturation likely explains the observation that first- and early second-trimester infections are associated with the greatest risks of fetal morbidity and mortality. In addition, PVB19 infection is associated with an increased rate of apoptosis in the villous trophoblast[279], and cellular infectivity likely also requires the presence of a co-receptor[307] (which may explain why some cells with the globoside escape PVB19 infection). With infection of the trophoblast, the virus crosses the placental barrier[306], and can thereby infect the rapidly expanding fetal erythropoietic compartment, which, in turn, can lead to severe fetal anemia due to erythrolysis, and in combination with hepatic necrosis, siderosis, and fibrosis, reduced plasma oncotic pressure, and congestive heart failure[308–310]. Fetal myocarditis and cardiac dysfunction

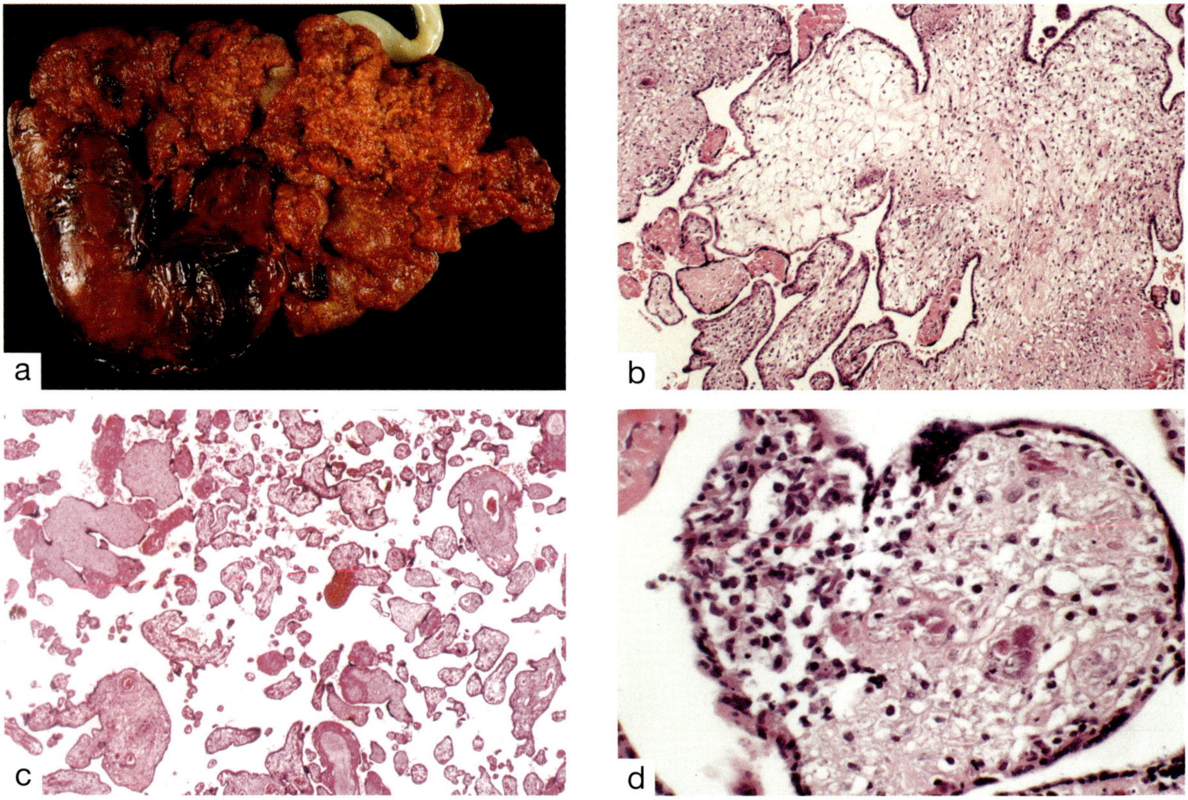

Figure 63 Cytomegalovirus (CMV) placentitis. (a) Maternal presentation of placental abruption led to rapid delivery of this case at 34 weeks of gestation. The infant was stillborn. The placenta is enlarged and boggy, likely contributing to the abruption; an acute retoplacental hematoma is present. (b and c) Examples of the histopathologic spectrum of CMV placentitis. (b) Proliferative lymphohistiocytic/lymphoplasmacytic villitis with bulky dysmature, villous edema, and CMV inclusions (central villi), as well as sclerosis of some villi (central left). (c) More chronic CMV villitis with definitive sclerosis of many villi. (d) Lymphohistiocytic villitis with CMV inclusions. (e) CMV villitis in placenta from preterm birth. (f) Sclerotic villus with hemosiderosis, 'tombstone calcifications' and CMV inclusions, and chronic villitis, from case of chronic CMV placentitis confirmed by immunoperoxidase stain for CMV. (g) Positive immunoperoxidase staining for CMV in nuclei of villous stromal Hofbauer cells

likely also contribute to the morbidity and mortality of PVB19.

Depending upon the gestational stage of onset, chronicity, and severity of infection, the placenta and cord may be markedly to mildly hydropic. The diagnostic feature of PVB19 is the presence of pale eosinophilic to lilac-colored intranuclear inclusions with chromatin margination in circulating abnormal giant pronormoblasts within the fetal vessels of the placenta (Figure 64a and b). While formalin fixation and hematoxylin–eosin stain do not clearly distinguish the basophilic normoblast stage of erythropoiesis, this stage is the last to undergo mitosis in erythrogenesis, and thereby enables replication of this single-stranded DNA virus. The normally greater nuclear size of this stage of the normoblast is exaggerated by PVB19 infection, inclusion formation, and maturational arrest, and while less differentiated stages are also infected, this stage is most easily seen microscopically. Newly infected cells will show single, tiny, dark, round central inclusions, but these can be difficult to detect[311]. Later non-lysed stages of infected normoblasts may also show eosinophilic inclusions and margination of their chromatin. Villitis is minimal, but chorionic villi are edematous, with prominent Hofbauer cells, and, on

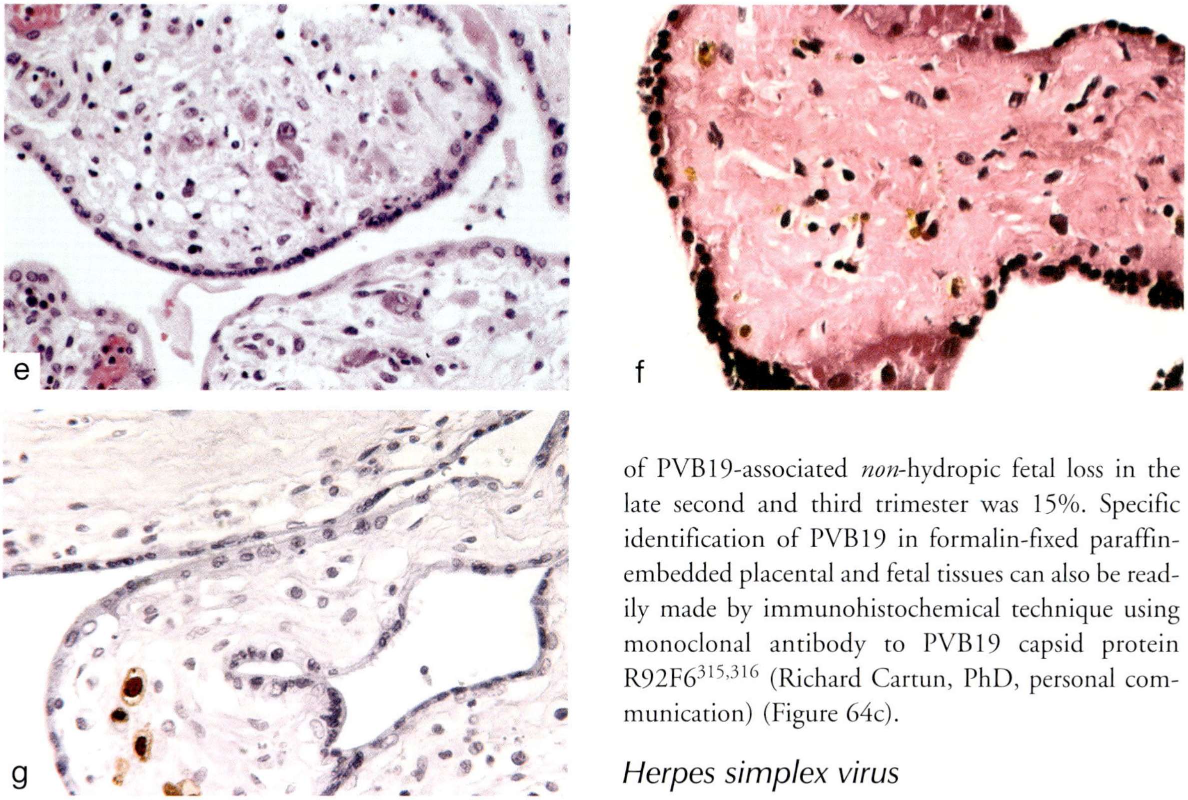

Figure 63 *Continued*

low-power view, erythroblastosis is usually striking. In placentas from gestations of resolving or resolved hydrops and live-born infants, the numbers of infected cells may be so low as to be histologically undetectable. Thus, a negative placental examination does not necessarily exclude PVB19 infection, and fetal normoblastemia (increased numbers of circulating nucleated orthochromic normoblasts) may be the only clue to its presence. Histologic and cytologic detection of PVB19 has been enhanced by *in situ* hybridization, electron microscopy, and polymerase chain reaction amplification (PCR)[312,313]. PCR is also particularly recommended for autopsy cases for which there is a high index of suspicion of PVB19 infection and inclusions are not evident[310,313]. It is also helpful in cases of fetal demise compromised by maceration. Of interest is that Tolfvenstam and colleagues[314] found that, by using PCR, the frequency of PVB19-associated *non*-hydropic fetal loss in the late second and third trimester was 15%. Specific identification of PVB19 in formalin-fixed paraffin-embedded placental and fetal tissues can also be readily made by immunohistochemical technique using monoclonal antibody to PVB19 capsid protein R92F6[315,316] (Richard Cartun, PhD, personal communication) (Figure 64c).

Herpes simplex virus

About 95% of intrauterine herpes simplex virus (HSV) infections represent acute ascending infections from the maternal genital tract, and most occur with intact membranes. *Hematogenous* spread of HSV probably results from marked maternal viremia. Ascending infections typically produce acute chorioamnionitis with amniotic necrosis and multinucleated giant cell cytopathy, with inclusions visible within amniocytes of the free membranes and fetal plate, and also of the umbilical cord. With time, chronic lymphoplasmacytic chorionitis, funisitis, and deciduitis may develop. Plasma cell-filled blisters may be seen on the amniotic surface and in great numbers in the subchorionic space[4]. In both the acute and the more chronic case of ascending infection, identification of suspected HSV inclusions can be confirmed by specific immunoperoxidase stain. In the uncommon instance of hematogenous transmission, scattered villous trophoblastic and stromal necrosis is seen, but there is generally a remarkable paucity to absence of an inflammatory reaction. Grossly, such lesions may be detectable as punctate

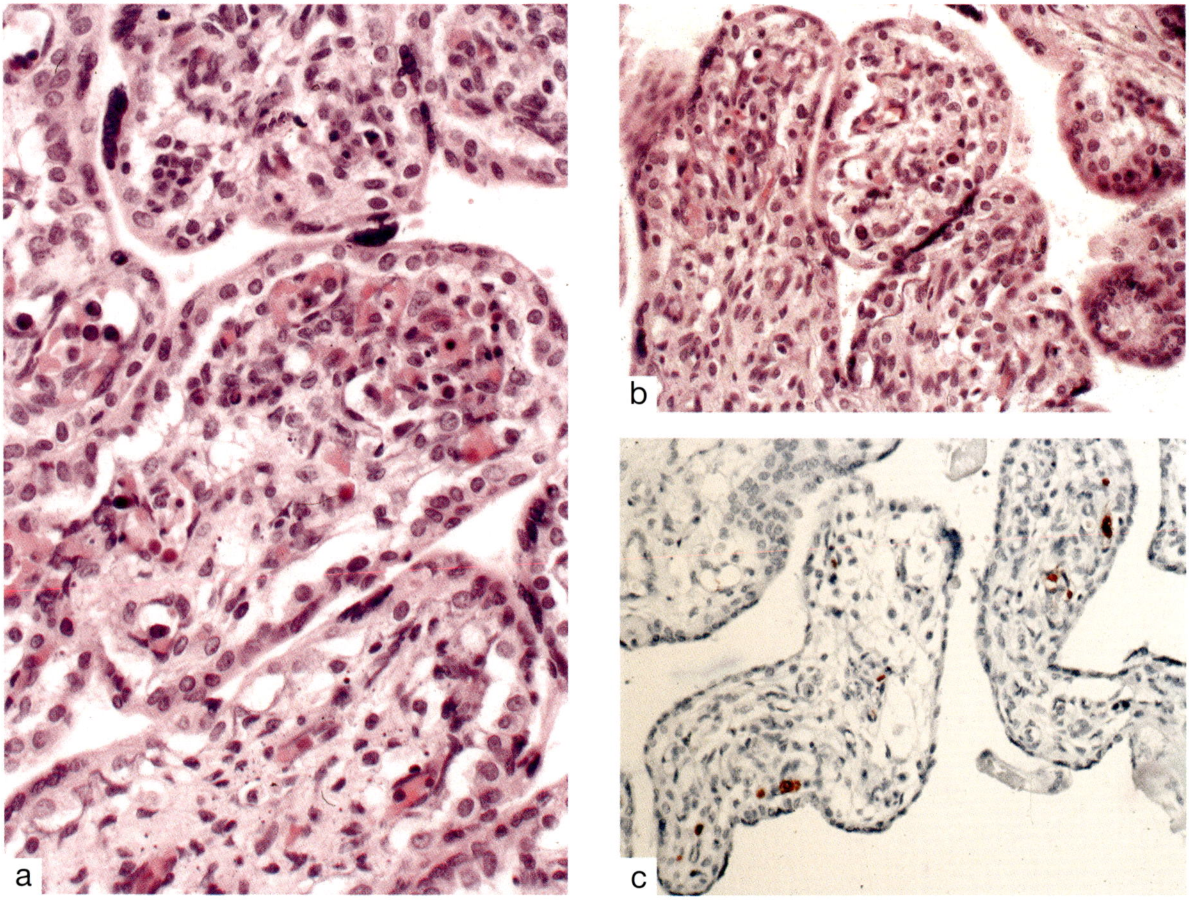

Figure 64 Parvovirus B19 (PVB19) infection. (a and b) Villous edema and erythroblastosis are present, the latter due to the viral proliferation within, and lysis of, immature fetal red cells. Several giant basophilic normoblasts are seen in the capillaries in the villus at the left margin of the photomicrograph, and many nucleated immature forms are seen in the villus at its right and in others. The inclusions of PVB19 are detectable as the abnormal, enlarged basophilic normoblast nuclei and as the reddish-purple inclusions in the nuclei of other red cells in the field. Higher-power photomicrograph shows several PVB19 inclusions in giant pronormoblasts (the size of a normal nucleated erythrocyte can be seen in the upper left of the field for comparison). Their coloration is variable on hematoxylin–eosin stain; inclusions with margination can appear darker as in the center of this field, or have the classic lighter glassy appearance. (c) PVB19 identified in fetal erythrocytes by immunoperoxidase stain using antibody against PVB19 capsid protein R92F6 (x200). (Courtesy of Richard Cartun, PhD)

foci of yellow-white necrosis if careful inspection of the placental cut surface is performed and/or a magnifying hand lens used; thus, the lesions resemble those of *Listeria* and syphilitic placentitis (see below). Microscopically, typical glassy intranuclear inclusions may be identifiable within trophoblasts, but immunoperoxidase stains are again useful adjuncts in these cases[4,126,298,317]. The umbilical cord may show HSV inclusions or positive immunoperoxidase staining in subamniotic mesenchymal cells[318] and necrotizing funisitis[319]. Chronic lymphoplasmacytic deciduitis has also been seen in transplacentally transmitted infection[320]. Schwartz and Caldwell[321] demonstrated a positive reaction for HSV in the decidual cells by using a DNA *in situ* hybridization technique. Of note is that coincident intrauterine HSV and CMV infection has also been reported[322].

In our experience, an accompanying history of maternal HSV infection is often lacking, and, in addition, the prepartum risk of ascending route of transmission may not always be appreciated. One of the authors (OF-P) has seen a case of HSV-caused intrauterine fetal demise at 33 weeks of gestation, for which a history of maternal genital infection had been documented early in the second trimester. The woman had been told that her fetus was not at risk, because HSV infection of the infant was due to passage through an infected birth canal. HSV placentitis in this case included histopathologic evidence of both ascending and hematogenously spread infection with HSV-positive cells in the amnion and in the villi (Figure 65); the latter may have represented sequelae of coincident or subsequent viremia.

Rubella

The incidence of congenital rubella syndrome (CRS), characterized by IUGR, microcephaly, microphthalmia and cataracts, deafness, cardiac defects, jaundice and hepatosplenomegaly, thrombocytopenia and anemia, interstitial pneumonitis, meningoencephalitis, and osseous changes[33,323], in the USA, is extremely low, at 0.01–0.08 per 10 000 live births[323], due to the rarity of maternal rubella infection during pregnancy. The latter is attributable to well-established immunization programs. However, many developed countries, including the USA[323,324], have documented regional increased rates of rubella infection and/or CRS due to an influx of seronegative and unvaccinated immigrants from developing nations[325–330]. Depending upon the geographic location, some 6–25% of women of child-bearing age in the USA have been estimated to be seronegative[331] and thereby at risk for contracting rubella during pregnancy. Therefore, the pathologist should consider rubella as a possible cause of chorionic villitis in patients belonging to increased-risk groups. The risk of CRS is about 100% if maternal infection occurs in the first trimester, but declines to 35% or less with infection between 13 and 16 weeks, and progressively attenuates thereafter as gestation proceeds[33]. Vaccination just prior to or during pregnancy is avoided, since the vaccine incorporates attenuated live virus, but it has not been found to affect pregnancy outcome or cause CRS in most studies[332].

Placental pathology of rubella shows some correlation with chronicity of maternal infection. More recent infection is associated with focal necrotizing villitis with endarteritis of the villous vessels; focal trophoblastic necrosis with or without neutrophilic infiltrate; and perivillous fibrinoid deposition. Eosinophilic inclusions may be present in the villous endothelial cells or trophoblast, and Hofbauer cell numbers may be increased[3,333], but these changes are not specific, nor present in all cases. Chronic changes include villous avascularity and sclerosis. Placentas from cases of periconceptional or gestational vaccination have historically not shown villous lesions, but decidual changes have been described[4].

Varicella

Primary maternal varicella infection during pregnancy, which is currently uncommon, will decline further with the vaccination programs established in recent years. The low numbers of affected pregnancies generally continue to term, without fetal/neonatal sequelae[4,33], but in some cases sequelae for the mother and fetus can be serious. Between 10%[334] and 33%[335] of pregnant women develop pneumonitis, and about 2% of these require ventilator support[334]. Congenital varicella infection (CVI), characterized by skin scarring and defects, segmental limb hypoplasia, cerebral cortical atrophy, hydronephrosis, chorioretinitis, and cataract formation can also result in neonatal death[336]. Rates of fetal or neonatal infection and death are related to the timing and severity of maternal infection; transplacental transmission rates of 83%, and 21% neonatal mortality rates, have been reported with maternal pneumonitis[4], whereas Enders and colleagues[336], found only a 0.6% overall rate of CVI. Infections occurring between 13 and 20 weeks of gestation are associated with the greatest risks of CVI (1.4%[337]–2%[336]. First-trimester infections are associated with spontaneous abortion (7.5%)[4] and CVI (0.4%)[336]). However, maternal infection after 20 weeks of gestation is rarely associated with fetal disease[335,338] unless the mother acquires acute infection just prior to delivery, with insufficient time to generate an antibody response; in these instances, the infant is at high risk for varicella

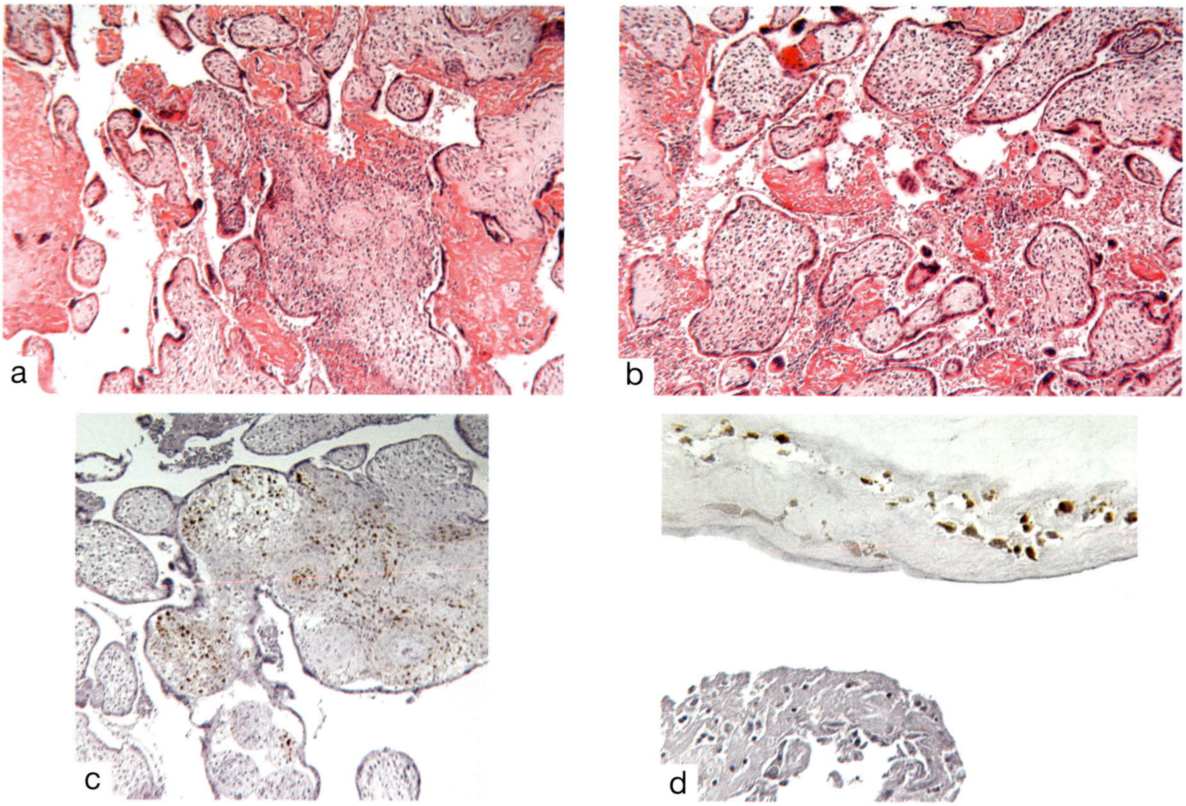

Figure 65 Herpes simplex virus (HSV) placentitis. (a and b) HSV chronic villitis with foci of necrosis and intervillositis and perivillous fibrinoid deposition. (c) Positive chorionic villous immunoperoxidase staining for HSV in this case. (d) Hematoxylin–eosin stains showed these HSV-immunopositive stained cells to be glassy and occasionally multinucleated, amniotic squamous cells incorporated into the basement membrane of the amnion. No non-specific staining is seen in the necrotic cells in the lower aspect of the field

infection, and disseminated visceral and central nervous system (CNS) disease.

Placental examination from gestations complicated by clinically diagnosed maternal varicella is often unrevealing. Very rarely, maternal varicella pneumonia may result in grossly detectable placental pathology: necrotic yellow punctate foci may be seen on the fetal surface and within the parenchyma; moreover, in these instances, the gross differential diagnosis includes *Listeria*, syphilis and herpes virus placentitis, so the finding is not specific. In the study by Qureshi and Jacques[335], only one placenta, from the delivery of an infant with clinically suspected congenital varicella, of the 19 available for review demonstrated extensive basal chronic villitis, and only two additional cases showed rare foci of chronic villitis; most of their studied cases showed no virus-associated histopathology. Microscopic examination, particularly of grossly necrotic or whitish foci, may reveal necrotizing granulomas with neutrophilic infiltration, and may include sites of giant cell transformation and deposition of intervillous necrobiotic debris (Figure 66). Milder forms of chronic inflammation may be seen, including chronic lymphohistiocytic villitis and villous thrombosis and atrophy. These milder findings are similar to those seen in villitis of unknown etiology (VUE) addressed below. Plasma cells may rarely be identified and chorioamnionitis may be present as well. Usually, however, there are no viral inclusions in the placental tissue, although inclusions were present in the decidual cells in the cases described by Garcia[339]. PCR and immunohistochemical stains

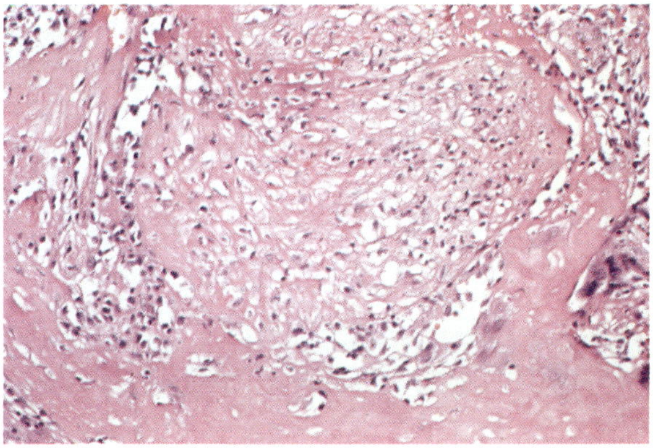

Figure 66 Granulomatous villitis due to varicella. Reprinted with permission from reference 335

for varicella antigen may be warranted to distinguish varicella placentitis from VUE[335]. A history of clinical suspicion is key to the likelihood of finding viral pathogens such as varicella (or non-viral pathogens, such as *Toxoplasma*, see below)[4].

Hepatitis

Vertical transmission of hepatitis A is rare, since viremia is of short duration, and while fetal infection may be manifested as ascites and meconium peritonitis, no placental pathology has been described for hepatitis A, or C or G. Hepatitis B, for which the carrier rate is high, is potentially a significant pathogen, but transplacental transmission is also uncommon, and infants have had upper-gastrointestinal ulcerations suggestive of enteral infection due to ingestion of virally infected amniotic fluid. The few correlative placental studies have shown prominent bilirubin staining of and entrapment by Hofbauer cells and focal synctiotrophoblast staining and necrosis, reflecting maternal hyperbilirubinemia, but no villitis or other diagnostic histopathology. This absence of inflammation is interesting given that immunohistochemical stains for hepatitis B surface antigen and hepatitis C core antigen have yielded widespread staining of trophoblast, Hofbauer, and villous capillary endothelial cells. The greatest risk of transmission to the infant occurs at delivery due to enteric contamination by maternal fluids[4].

Coxsackie and ECHO viruses

While these viruses are common infectious agents with serious sequelae in the neonatal period, infection during gestation has generally been observed to be of little to no consequence to the fetus. However, there are reports of transplacental infection with both Coxsackie and/or ECHO (enteric cytopathogenic human orphan) viruses, with fetal loss and fetal hydrops and myocarditis[3,4,340], and virus has been isolated from the placenta in some of these cases[341]. The placentas, when examined, have shown no pathology to dense perivillous fibrinoid deposition similar to that seen in maternal floor infarction/ massive perivillous fibrinoid deposition (see above section in this chapter) and villous necrosis[342], or chronic villitis and intervillositis similar to VUE (see below)[343]. Recently, Nuovo and colleagues[344,345] have found striking incidences of enteroviral/ Coxsackie viral staining in trophoblasts and Hofbauer cells by use of immunoperoxidase methods in placentas from cases of perinatal death, or from deliveries of infants with neonatal idiopathic respiratory distress or CNS dysfunction. The placental histopathology was non-specific, but they concluded that immunocytochemical detection of Coxsackie virus in fetal and/or placental tissues from test cases, in the absence of its detection in controls, was evidence of intrauterine Coxsackie infection as the cause of these adverse outcomes. Their report is of particular concern because, of the 76% of their placentas that had immunohistochemical and/or histopathologic features of intrauterine infection, viruses were detected in 67.4% of the cases (bacteria in 32.6%), and nearly half of these (22/46 cases) were determined to be due to Coxsackie virus. These findings have significant implications if further investigations confirm these investigators' observations, especially in cases in which there are non-specific placental histopathologic features.

Villitis of unknown etiology

The presence of inflammatory infiltration of terminal villi can occur without any demonstrable infectious etiology. Altshuler[346] labeled this entity 'villitis of unknown etiology' (VUE), and it is a diagnosis of exclusion. VUE occurs in 5–10% of consecutively examined placentas[4], but incidences of up to 34% have been reported[347]. It is present in 3–18% of *term* placentas[348], but is less common in placentas from gestations of < 32 weeks in duration[250]. Its variable incidence likely reflects placental tissue sampling, since it is most often focal or patchy in its distribution. Also, its rate varies with the maternal–fetal/neonatal population studied; as noted below, it is more frequently identified in placentas from gestations complicated by intrauterine fetal demise or IUGR[349] and/or hypertension[350].

While there is no consistent association between the presence of VUE and low placental weight and/or pallor, placentas with VUE are often relatively pale and small. Occasionally, there may be parenchymal mottling, and, rarely, scattered, punctate, firm, white lesions may be grossly detectable (personal communication, R. Baergen, MD). Microscopically, VUE exhibits a broad histomorphologic spectrum[4,29,126], and essentially all of the patterns described under the classifications of villitis, above, have been seen. In addition it may be focal or diffuse in distribution, and range from mild to severe in inflammatory intensity[351,352]. Low-power scan is especially helpful in distinguishing VUE from other villitides, since VUE characteristically involves the basal and subchorial terminal villi (Figure 67a and b), and spares the stem villi and the middle parenchymal zone. Also, unless unusually diffuse, VUE usually involves less than about 5–10% of the villi[29], and the intervening villi are usually entirely unremarkable. Most commonly, VUE is characterized by a proliferative lymphocytic or lymphohistiocytic villitis (Figure 67c), and there may be some component of stromal destruction and/or villous necrosis and atrophy (Figure 67d). However, focal necrotizing, granulomatous, cicatrical, and/or reparative villitis have also been noted. Plasma cells are not seen, and a significant neutrophilic inflammatory component, stromal dystrophic mineralization, or fibrosis is unusual[4,29,126]; the presence of these, particularly of neutrophilic inflammation[29] or plasma cells and fibrosis, warrants exclusion of an infectious process (see above discussions of *Listeria*, syphilis, CMV, and HSV). Scattered collections of mononuclear cells may be present in the intervillous space, and occasional perivillous fibrinoid deposition and villous agglutination may be seen. The decidua basalis typically shows chronic non-specific deciduitis, with or without necrosis[3,4]; plasma cells are found in a third of cases[29]. Associated chronic chorioamnionitis was commonly associated with VUE in the studies by Gersell[249] and Jacques and Qureshi[353], although Redline[29] has found it unusual. Funisitis, however, is not seen. Finally, degenerative changes localized to the vicinity of an infarct may resemble VUE, but such changes should be not be confused with VUE.

VUE has been associated with poor pregnancy outcome and IUGR in a number of studies[126,349,351,352,354–357]. It also has been found to have a high risk of recurrence (~ 10–25%)[351,358], as well as a risk of pregnancy loss, in instances of recurrent VUE[358]; Redline and Abramowsky[358] found a 17% recurrence risk of VUE and a 60% rate of reproductive loss in their cohort of patients with recurrent villitis. Chronic villitis/VUE may also be responsible for discordant growth in dichorionic twins[353,358–360]. However, it has long been appreciated that the severity of the villitis in VUE and/or its pattern of distribution are not fully predictive of the association or severity of IUGR seen with VUE[4]. In some cases, absolute reduction in villous tissue appeared to be a potential explanation, but IUGR was also seen in cases with minimal VUE. Sampling and/or coexistent placental ischemia appeared at least partly to explain these cases of IUGR and intrauterine fetal demise[349,350]. The extent of histologic sampling of the placenta will also affect the frequency of diagnosis of VUE, and Khong and colleagues[361] have reported a lack of interobserver concordance among experienced pathologists. However, studies have indicated that some histomorphologic patterns are more predictive of fetal morbidity and mortality. Labarrere and Mullen[362] noted that VUE with fibrinoid and trophoblastic necrosis and striking massive chronic intervillositis (largely monocytes and some lymphocytes) was highly associated with IUGR, but some of their cases also showed decidual atherosis; they

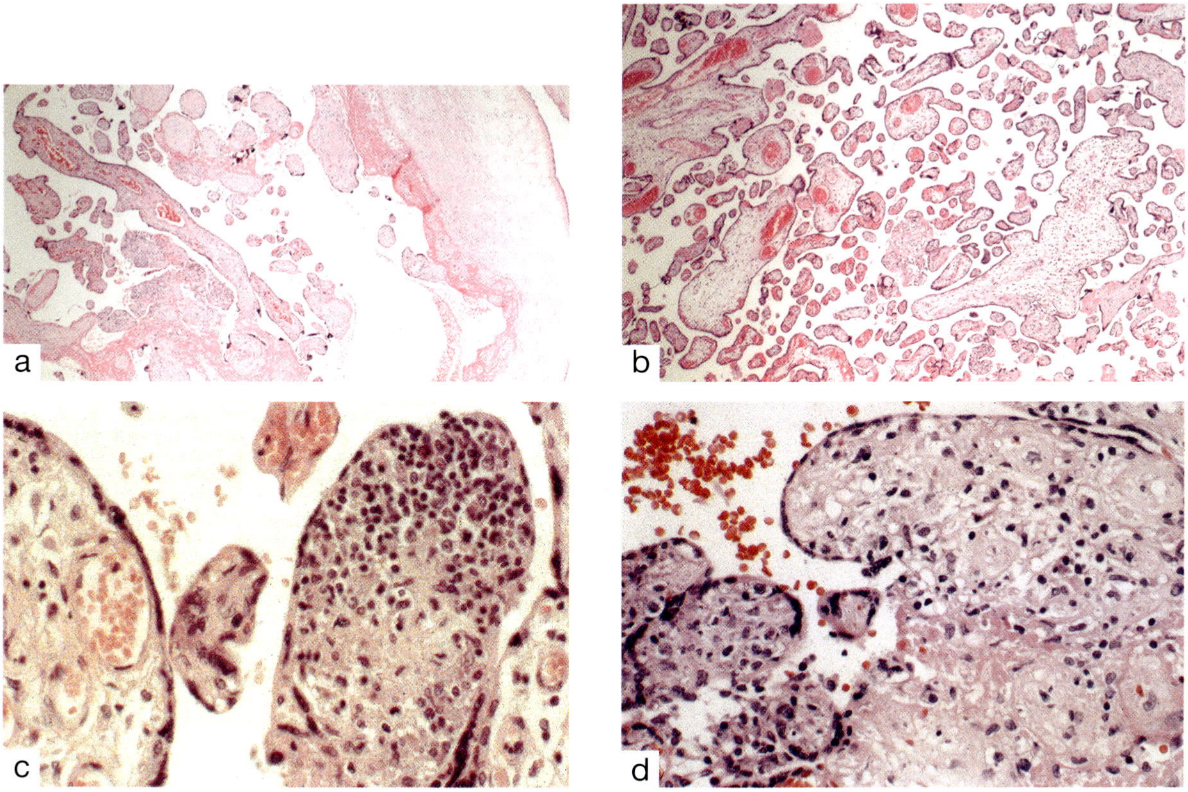

Figure 67 Villitis of unknown etiology (VUE). (a) VUE characteristically involves scattered subchorial and basal terminal villi, sparing stem villi and usually mid-zonal parenchymal viili. (b) The patchy distribution of VUE is best appreciated at low power. In this photomicrograph, it affects a few terminal villi in the center and upper right field. (c) Proliferative VUE characterized by lymphohistiocytic infiltrate. (d) VUE with stromal destruction, necrosis, and villous atrophy

termed this form of VUE an 'extreme variant'. Redline[29] has noted that when 'focal VUE' (focal defined as VUE involving < 5% of the villi) is limited to a few clusters of villi on a single slide of the placental parenchyma and/or to the basal villi (focal and basal villitis, respectively), risks of IUGR, chronic fetal monitoring abnormalities, and cerebral palsy are not increased. However, diffuse, severe VUE (generally < 50% involvement with intervening areas of normal villi) is often accompanied by significant intervillous fibrinoid deposition and is associated with increased rates of preterm delivery, IUGR, intrauterine fetal demise, and recurrent pregnancy loss. The extensive fibrinoid deposition presumably interferes with adequate transport of nutrients across the trophoblast. In unpublished studies, he has observed that, in addition to diffuse, severe VUE, VUE with primary and secondary stem villous vasculitis (which can lead to FTV) (see Chapter 9, section on 'Fetal thrombotic vasculopathy') is also associated with increased risks for cerebral palsy in term infants.

There is mounting evidence that VUE is an immunologically mediated process suggestive of host versus graft response. The inflammatory infiltrate in VUE has been characterized, by immunohistochemical stains, to consist largely of macrophages (CD68 positivity) with few T-cell lymphocytes (CD3/CD4 positivity)[347,349,363,364]; B cell differentiation, natural killer cells, and esosinophils have not been found. T cells constitute the infiltrate in chronic chorionitis, as well[353]. Intravillous T-lymphocytes have been determined to be of maternal origin using *in situ* hybridization with X and Y chromosome-specific probes and immunostaining for CD3 and CD45 on

VUE placentas from male infants[349]. Labarrere and Faulk[365] also found that the majority of intravillous mononuclear cells were of maternal origin, in their study using double-antibody immunohistochemical staining for human leukocyte antigen (HLA)-D and HLA-DRw 52 in placentas with maternal–fetal mismatch. The early findings by Labarrere and Mullen[362] were also highly suggestive of an intense immunologic response, and Doss and colleagues[348] have noted that the histopathologic similarities of the maternal inflammatory cells in VUE and marked chronic intervillositis (see below) suggest that a similar immunologic mechanism may underlie both processes. The vast majority of investigators have excluded an infectious etiology for VUE and favor immunologic host-versus-graft (allogenic rejection) process. Whether other mechanisms may be operative is unclear, but this apparent process of maternal rejection may also involve complement-fixing immune complex formation[363,366]; defective blocking factors[366]; cytotoxic antibodies directed against villous trophoblasts and lymphocytes in association with maternal antiphospholipid syndromes[367]; or increased avidity of blood monocytes for syncytial cells upon cytokine-mediated activation of surface intercellular adhesion molecule (ICAM) type 1[368].

Massive chronic intervillositis

As noted above, when VUE with fibrinoid is present, a marked chronic inflammatory infiltrate may also be present in the intervillous space[362]. It may be a result of ulceration of the trophoblastic lining, since VUE is associated with increased, unexplained MSAFP levels[4]. However, an inflammatory infiltrate in the intervillous space may also occur in the essential *absence* of villitis. The presence of striking and usually predominant mononuclear intervillositis is referred to as 'massive chronic intervillositis' (MCI)[348,369], and is characterized by diffusely dispersed intervillous aggregates of histiocytes (monocytes) amidst scattered lymphocytes and occasional neutrophils and increased perivillous fibrinoid deposition (Figure 68). It has been particularly associated with IUGR, fetal demise[369], and recurrent abortion[348]. As stated above, it may represent an extreme variant of VUE. Maternal conditions associated with MCI included pre-eclampsia, hypertension, substance abuse, systemic lupus erythematosus, and diabetes. The etiology of MCI is not known, but: the intervillous masses of monocytes (α-1-antichymotrypsin positive, lysozyme positive) and the overlap in the populations of these cells with those in VUE; the IUGR; the underlying presence of maternal autoimmune conditions in some cases; the high risk of recurrence; and the elevated MSAFP are compatible with the maternal host-versus-graft rejection process and a similar pathogenesis for VUE and MCI[348]. However, an inflammatory response to an infectious pathogen cannot be excluded[368]. As stated above, under infectious villitis, malaria has also been associated with intense intervillositis[370].

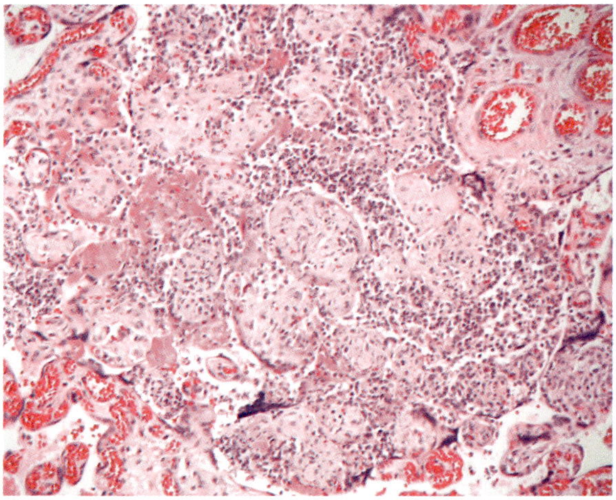

Figure 68 Massive chronic intervillositis. The intervillous space is heavily infiltrated by masses of lymphocytes and monocytes, with occasional neutrophils and increased perivillous fibrinoid deposition

Poliomyelitis, mumps, influenza, and parainfluenza viruses

While virus has been isolated from the placenta in some cases of maternal infections with these agents, the placentas have either not been described or placental lesions have not been identified[4].

Infectious mononucleosis

In abortions occurring in association with maternal infectious mononucleosis, villitis with lymphoplasmacytic infiltration, endothelial damage, and necrosis of trophoblasts, and deciduitis have been described[371]. It is not certain whether these lesions were related to Epstein–Barr virus.

Vaccinia and variola minor

These viral pathogens are included for completeness' sake, but since the eradication of smallpox, such infections have not been reported. Focal necrotizing villitis with neutrophilic inflammation and membranous necrosis have been described in vaccinia infection of the placenta, but since the 1960s these rare cases have occurred as complications of maternal vaccination during pregnancy[3,4]. Similarly, rare cases of necrotizing granulomatous villitis were reported with variola minor (a mild form of smallpox occurring previously in South America and western Africa).

Human immunodeficiency virus

Mother to child transmission (MTCT) Rates of MTCT of HIV in untreated women include intrauterine, intrapartum, and peripartum transmission, and vary from 14 to 48%[372]. With intensive use of antiviral therapy of the mother during pregnancy and labor, and of the newborn, in the USA, the transmission rate has been brought down from 22.6–25%[373,374] to 7.6%[373].

Timing of MTCT MTCT occurs chiefly in the intrapartum (15–25%)[33] and peripartum periods (40–80%)[375], with highest risks of peripartum transmission associated with preterm birth and prolonged membrane rupture[33]; breast-feeding is associated with 10–29% increased risk of MTCT[376,377]. Thus, intrauterine infection prior to the peripartum period is the least frequent mode of transmission. Mwanyumba and colleagues[378] found a 6.0% rate of transplacental infection, but even higher rates of 25–40% are indicative of the significant protective effect of the placental barrier[379].

Risk factors for MTCT High maternal viral load is the most important risk factor[378,380]; viral strain may also be a factor[378,381]. Chorioamnionitis has been an important factor identified in six[378,382–386] of seven clinicopathologic studies; Schwartz and colleagues[387] did not demonstrate an increased risk of perinatal HIV transmission with chorioamnionitis. Co-infection with bacterial, other sexually transmitted, CMV[378,379,388], or malarial pathogens[389,390] also increases the risk. Co-infection may contribute to the increased risks of MTCT associated with chorioamnionitis, but the presence of HIV-infected genital tract secretions and ascending infection may also be responsible[378,379]. It is interesting to note that although malaria with high-density parasitemia increases the risk, controlled malaria may be protective because it generates a generalized immune response[391].

Mechanism of MTCT The main mechanism is the direct intrapartum and peripartum exposure of the infant's skin and mucous membrane (with possible abrasions) to genital secretions and maternal blood containing HIV. Factors related to the low rate of intrauterine transplacental transmission and/or relative trophoblastic resistance to HIV include:

(1) Lack of class I HLA necessary for transfer of HIV from maternal lymhocytes[379];

(2) Lack of trophoblastic CD4 antigen in some investigators' studies;

(3) Low level of HIV chemokine co-receptors CCR5 and CXR4[277];

(4) Leukocyte inhibitory factor receptor expression up-regulation in infected trophoblasts that inhibits HIV replication[392];

(5) Increased rate of apoptosis[393];

(6) Low virion production in HIV-infected trophoblasts that appears to be related to the high rate of internalization of p24 within cytoplasmic endosomes[394].

The latter two observations suggest that the placenta may also act as a 'sink' for HIV, and prevent its transmission to the fetus. Furthermore, high circulating levels of β-hCG during pregnancy may inhibit viral replication[395]. Successful viral entry into the placenta has recently been linked to the HIV-presenting role of dendritic cell-specific binding lectins DC-SIGN and DC-SIGNR[377,396,397] and leukocyte-specific integrin LFA-1, which enhances T-cell lymphocyte-to-placenta adherence[277].

Placental pathology Placental changes in HIV are neither specific nor uniform. In a large number of cases the placenta is grossly and microscopically normal[4]. Chorioamnionitis occurs in 8–60% of cases[378,398]; low fetal : placental weight ratio[399] and coarse, cellular or hypovascular villi are non-specific findings[400]. Other placental findings include deciduitis, Hofbauer cell hyperplasia, villous edema and dysmaturity, chorangiosis, increased perivillous fibrin(oid) deposition[378,399], and funisitis[387]. Chorionic villitis is extremely rare[378].

Evidence of HIV in the placenta includes:

(1) Presence of retrovirus-like particles in the trophoblast on electron microscopy[400];

(2) Positive reaction for immunoperoxidase stain using antibody against HIV-p24[398,401] in the trophoblast and/or Hofbauer cells and endothelial cells[401] and for *in situ* hybridization[398];

(3) *In situ* PCR labeling for HIV in the trophoblast, Hofbauer cells, and endothelium[379,402].

The proportion of cases in which HIV can be demonstrated is variable among the different series, and a combination of techniques may increase sensitivity[395]. HIV seems to be present in the placentas of HIV-infected pregnant women more commonly than suggested by earlier results[379].

Fungal infection

The partial immunodepression during pregnancy potentially places the mother at increased risk for infectious agents requiring cell-mediated immunity. However, with the exception of candidal infections, most types of fungal infections are very uncommon in otherwise healthy women.

Candidal infection

These are essentially ascending infections, due to cervicovaginal candidiasis. Risk factors include oral contraceptive use, antibiotic therapy, maternal diabetes[4], cervical cerclage[403], and retained intrauterine contraceptive device[4,404–406]. The majority of infections are due to *Canidida albicans*, but *C. parasilosis* and, rarely, *C. tropicalis*, *C. glabrata*, and other species have been identified[4,407]. Acute chorioamnionitis and funisitis are the characteristic lesions seen in candidal infections[4]. As stated in Chapter 12, section on 'Acute chorioamnionitis', and in Chapter 11, punctate yellowish lesions of the cord, sites of subamniotic microabscesses, and necrotizing funisitis (NF) are often due to candidal infection. Candidal necrotizing funisitis is linked to gestationally dependent risks of perinatal mortality; the highest risks for fetal and neonatal demise are associated with extreme preterm delivery, and, while the infants are infected, there are minimal risks of mortality at term[406]. Fungal pseudohyphae are often difficult to identify on routine hematoxylin–eosin stain, and the use of silver stains, such as Gomori methenamine silver stain, is strongly recommended. However, if gross punctate yellow cord lesions or histologic subamniotic microabscesses typical of *Candida* species infection are identified on routine stains, the neonatologist (and/or obstetrician) should be notified immediately of the potential for this fungal infection. Delay of notification may compromise initiation of critical clinical evaluation, and the pathologist should not wait for receipt of confirmatory stains in this instance, since the mortality of NF is high in the preterm infant.

Villitis with candidal infection has only been reported twice. The case of abortion reported by Bittencourt and colleagues[404] was associated with a retained intrauterine contraceptive device, and the placenta showed strong evidence of maternal fungemia with focal chorionic villous necrosis, chronic villitis, intervillous abscesses, and umbilical venous fungal invasion. Rivasi and associates[408] found that one of their four cases of candidal infection showed chronic villitis, but there was no evidence of systemic maternal or fetal infection. They postulated that the villitis represented spread to the villous tree from chorioamnionitis.

Coccidioides immitis and *Paracoccidioides brasiliensis*

Approximately 80 cases of gestational coccidioidomycosis have been reported over the past 50 years, and the overwhelming majority of cases have shown the infection to be limited to the placenta and/or no evidence of neonatal infection. These observations are further evidence of the significance of the placental barrier. The placenta has typically shown multifocal necrotizing villitis with moderate to extensive perivillous fibrin(oid) deposition, a marked acute inflammatory response around spherules of *Coccidioides immitis*, patchy placental infarction, or tuberculoid granulomas[3,4,409]. The cases of neonatal infection for which the placenta was negative have suggested that intrapartum exposure may also play a role[4] in perinatal transmission.

There is a single case report of intrauterine *Paracoccidioides brasiliensis* infection[410] occurring in a woman who had received antifungal treatment, prior to pregnancy. The placenta showed numerous *P. brasiliensis* yeast forms in the intervillous space entrapped within a mononuclear infiltrate, and there was damage of the trophoblastic layer. The infant was preterm but not infected, and had antibodies to the organism.

Blastomyces dermatitidis

In their retrospective 20-year review of endemic blastomycosis, Lemos and colleagues[411] identified only three pregnancies complicated by *Blastomyces* with an additional 17 found on review of the literature. Eighteen babies were live-born and unaffected, but two had transplacental infection and were stillborn, one delivered of a woman with untreated blastomycosis. The placentas showed non-necrotizing granulomas and chronic villitis in the cases of transplacental infection, but no diagnostic changes in the remaining placentas.

Histoplasma capsulatum

Only four cases have been documented[412,413], attesting to its very rare occurrence during pregnancy, even in endemic areas. Only one documented case of transplacental transmission has been seen[413]. Placentas in three examinations showed no fungal elements or diagnostic pathology, including one from a case of maternal–fetal death in which the pregnancy was also complicated by maternal diabetes, and one from which the mother had meningoencephalitis[412]. In the fourth case, the placenta showed intracytoplasmic clusters of yeast morphologically consistent (by hematoxylin–eosin, Grocott modification of Grocott–Gomori methenamine silver, and periodic acid-Schiff stains) with *Histoplasma* in Hofbauer cells of the stem villi and trophoblast[413]. The live-born preterm infant from this gestation was infected, but was successfully treated, despite a 5-week delay in onset of therapy.

Mucor and *Zygomycetes*

A single case of Zygomycetes-like fungal infection of the placenta has been reported in the English literature[414]. Zygomycetes-like organisms were morphologically and incidentally diagnosed in this placenta; abundant hyphae were seen in the free and chorionic plate membranes and cord, but no inflammation, thrombosis, or necrosis was present.

Other fungal agents

Kida and colleagues[415] have described the presence of colonies of *Cryptococcus* species in the intervillous spaces in the placentas from a woman with autoimmune deficiency syndrome (AIDS), who died of disseminated cryptococcosis. Similar findings were seen in the placenta from a woman with systemic lupus erythematosus, who had been treated with steroids[416]. In neither case were there intravillous organisms or villitis. *Apergillus niger* has been reported to result in prominent granulomatous villitis and intervillous organisms[3] but no transplacental transmission. However, Klock and associates[417] found no placental or fetal pathology despite maternal death, in their case of disseminated aspergillosis.

Parasitic infection

Transplacental transmission of *Trypanosoma cruzi* infection (Chagas' disease occurring in South

America) has been described[418]. Placentas are frequently enlarged and hydropic. Large numbers of amastigotes are commonly seen in the Hofbauer cells and amniocytes. Chronic villitis with granulomatous reaction and fibrosis is present. The intervillous spaces show fibrin deposition and accumulations of mononuclear cells. Schistosomiasis occurring in the Far East and Africa can involve the placenta. Ova may be present in the villi and/or the intervillous spaces. An inflammatory reaction is usually absent. Congenital malaria has been described in tropical countries with endemic incidence of the infection, but transplacental transmission is surprisingly rare. Evidence of plasmodial organisms in the maternal RBCs in the intervillous space does not equate with fetal infection. The organisms can be demonstrated in the smears made from the placenta and in the maternal RBCs in the intervillous spaces, but fetal parasitemia has not been identified in the placenta (Figure 69). Lymphomononuclear infiltration of the villi may be present, but the characteristic features are large aggregates of macrophages and fibrin deposition in the intervillous space. Abundant malarial pigment (derived from breakdown of hemoglobin) is deposited in these macrophages, fibrin, and to some extent in the villous Hofbauer cells, and imparts a dark brown to black color to the placental cut surface[3]. Massive chronic intervillositis suggesting a strong maternal immune response and with near obliteration of the intervillous space by monocytes is an infrequent finding. However, it is more common in primiparous women with malaria, and is linked to poor fetal outcome and low birth weight[370]. The study by Sugiyama and co-workers[419] suggests that intercellular adhesion molecule-1 on monocytes in the intervillous space contributes to intervillous leukocyte infiltrations and sequestrations of parasitized erythrocytes in mononuclear and fibrin(oid) masses. Such sequestration from trophoblasts and villi may contribute to the low rate of transplacental malarial infection. Since plasmodia have not been demonstrated in the villi, it is not clear how the organisms spread across the placenta. It appears that fetal infection occurs via the transfer of maternal blood to the fetus – a phenomenon that is rare[4].

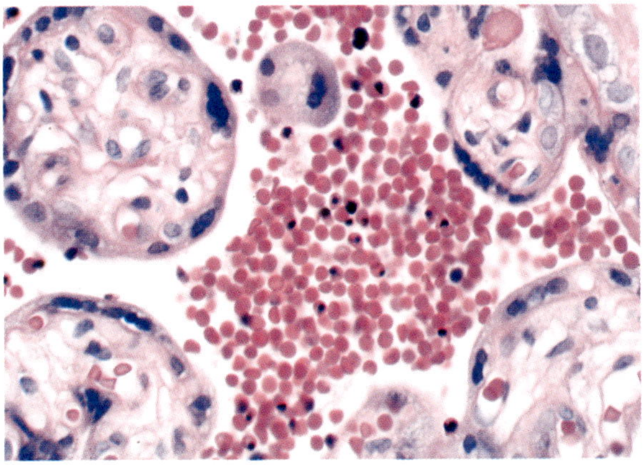

Figure 69 Malarial parasites in the maternal red blood cells (RBCs) in malaria. Note that there are no parasites in the fetal RBCs in the villous capillaries (hematoxylin–eosin, x400)

Toxoplasma gondii is the most important parasitic placental infection in Western countries. The placenta shows involvement of varying severity[420]. There may be mild lymphoplasmacytic infiltration of villi; granulomatous lesions characterized by foci of villous necrosis with mononuclear and giant cells; or necrotizing villitis with acute inflammatory reaction. The role of apoptosis is unclear, but it appears that infection slows the rate of apoptosis in the trophoblast[421]. Although both free and encysted forms of the organisms can be present, the latter are more common. Chronic NF in the absence of the features of candidal infection but with villitis should prompt rigorous search for the cysts. They can be identified in the chorionic villi (Figure 70), but are often more easily detected in the relatively acellular background of Wharton's jelly of the umbilical cord, appearing as isolated cysts, since they elicit little adjacent inflammatory response. Immunoperoxidase stains for *T. gondii* are highly useful in these settings.

NON-TROPHOBLASTIC TUMORS OF THE PLACENTA

Gestational trophoblastic diseases (partial and complete hydatidiform moles, invasive hydatidiform mole, choriocarcinoma, placental-site trophoblastic

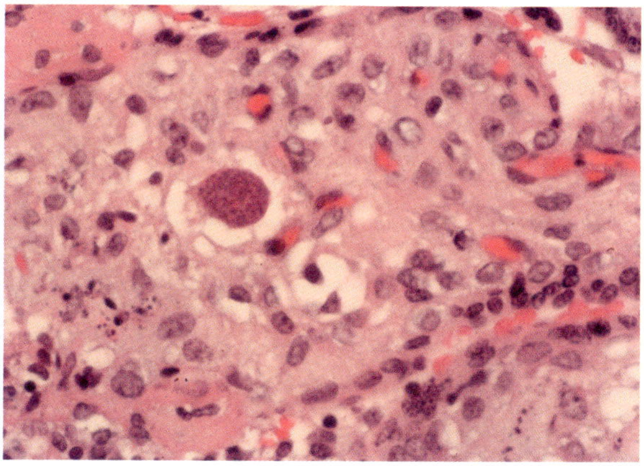

Figure 70 Cyst of *Toxoplasma gondii* in a villus without inflammatory reaction. This emphasizes the need for search for causative organisms in both inflamed and non-inflamed villi in infectious villitis (hematoxylin–eosin, x400)

tumor, miscellaneous lesions such as exaggerated placental site, placental-site nodule, and unclassified trophoblastic lesion) generally fall into the realm of gynecologic pathology, and are not addressed in this book. However, we do very briefly address the lesion *intraplacental* choriocarcinoma because of the interpretive problems associated with findings of cellular proliferation and atypia in some cases of chorangioma. The primary non-trophoblastic tumors of the placenta are the tumorous villous vascular proliferations (chorangioma and chorangiomatosis)[144,422], and the rare hepatocellular adenomas, teratomas, and so-called intraplacental smooth muscle tumors. Secondary, metastatic tumors of maternal and fetal origin can also occur.

Villous vascular 'tumors'

Chorangioma

General The term 'chorangioma' (placental hemangioma) is fairly fixed in placental terminology, but chorangiomas are histologically and behaviorly probably better classified as hamartomas of the villous tree, rather than true neoplasms. They have not been identified in first-trimester abortuses or placental tissues from gestations of less than 24 weeks' duration, and they are generally very small, and located in the peripheral and subchorionic placental parenchyma. The exact classification of these lesions remains unresolved since no clonality studies have been performed[3].

Incidence Chorangiomas are the most common 'tumor' of the placenta, with a generally accepted, estimated occurrence of 1% in term placentas[423]. Chorangiomas are more common in placentas from high-altitude gestations (rates of 2.5–7.6% to as high as 22.7% have been reported[4]), and, in these instances, they are accompanied by features of placental ischemia or circumvallation (see section on 'Extrachorial placentas', this chapter). Chorangiomas have also been seen more frequently in conjunction with pre-eclampsia[4], advancing maternal age (especially age over 30 years), primiparity, maternal hypertension, and gestations with female fetuses[429], and with twin and multiple gestations[144,424,425]. However, their occurrence is not increased in gestations complicated by maternal diabetes mellitus[144,422,424]. Chorangiomas may also be seen in connection with Beckwith–Wiedemann[426] (see above section on 'Large placenta') and Wolf–Hirschorn[427] syndromes.

Gross features Chorangiomas are characteristically small (often 0.5 cm in diameter or less), well-circumscribed, nodular lesions of the fetal plate and marginal parenchyma. In the study by Guschmann and colleagues[424], 55% were localized to the subchorial zone. The lesions may be easily overlooked, grossly misidentified as intervillous thrombi, or misinterpreted as representing sites of chorionic villous infarction. Their macroscopic features and the limitations of placental parenchymal sampling probably account for their broad range of reported incidences cited above; histologic examination of numerous sections increases their detection. Grossly identifiable chorangiomas usually have firm, deep-red, fleshy cut surfaces, but, since they are perfused by the fetal circulation, thrombosis and autoinfarction may occur and be evidenced by a variegated appearance of hemorrhage, yellow-tan discoloration, necrosis, fibrosis, and gritty mineralization. Larger chorangiomas typically bulge from the fetal surface or displace villous parenchyma, and examination may reveal a vascular pedicle arising from the inferior aspect of the

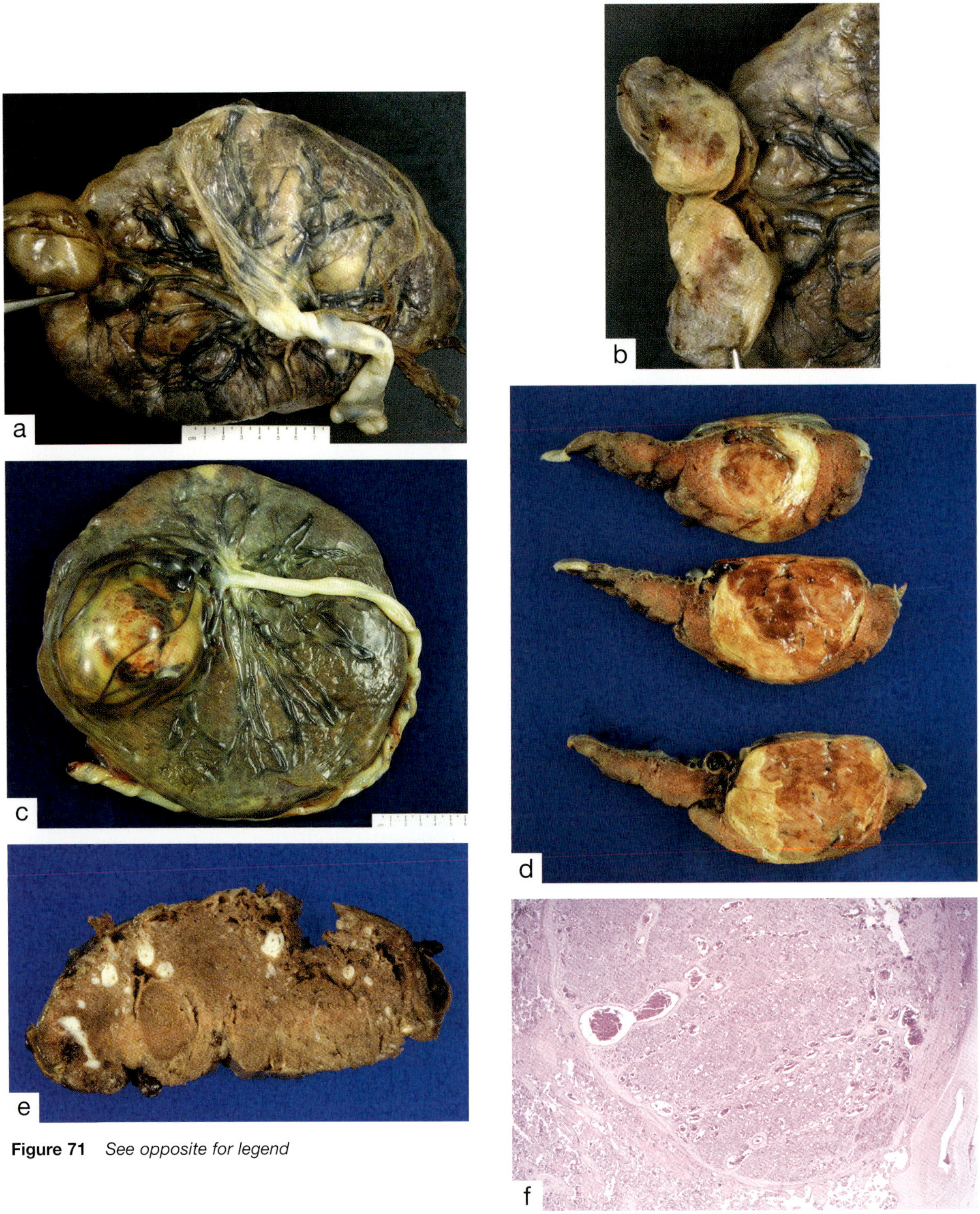

Figure 71 *See opposite for legend*

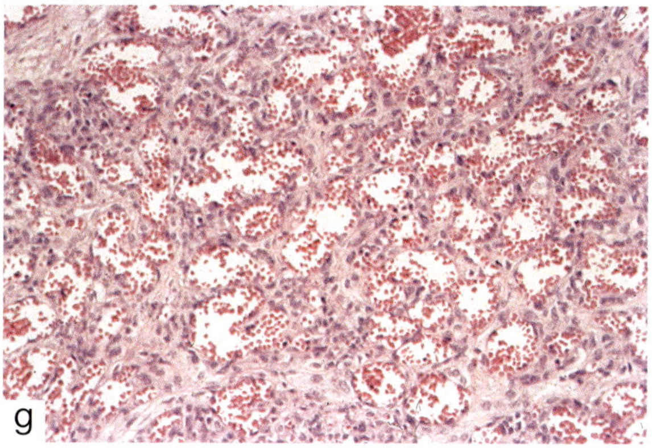

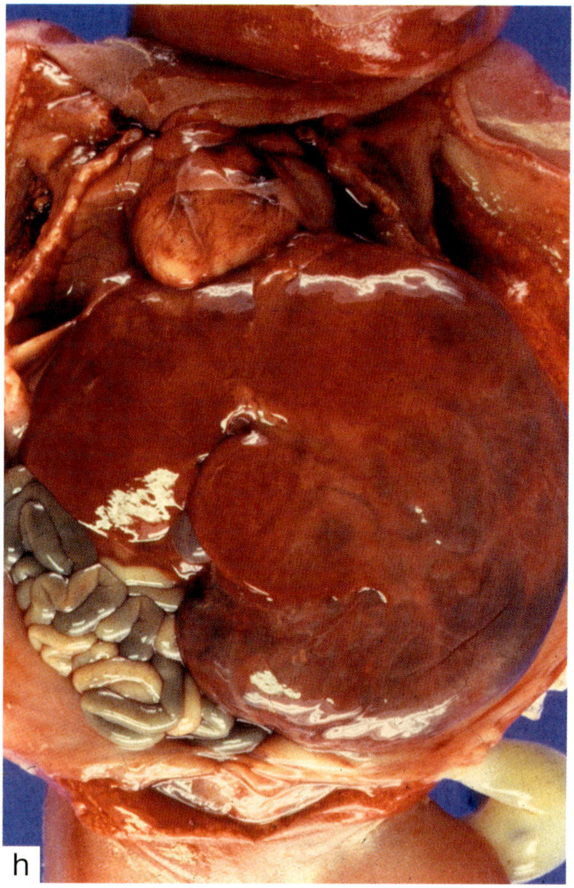

Figure 71 Chorangioma. (a) This is a 4.3-cm chorangioma with features typical of larger detectable lesions. It is subchorial, peripheral, multinodular, bulging, firm, and supplied by prominent chorionic plate feeder vessels. (b) Its fixed cut surface shows firm, tan, congested tissue with areas of hemorrhage, autoinfarction, and necrosis. (c and d) The fresh, intact gross specimen and cut surfaces of a central, 12-cm, giant chorangioma, which resulted in fetal hydrops, are shown for comparison with (a) and (b). (e) Cut surface of a placenta with multiple, small chorangiomas, nearly all of which have autoinfarcted, is shown. (f) Low-power photomicrograph shows subchorionic chorangioma with expansive proliferation of villus by vascular lesion and clear demarcation of the mass from the adjacent chorionic villi. (g) Typical appearance of capillary-type pattern of proliferation in chorangioma. (h) Intrauterine fetal demise at 24 weeks of gestation due to fetal hydrops associated with placental chorangioma (4.5 cm) but also a massive hepatic angioma was identified. (Case consultation from Catherine Craven, MD, University of Utah, Salt Lake City, UT, to Ona Faye-Petersen, MD)

chorionic plate. Single large-to-massive lesions (up to 16 cm)[3,422,428–434] and extensive chorangiomatous involvement (including 8–10-cm nodules with a 1500-g aggregate[434] scattered throughout the placenta) have been reported[4,144] (Figure 71a–e).

Histologic features The lesions are composed of excessive proliferations of small fetal vessels embedded in scant connective tissue and covered by trophoblastic epithelium. They appear to represent expansions within a single villous structure (Figure 71f and g). Capillary proliferations characterize smaller and microscopically detected chorangiomas. However, larger lesions may exhibit a histomorphologic variation that includes capillary, cavernous, hypercellular, endotheliomatous, hyalinized, or fibromatous fields. As above, sections of subchorionic lesions may reveal the presence of large 'feeder' vessels from the chorionic plate and a villous stromal component. Those found near the cord insertion site may be relatively myxomatous, due to the incorporation of Wharton's jelly[4]. Acute or chronic thrombosis, infarction, hemosiderosis, and dystrophic mineralization may also be seen, particularly in chorangiomas measuring several centimeters in dimension.

Significance Small and solitary and even small and multiple chorangiomas are usually of no clinical significance. Gestational complications are associated with large (≥ 5 cm) and multinodular lesions. Complications reflect that chorangiomas form sponge-like sequestrations of fetal blood, and presumably act as peripheral arteriovenous shunts because their vascularity is not matched by a proportionate increase in villous surface area for exchange. Complications include: microangiopathic anemia due to their labyrinthine structure, cardiomegaly, non-immune hydrops (due to loss of protein in the lesional interstitium), fetal growth restriction, polyhydramnios, pre-eclampsia; toxemia of pregnancy; preterm delivery; placental abruption; dystocia; perinatal thrombocytopenia and/or disseminated coagulopathy; spontaneous (fetomaternal) hemorrhage; and fetal death[3,4,311,422,425,432–439]. Preterm birth and/or polyhydramnios are the most common gestational risks identified[424,425,429,438], and non-immune hydrops, intralesional vascular rupture or fetomaternal hemorrhage, and disseminated intravascular coagulation are the most significant risk factors for intrauterine fetal demise[4,422,425,432,439]. Rates of fetal demise range from 40%[428] to about 66%[439]. Because of these complications, ultrasonographic surveillance of large chorangiomas has been recommended[429,439].

The occurrence of spontaneous thrombosis of feeding blood vessels resulting in infarction and shrinkage of chorangiomas and clinical improvement of the fetus has led to the successful fetoscopic or ultrasonographically guided ablation of feeder vessels[428,440] and application of laser therapy[441]. Amnioreduction[425,429] and intrauterine fetal transfusion[435] have also been successfully used.

Recurrence of multiple chorangiomas in a subsequent pregnancy has been reported; isolated chorangiomas are not known to recur[4,442]. Coincident presence of hepatic angioma and cutaneous angiomatosis in infants, who were not otherwise known to have Beckwith–Wiedemann syndrome, has been reported in rare instances[3,443–445] (Figure 71h).

Pathogenesis The pathogenesis of chorangioma is unclear. As discussed in Chapter 9, and in Chapter 8's section on 'Lesions due to disturbances of maternal blood flow', the peripheral and subchorionic regions of the placenta are normally relatively hypoxic. These observations and chorangioma's increased incidence in conditions associated with high altitude, pre-eclampsia, and hypertension have led investigators to favor hypoxia-induced reactive hyperplasia and/or hamartomatous, stem villous maldevelopment as the pathogenetic origin of chorangioma, over that of primary, early embryofetal, neoplastic proliferation[4,144,422]. The potential hypoxia-induced excessive angiogenesis is potentially stimulated by vascular endothelial growth factor, placental growth factor[446], angiopoietin growth factors, and possibly platelet-derived growth factors[447]. A relationship between the development of chorangioma and infantile hemangiomatosis may also be possible, since juvenile cutaneous hemangiomas have been found to express *placenta*-associated vascular antigens Fc γ RII, Lewis Y antigen, merosin, and GLUT1, a glucose transporter normally present only in endothelial cells with blood–tissue barrier function (i.e. brain and placenta)[448].

Special considerations: atypical hyperplasia in chorangioma The overwhelming majority of chorangiomas pose little diagnostic challenge. However, to date, a handful of lesions have been reported to exhibit solid-appearing areas of endothelial hypercellularity that also show sufficient nuclear atypia, mitoses, and focal necrosis to suggest the presence of malignancy or 'chorangiosarcoma'. While none of these has been identified to invade adjacent placental tissue or metastasize to the mother or baby, cautious follow-up of the mothers and infants in these cases of 'atypical cellular chorangioma' has been advised[449]. In addition, two cases of chorangiomatous lesions showing combined vascular and trophoblastic hyperplasia with trophoblastic atypia, sufficient to warrant a diagnosis of 'chorangiocarcinoma', have been documented[450,451]. As in the isolated cases of atypical cellularity of the endothelial component, neither of these lesions was associated with maternal or infant metastasis or morbidity.

The rarity of these reports suggests that such atypical cellular proliferations, in chorangioma, are exceedingly unusual. However, it is discussed herein, because two recent reviews have revealed that striking trophoblastic hyperplasia, reminiscent of malignancy, is probably more common than the literature has suggested. Khong[446] found it in 65% (15/23) of chorangiomas in his series, and Ogino and Redline[144] found trophoblastic hyperplasia in 50% of their cases, with nearly 14% (5/36) exhibiting moderate hyperplasia that was highly monoclonal antibody 1 (MIB-1) immunostain-positive for Ki-67 antigen (a marker of cell proliferation) in representative samples. The trophoblastic proliferations in the series by Khong[446] exhibited multilayered and filigreed patterns with nuclear atypia, abundant mitoses, and/or focal necrosis of the syncytiotrophoblast and cytotrophoblast. He further demonstrated that chorangiomas bearing these neoplastic-appearing trophoblastic proliferations had a significantly higher proliferation index by MIB-1 immunostaining than did their unexceptional counterparts, and showed an immunohistochemical staining pattern comparable to *choriocarcinoma* of malignant trophoblastic disease (positive anti-human placental lactogen (hPL), human chorionic gonadotropin (hCG), and placental alkaline phosphatase (PLAP) staining). However, none of the cases that he or Ogino and Redline[144] identified demonstrated placental villous invasion or free masses of choriocarcinomatous tissue in the maternal space, histopathologic features associated with frank malignancy and true *intraplacental choriocarcinoma* (also termed 'placental choriocarcinoma' or 'choriocarcinoma-*in-situ* of the placenta'). In addition, none could be linked to coincident maternal or infant metastatic disease or later occurrence of malignant gestational trophoblastic disease. Nevertheless, because of the metastatic potential of intraplacental choriocaricinoma[452–454] and the possibility proposed by Jaunaix and colleagues[450] that their case of chorangiocarcinoma represented a 'missing link' between chorangioma and placental choriocarcinoma, Khong[446] proposed that the term 'chorangioma with trophoblastic proliferation' be applied to lesions with suspicious-appearing atypia and proliferation, and that their identification should prompt close clinical follow-up of the respective mothers and infants.

Chorangiomatosis

This term refers to placentas with multiple chorangiomas[422]. However, Ogino and Redline[144] have applied 'chorangiomatosis' more specifically to describe chorangioma lesions in which capillary and stromal proliferations 'permeate normal villous structures' instead of forming the centrally expanding, nodular configurations of capillaries and stromal structures that characterize routine chorangiomas. They determined that it differed morphologically from chorangi*osis* because chorangiosis involved *terminal* villi, was not seen before 32 weeks, and was more common after 37 weeks; in chorangiosis, capillaries are numerous and closely approximating (see 'Chorangiosis' in section on 'Abnormalities of villous blood vessels' in Chapter 9). Chorangiomas and chorangiomatosis involve more proximal elements of the villous tree, show presence of perivascular, muscle-specific actin cells, stromal collagenization and lattice-like reticulin, increased stromal cellularity, and associated increased spacing between capillaries. In their study of 75 cases of chorangioma, they found 39 that demonstrated a permeative pattern of capillary and stromal proliferation and determined that distinguishing chorangiomatosis, as they defined it, had significant implications. A diffuse, multifocal pattern in the placenta (Figure 72 a and b), in contrast to 'focal' or 'segmental' patterns (Figure 72c–f), was associated with extreme prematurity (delivery at < 32 weeks of gestation), congenital malformations, and fetal growth restriction. They also concluded that diffuse multifocal chorangiomatosis (Figure 72 a, a-1 and b) was associated with delayed villous maturation, avascular villi, and placentomegaly, and had its onset earlier in gestation than did the other forms. In contrast, they proposed that routine chorangiomas and localized focal and segmental forms of chorangiomatosis represented lesions of immature stem villi. Of note, however, is that they found both chorangioma and all forms of chorangiomatosis associated with pre-eclampsia, preterm delivery between 32 and 36 weeks, and/or multiple gestations.

Given the different applications of the word chorangiomatosis and its seeming overlap with features of what has been identified as 'mesenchymal dysplasia of the placenta'[159,455,456] and the difficulties that can be encountered in applying the diagnostic

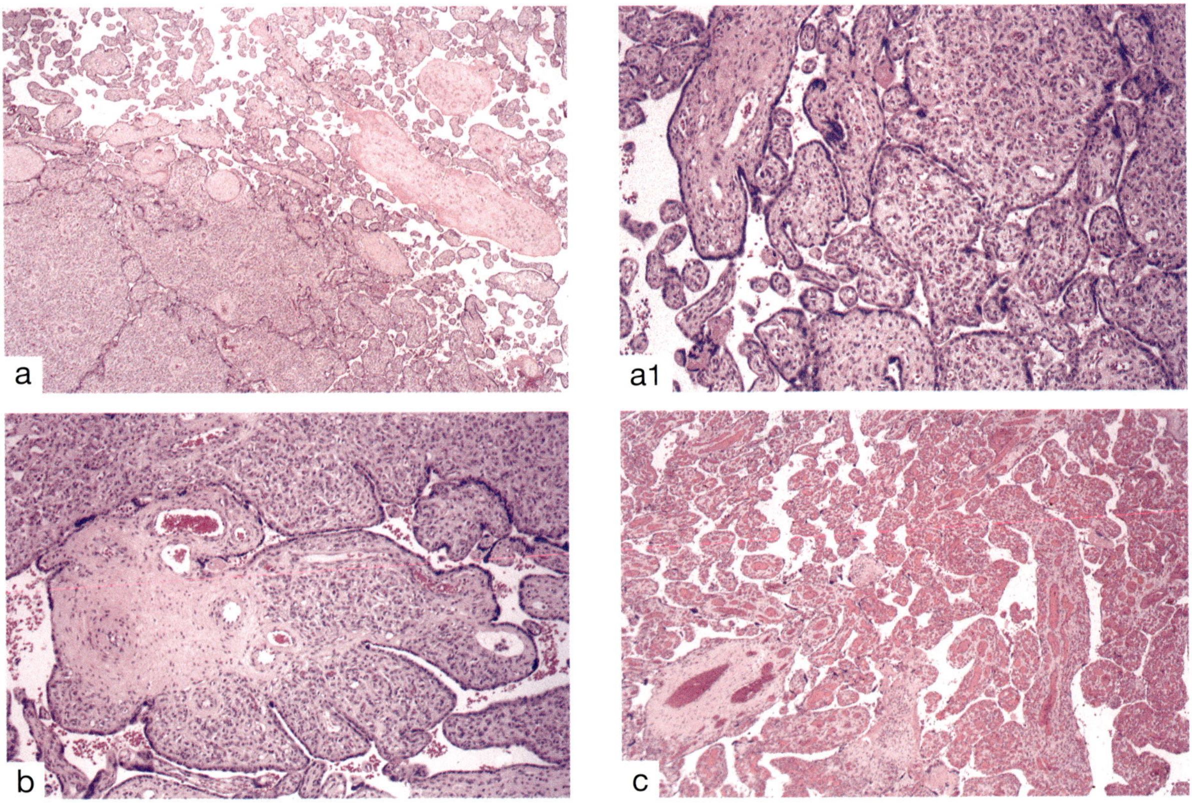

Figure 72 Chorangiomatosis, as defined by Ogino and Redline144. A permeative pattern of capillary and stromal proliferation into villous structures is seen. Also several levels of the villous tree are involved. In neither the diffuse multifocal nor the localized segmental form is there always a discrete transition between normal and abnormal villous tree, although generally clear differences can be seen at low power between affected and unaffected villi. (a, a-1, and b) The diffuse, multifocal pattern involves numerous sites thoughout the placenta. Involved portions of the villous tree are very bulky due to extensive proliferation of capillaries and stroma in large villi. This pattern was associated with higher risks of perinatal morbidity and mortality. (c and d) Localized segmental chorangiomatosis involves presumably the more distal, immature intermediate villi, and far fewer segments of the villous tree. The proliferations are similar to chorangiosis, but, in addition to the terminal villi, the more proximal intermediate villi are also involved, as seen here. (e and f) Immunoperoxidase stain for muscle-specific actin (MSA) (e) and reticulin stain (f) reveal the presence of pericytes and reticulin in the abnormal villi, respectively; these features again distinguish chorangiomatosis from chorangiosis, which is MSA-negative and does not show a multifibrillar lattice-work type of distribution of reticulin. (Material supplied by Raymond Redline, MD, Case Western Reserve University Hospital, Cincinnati, OH)

criteria of chorangiomatosis[457], it may be prudent to accompany any use of the term chorangiomatosis, in a surgical pathology report, with a clarifying definition.

Hepatocellular adenoma

The hepatocellular adenoma is an extremely rare, incidental, non-trophoblastic tumor that is a well-circumscribed, 1-cm or less in size, encapsulated, subchorionic, or villous nodule. It consists of tissue resembling fetal liver, with immature hepatocytes in aggregates or thick cords punctuated by small islands of erythropoiesis in sinusoids, but differs from a heterotopia because it lacks bile ductules, portal tracts, and central veins. It is believed to develop from displaced hepatocytes that have migrated, via the primitive yolk sac, to the placenta, during early embryogenesis. It must be distinguished from cytotrophoblastic cell islands, heterotopic fetal adrenal

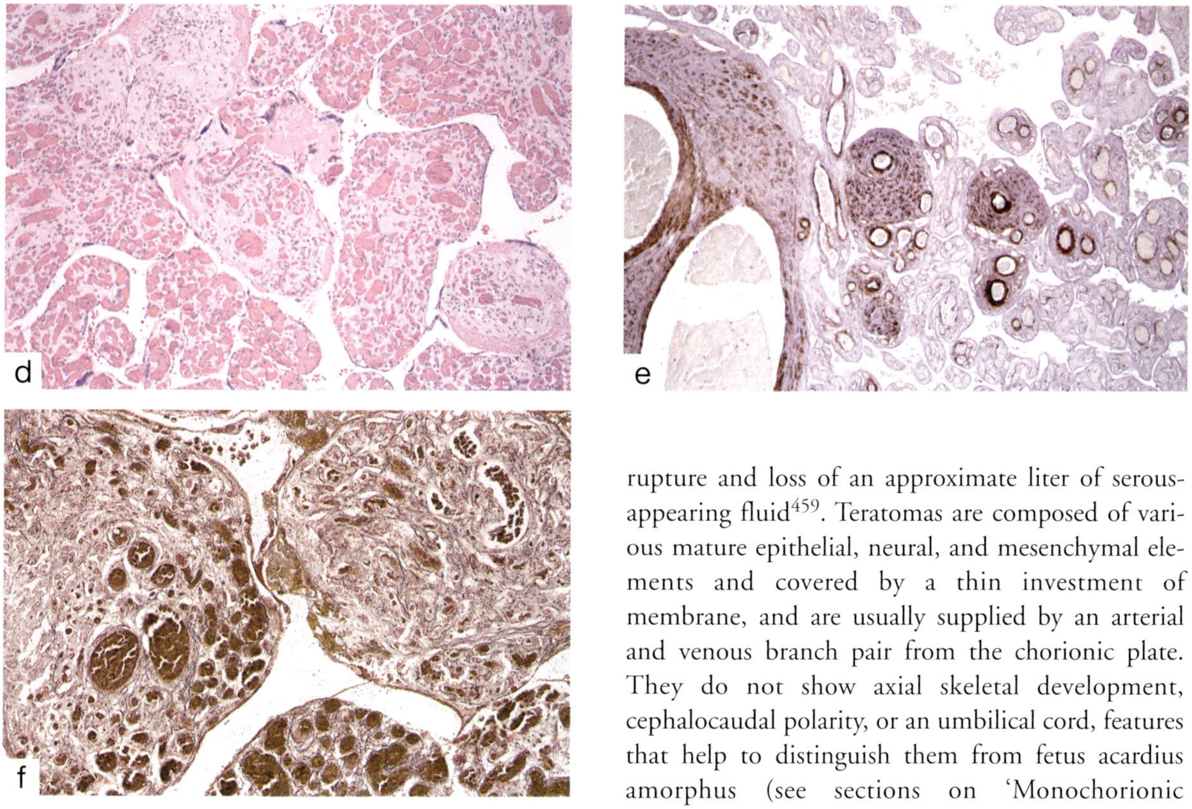

Figure 72 *Continued*

cortical rests, teratomas, and maternal or fetal metastatic foci (see below)[458].

Teratoma

Teratomas of the placenta are also extremely rare; about 21 cases have been reported. The tumor is a well-circumscribed, solid, round to oval mass that lies between the amnion and chorion on the fetal surface or in the membranes at the placental margin. Its location appears to suggest its probable origin from germ cells developing in the dorsal wall of the yolk sac that have migrated abnormally into the umbilical cord to the placental surface. (Teratomas of the umbilical cord have also been reported.) Reported dimensions have ranged from 2.5 to 11 cm[3,459,460], but the largest may have been of even greater dimension *in situ*, since delivery of the placenta resulted in tumor rupture and loss of an approximate liter of serous-appearing fluid[459]. Teratomas are composed of various mature epithelial, neural, and mesenchymal elements and covered by a thin investment of membrane, and are usually supplied by an arterial and venous branch pair from the chorionic plate. They do not show axial skeletal development, cephalocaudal polarity, or an umbilical cord, features that help to distinguish them from fetus acardius amorphus (see sections on 'Monochorionic monoamniotic placenta' and 'Acardiac twin' in Chapter 15). However, a few examiners have stated that such distinction is artificial and hold that teratomas really represent failed twin or multiple gestations[3,4]. While this issue of origin may remain unresolved, gestations with fetus acardius amorphus are frequently associated with congestive heart failure in the normal fetus, polyhydramnios, and premature labor. Placental teratomas are nearly always associated with normal pregnancy outcome and fetal development. A single case of maternal death and placental teratoma has been reported. Maternal death was due to amniotic fluid embolism (AFE), following a cesarean section delivery performed for premature rupture of the membranes and fetal distress, at 34 weeks of gestation. AFE is a known risk associated with cesarean section (see section in Chapter 12), but the potential roles of the 11-cm placental teratomatous mass, described above, in the onset of preterm labor, or tumor fluid volume, in the content and entry of amniotic material into the maternal circulation, were not discussed[459].

Intraplacental smooth muscle tumor

This lesion has been identified in three case reports as a smooth muscle tumor of the maternal surface with gross finger-like extension into the neighboring placental parenchyma, and cellularity, mitotic rate, and histopathology suggestive of malignancy[461–463]. Sadly, the two most recent reports document the same 6-cm tumor found in the placenta of a healthy male term infant written from the respective perspectives of the pathologists and clinicians involved in the case. The report by Ernst and colleagues[462], published first, is superior in content and scientific substantiation. The tumor, while it appeared to be arising from within the placenta and had ultrasonographic and gross features compatible with a chorangioma, was concluded to be a uterine leiomyoma, that had become incorporated in the base of the placenta, by use of polymerase chain reaction for the Y chromosome; Y chromosome was identified in the placental tissue but not in the tumor. The woman underwent a postpartum hysterectomy and pelvic node dissection; the lymph nodes were negative[463], and only two tiny subserosal uterine leiomyomas were identified[462]. The report by Tapia and associates[461] also describes a markedly similar basal mass embedded within placental parenchyma, and *intramembranous*, but otherwise comparable, smooth muscle tumors were reported by Misselevich and colleagues[464] and Tarim and co-workers[465]. Tapia and associates[461] and Misselevich and colleagues[464] favored a placental origin of their tumors, but their cases were not evaluated using molecular techniques. Tarim and co-workers[465], however, confirmed the uterine origin of their mass, again by using the PCR technique for the Y chromosome. The leiomyomatous masses identified by the two earlier groups[461,464] could represent proliferations of the mural component of stem villous vessels, but they more likely represent a pedunculated extension of a leiomyoma of the uterus (possibly even metaplastic endometrial origin)[462]. The differential diagnosis of the so-called intraplacental smooth muscle tumor includes chorangioma, of course, and placenta accreta (see above section on 'Placenta accreta' in this chapter).

Metastatic tumors

Metastatic tumors of maternal origin

Maternal malignancy during pregnancy is uncommon, and placental metastases from maternal malignancies are rare and are generally associated with disseminated maternal disease. Maternal melanoma and breast cancer (Figure 73) are the most frequently recognized tumors. Melanoma is most common likely because it affects young individuals and because of its high risks for hematogenous spread, in contrast to cervical cancer, which is primarily spread by lymphatic involvement[3]. Pregnancy *per se* does not alter the incidence or course of maternal melanoma[466,467]. To date, melanoma is the only malignancy to exhibit frequent villous invasion[3] and spread to the fetus; placental involvement is associated with a 22%[467] to 25%[468] risk of fetal metastasis. Such spread is almost uniformly fatal; there are nine reports of intrauterine metastasis to the fetus, with death in infancy occurring in all but one affected baby[3,467]. Of note is that metastatic melanoma may be grossly detected as dark-brown or black lesions in the placental parenchyma. Other tumors have escaped detection since tumors other than melanoma have rarely exhibited villous invasion. Single case reports of gastric, adrenal, tracheobronchial and squamous neck carcinomas, and thigh myxosarcoma and Ewing's sarcoma of bone, and two cases of breast carcinoma, have been reported[3].

The remaining cases of tumors identified as maternal metastases to the placenta have shown involvement limited to the maternal space, and there is some debate as to whether such restriction to the maternal blood merits the term 'metastasis'. However, the lack of villous attachment or invasion may reflect sampling, and the fact that the tumor cells are often present in aggregates or sheets suggests that tumor growth is occurring within the intervillous space[3]. The unique blood flow patterns may provide sluggish, sequestered spaces that facilitate tumor replication. The role of the placental barrier is unclear, but placental 'metastasis' to the intervillous space has been identified for a variety of solid tumors, with breast[3,469,470] and lung[3,471] being the

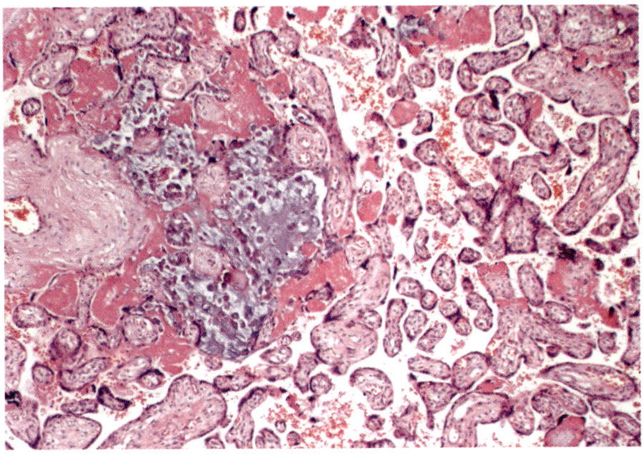

Figure 73 Metastatic maternal breast adenocarcinoma to the placenta. Tumor cells are present in the intervillous space and adhere to, but do not invade, the surfaces of the chorionic villi. Mucicarmine stains were performed and were positive

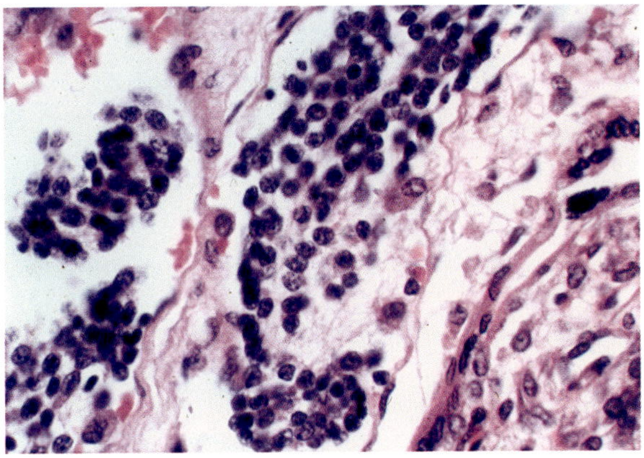

Figure 74 Metastatic fetal neuroblastoma tumor cells present in the villous capillaries in congenital neuroblastoma. Note that their presence is restricted to the lumina of the capillaries (hematoxylin–eosin, x400)

most common. Rare reports have included pancreatic[3,469], ovarian, primitive neuroectodermal[472], and medulloblastoma[3] tumors. One case with extensive placental involvement by a poorly differentiated, metastatic adenocarcinoma of unknown primary site resulted in fetal demise and postpartum maternal death[473]. Hematologic malignancies, including lymphoma[474], have been reported, but leukemic aggregations[475] are probably far more common than documented. In no case has placental involvement been reported to herald the recognition of an occult maternal malignancy.

Metastatic tumors of fetal origin

Fetal neuroblastoma[476–478] (Figure 74), hepatoblastoma[479,480], sacrococcygeal teratoma[481], and leukemia[3] have been identified within fetal blood vessels in the placenta. One such case included primary recognition and early diagnosis of a congenital primitive epithelial tumor of the liver[455]; such recognition and evaluation of fetal metastatic tumor within the placenta may obviate needs for further or invasive diagnostic procedures in the infant[477,480]. Concordant congenital leukemia[482] and some cases of concordant neuroblastoma[483] in monozygotic twins likely represent cases of metastatic spread from one twin to the other via placental anastomoses. Similar placental anastomotic spread has been postulated for the development, in late childhood, of T-cell malignancies of identical clonality in a pair of monozygotic twins[484] (see section on 'Twin placentas' in Chapter 15). The detection of malignant cells in fetal vasculature of the placenta, therefore, has special significance.

11

Lesions of the umbilical cord

The umbilical cord contains two arteries and a vein, which are embedded in Wharton's jelly, composed of a mucoid ground substance and a network of fibroblasts. Wharton's jelly protects the blood vessels from mechanical trauma. The umbilical cord is covered by amniotic epithelium. The umbilical arteries have a two-layer muscle coat that is contracted, giving the vessels an undulating appearance on histologic sections. The umbilical vein shows a less compact muscle coat (Figures 10 and 11). The umbilical vessels are arranged in a spiral fashion, with the cord usually twisting to the left. Absent twist has been associated with poor outcome including stillbirth[485], and absent or right twist has been associated with single umbilical artery[486]. When the vessels are longer than the cord, the vessels fold, forming so-called false knots, which are of no clinical significance (Figure 75). Absence of the cord (limb–body wall complex or body stalk anomaly) is extremely rare and is associated with markedly malformed fetuses (see below in Chapter 12, discussion of 'Amniotic disruption sequence')[487].

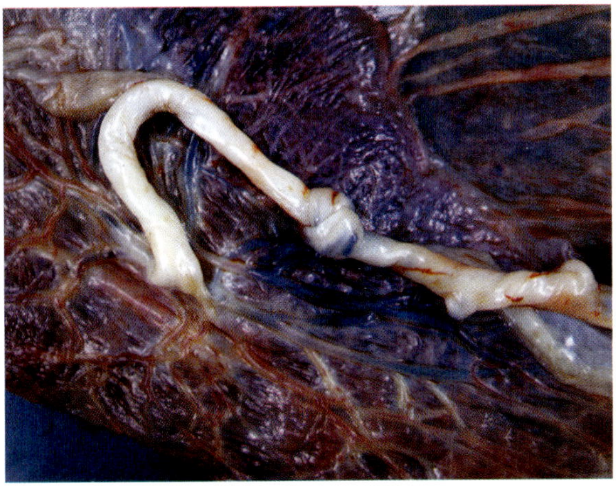

Figure 75 False knot in cord. False knots, varices, or excessively long loops of the umbilical vein bulge from the surface of the cord. Two are seen in this cord segment, on the right, along with a true knot of the umbilical cord (see also Figure 80 and associated text)

SHORT AND LONG UMBILICAL CORDS

Umbilical cord length cannot be ascertained with certainty by the pathologist, because a portion of the cord may not have been submitted to the laboratory. A normal cord length at term ranges from about 50 to 60 cm. In a large study by Naeye, umbilical cord length was measured from 20 to 47 weeks' gestational age. Average umbilical cord length was 32.4 cm at 20–21 weeks, 50.2 cm at 32–33 weeks, 55.6 cm at 36–37 weeks, and 59.6 cm at term[488]. There are problems associated with both abnormally long and abnormally short cords. An abnormally long cord over 75 cm is vulnerable to fetal entanglement (including nuchal cord), knots, prolapse, and compression, and may have formed due to increased

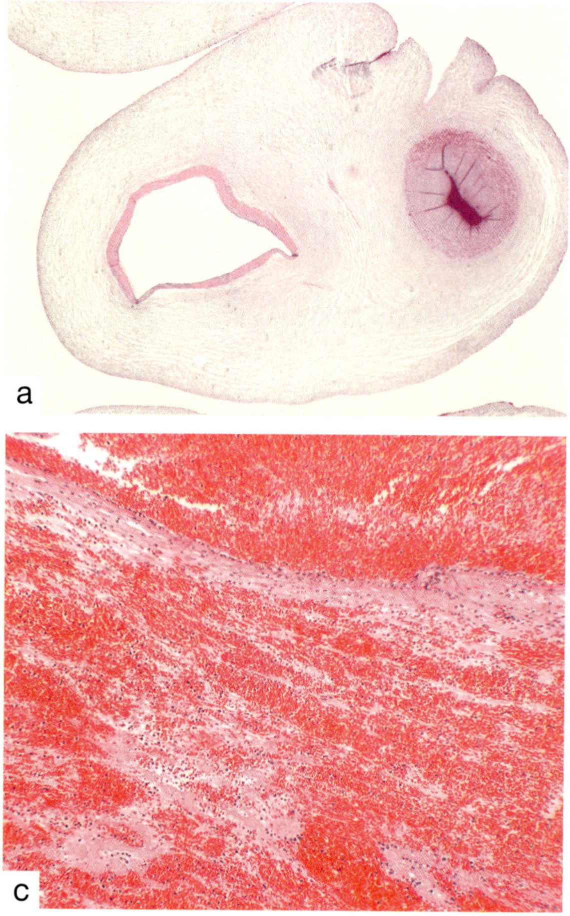

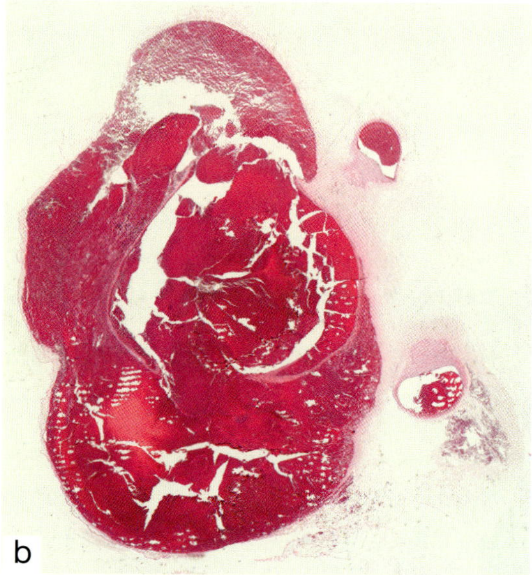

Figure 76 (a) Single umbilical artery. Cross-sections showing the single artery on the right, and the vein on the left. (Erroneous diagnosis of single umbilical artery may occur if transverse sections of cord do not include an essentially circumferential coat of amnion or show significant gaps in Wharton's jelly.) Deeper sections confirmed the absence of a second artery in this case. (b) This transmural section shows an acute rupture of the umbilical vein with dissection and hematoma formation within Wharton's jelly. This is from a 38-week gestation stillborn delivery in which the dissecting hematoma accounted for the intrauterine fetal death. There was a diffusely hemorrhagic segment of umbilical cord that measured 20.5-cm in length and up to 2.5 cm in diameter. The 2.5-cm dilated portion revealed dilated blood vessels and acute thrombus. The results from dissecting the hematoma and sections included in the sample are seen in this low power photomicrograph. (c) Higher-power magnification of the rupture site shows there is fibrin deposition both within and beyond the residual wall of the vessel. This finding is an important diagnostic feature that distinguishes incidental traction hematoma from real pathologic hematoma in the cord. (case contributed by Dan Pankowsky, MD, Summit Medical Center, Nashville, TN)

activity of the fetus. The significance of nuchal cords is unclear. Nuchal cords, even multiple, were not shown to be associated with significant adverse neonatal outcome in one study[487,489], but were felt to be significant in another[490]. Adverse neurologic sequelae have been associated with abnormally long cords[26]. An abnormally short cord, one less than 30–40 cm, is prone to traction during labor, with the risk of impaired circulation, cord rupture, or abruption, and can be due to decreased fetal movement, itself a potential indicator of fetal illness.

SINGLE UMBILICAL ARTERY

Single umbilical artery (SUA) is the most common congenital anomaly of the placenta (Figure 76a). The incidence of SUA is up to 1% of pregnancies[491]. Careful gross examination, and preparation of microscopic sections with full cross-sections of the cord from relatively non-spiraled areas, are necessary to appreciate this finding. The second umbilical artery may be absent or atrophic with a remnant present. SUA is associated with congenital anomalies in about 30% of cases[492]. Chromosomal abnormalities, as well as genitourinary, gastrointestinal, musculoskeletal, cardiovascular, and CNS anomalies, may be seen[493]. SUA is increased in incidence among twins, and there is an increased risk of prematurity, IUGR, and perinatal mortality with SUA[491,494].

SUPERNUMERARY UMBILICAL VESSELS

Care must be taken not to mistake duplicate lumens of a single tortuous vessel for a supernumerary vessel; however, an extra umbilical artery or vein can occur. Normally, the right umbilical vein regresses in the second month of fetal life, but may rarely persist[495]. Earlier reports suggested an increased incidence of congenital anomalies, and these should certainly be looked for; however, it has more recently been suggested that a four-vessel cord is not always an ominous finding[496]. Sections of the cord should also be taken at least 1.5 cm above the insertion site of the cord to avoid sectioning cord vessel branches or Hyrtl's anastomosis between the arteries[4].

VARICES AND ANEURYSMS

Aneurysms of the arteries are rare[497]. These lesions can be seen either in the umbilical cord vessels, or in the fetal vessels on the chorionic plate. Varices are also called false knots, and arise when the length of the umbilical vein exceeds the cord length. Varices and aneurysms may be subject to thrombosis or bleeding. Aneurysms may occur in association with SUA. Varices need to be distinguished from chorionic cysts with hemorrhage, and from vascular malformations. These lesions can be detected prenatally by Doppler ultrasound evaluation of flow patterns[493].

THROMBOSIS OF UMBILICAL CORD VESSELS

Thrombosis is usually secondary to mechanical factors leading to cord compression, such as velamentous cord insertion, knots, entanglement by amniotic bands, stricture, torsion, long or short cord, iatrogenic injury from cord sampling or transfusion, varices, and aneurysms. Thrombosis may also be associated with obstetrical complications such as acute chorioamnionitis, malpresentation, multiple gestation, precipitate delivery, or abdominal trauma; with maternal diabetes; and with fetal conditions such as hydrops fetalis or fetomaternal hemorrhage. Thrombosis may also be a reflection of a hypercoagulable state, such as a thrombophilia, in which case thrombi may also be seen in chorionic plate and stem villous vessels. An underlying etiology may not be found. Thrombi are more common in the umbilical vein than in the arteries. If of long duration, calcification may be seen. Fetal death may result from occlusion. A particular risk in thrombophilia is that venous thrombi may embolize to the fetus, where they can pass across the foramen ovale and lead to infarcts of vital organs, including the brain (paradoxical embolization)[498].

HEMATOMA AND RUPTURE OF UMBILICAL CORD VESSELS

Most hematomas of the cord are small and inconsequential. Spontaneous cord hematoma has been estimated to occur in 1/5000 deliveries[499]. Rarely, cord hematomas may be diagnosed on prenatal ultrasound, and a rare case has presented with lack of fetal movements and an abnormal non-stress test[500] or stillbirth (Figure 76b and c). Iatrogenic hematomas may be due to cord sampling or traction at delivery; hence, the timing of the hematoma is important. In some cases, more significant hematomas may occur with cordocentesis (see Figure 114), although most of these hematomas are of no significance[501]. Rupture of umbilical vessels may lead to significant hematoma formation in association with velamentous insertion, short cord, long cord, cord prolapse, aneurysm, or varices, and significant blood loss can lead to fetal morbidity and mortality. The pathologist cannot assess the volume of blood loss, but the size of the hematoma should be included in the report.

CALCIFICATION OF UMBILICAL CORD VESSELS

Luminal calcification of cord vessels may be seen with old thromboses. Calcifications in the wall of the vessel or in the Wharton's jelly may occur (Figure 77), and may be associated with intrauterine infection, strictures, hematomas, or meconium exposure[502,503]. Unremarkable calcification of embryologic cord remnants can also occur (see below, 'Embryonic remnants of the umbilical cord').

ABNORMAL INSERTION OF THE UMBILICAL CORD

The umbilical cord is normally inserted on the fetal surface, in a central, paracentral, or paramarginal position. The cord can also insert marginally into the disk (battledore placenta), which is usually of no significance, clinically, but may rarely be associated with stillbirth or growth restriction[491]. The umbilical cord may also insert in a velamentous fashion, into the membranes, which poses significant risk (Figures 46a and 78). In a velamentous insertion, the cord vessels at the insertion traverse the membranes and are unprotected by Wharton's jelly, and are exposed to the risk of compression and rupture during delivery. Thrombosis is also a risk (Figure 46a). If the exposed vessels overlie the cervix, the condition is termed vasa previa (Figure 78), and rupture of the vessels, clinically perceived as vaginal bleeding in the mother, may lead to fetal exsanguination. The frequency of velamentous insertions is increased in mothers who smoke cigarettes, and with advanced maternal age, maternal diabetes, multiple births, SUA, infants with anomalies, and pregnancies achieved by *in vitro* fertilization[491]. Another abnormality is furcate insertion (Figure 79), where the position of the insertion is normal, but the vessels lose their protection of Wharton's jelly above the insertion site, and divide above the fetal surface. These vessels are vulnerable to compression, rupture, and thrombosis, as well.

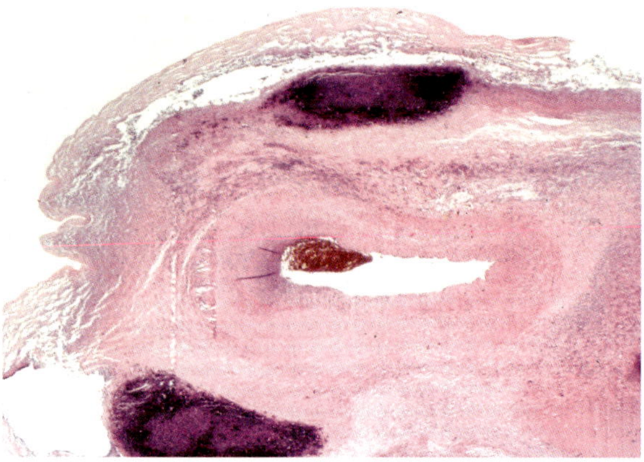

Figure 77 Calcification in the umbilical cord can result from many causes. In this case, necrotizing funisitis due to severe chronic candidal infection resulted in arc-like calcifications of the necrobiotic debris that accumulated within Wharton's jelly between the vessels (arteries in this photomicrograph) and the amniotic surface. The cellular and inflammatory debris resulted from interactions between fetal neutrophils migrating out toward the amniotic surface and the invasive fungal organisms they encountered. Arcs of inflammatory response and debris remain visible

KNOTS IN THE UMBILICAL CORD

There are two types of umbilical knots, false knots and true knots (Figures 75 and 80). As mentioned above, false knots result from focal redundancy, branching, or ectasia of the vein, or focal accumulation of Wharton's jelly, and are of no clinical significance. True knots represent entangled loops of cord that may be tight or loose, occurring in 0.3–2.1% of pregnancies[504]. They are more likely to occur with excessively long umbilical cords, polyhydramnios, or with a small fetus, and between twins in monoamniotic twin pregnancies[505], and generally form prior to the third trimester, when there is sufficient room for the fetus to pass through a cord loop, forming the knot. Potential sequelae, which include edema, congestion, and thrombosis, relate to the tightness of the knot. Arias and Heinonen found a four-fold risk of stillbirth in their series[504], while Sornes reported a ten-fold increased risk[506] (see Figure 80). Normal blood pressure in the umbilical vein is 10 mmHg. In

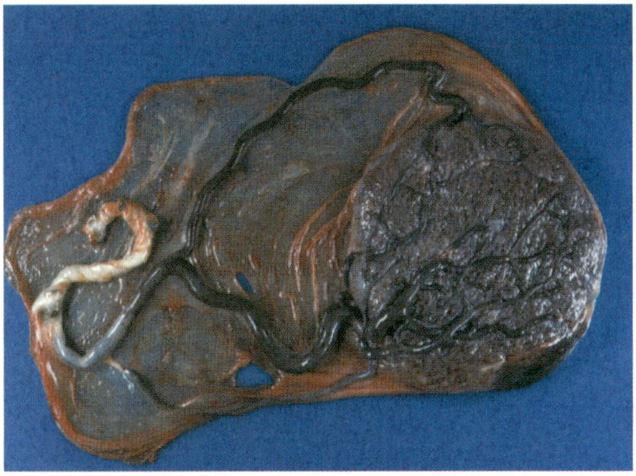

Figure 78 Velamentous cord insertion. Extensive intramembranous insertion of the cord vessels is present in this example. The vessels passed over the cervical os, in situ (vasa previa) (see also Figure 46a)

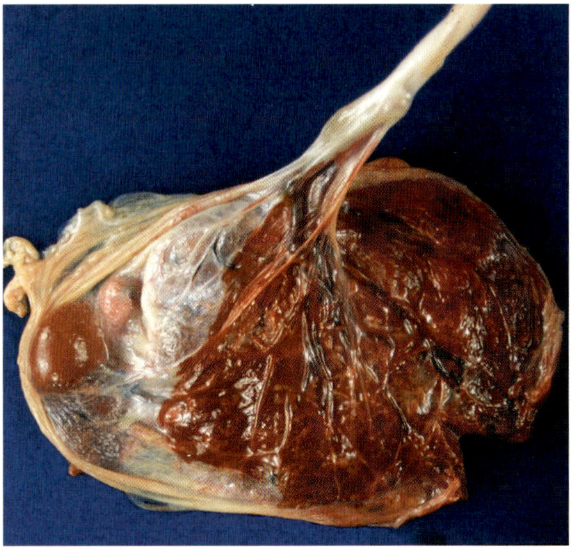

Figure 79 Furcate paramarginally inserting umbilical cord. The cord vessels divide in a sheath of amnion without protection of Wharton's jelly about 5 cm above the insertion site. There is an incidental subamniotic extravasation of blood that partially obscures the vascular ramifications, but they were intact and no hemosiderosis or thrombosis was detected. A small accessory lobe is present on the left

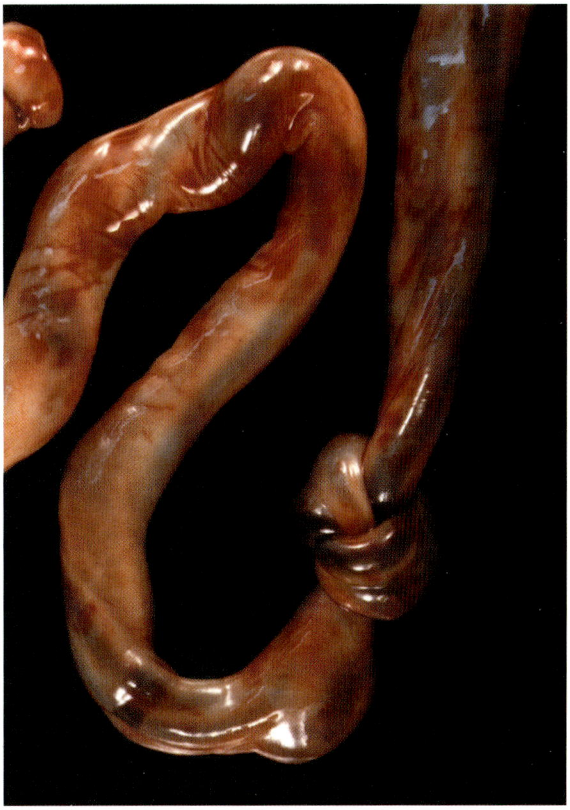

Figure 80 True cord knot. Intrauterine fetal demise occurred due to true cord knot. This is a tight true knot, which upon sectioning showed dilatation and acute occlusive thrombosis of the dilated umbilical vein on the placental side of the knot (inferior aspect of knot in picture). Note the flattening of the cord segment involved in the knot. The cord is otherwise edematous; its red-brown discoloration reflects the changes of maceration. The bulbous formation at the inferior pole is a false knot and not due to dilatation of the vein. (refer also to Figure 75)

in vitro experiments, a pressure of 100–110 mmHg is required to overcome the resistance in a tight knot caused by a 100-g weight[507]. Grossly, if the knot is tight, there may be cord edema, with distention of the umbilical vein, on the placental side of the knot. Presumably, fetal arterial pressure remains sufficient to perfuse the artery and bypass the obstruction for a time, but, in a tight knot, the vein is compressed and obstructed, and dilates. Histologically, there may be correlative thrombosis or thrombotic occlusion of the vein. The fetal side may show arterial thrombosis. Cord sections should be taken through the knot, and on either side, with notation as to which side. In the absence of gross or microscopic evidence of obstruction to venous flow, the knot should be interpreted as clinically insignificant.

TORSION OF THE UMBILICAL CORD

The normal cord is spiraled, usually in a counter-clockwise direction (with the orientation of the fetus facing the chorion plate), and coiling is established very early in gestation[4]. It has been suggested that the spiraling is secondary to fetal movements. Torsion, which is a localized rigid spiraling, as well as diffuse excessive twisting of the cord (Figure 81), is a rare association with fetal demise. The etiology of fetal death with excessive spiraling is uncertain, but it has been theorized to be more common in excessively long cords. Machin and colleagues[508] reported a series of excessively coiled cords, defined as over one coil/5 cm or 0.2 ± 0.1 coils/cm. Thirty-seven per cent of the overcoiled cords were associated with demise, 14% with fetal intolerance to labor, and 10% with IUGR. In torsion, a localized constriction may be seen, and it is usually at the fetal end. The cause is unknown, but cord stricture (see below) and long cord are predisposing factors. Obstructed blood flow leads to fetal morbidity and mortality. Based on cases of recurrent torsion with fetal death, it has been postulated that there may be a genetic component in some cases[509].

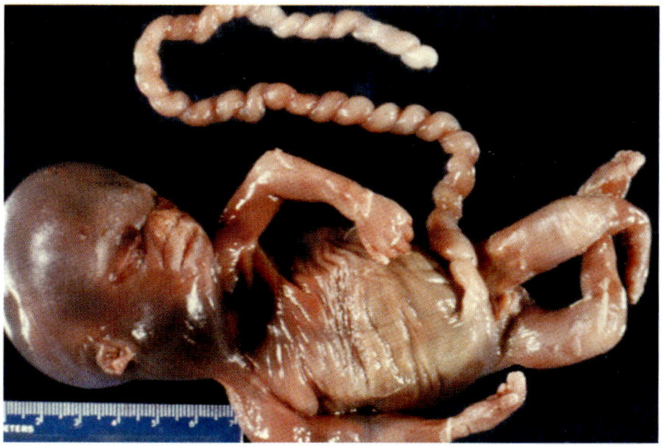

Figure 81 Excessive cord coiling (cord torsion) associated with fetal demise

STRICTURE OF THE UMBILICAL CORD

Torsion is often associated with a segmental stricture, with narrowing at the fetal end a common finding in macerated fetal demises, particularly in the second trimester. It has long been controversial whether this narrowing is a postmortem finding or the cause of demise. Features that have been suggested as evidence that the stricture is pre-mortem include the presence of the finding in some live-borns and fresh stillborns, the presence of recent thrombosis in some stillborns, and a history of decreased fetal movements prior to the demise[510]. Sections should be taken through the narrowed area, as well as on either side of the stricture if along the cord, or on the placental side if the stricture is at the umbilicus. Edema, congestion, and thrombosed vessels may be seen at the point of stricture, and this area should be assessed histologically, since they favor pre-mortem torsion. In addition to a possible relationship to long cords, focal deficiency of Wharton's jelly has been suggested as a cause of stricture.

EDEMA OF THE UMBILICAL CORD

Cord diameter is usually about 1.0–1.4 cm in the third trimester. Edema of the cord may be segmental, forming a pseudocyst, or diffuse. Focal lesions may occur in association with funisitis or near a hematoma. The edematous cord has a swollen, pale, translucent appearance on the external (Figure 82) and cut surfaces. In rare instances, the cord may be enlarged to as much as 5 cm in diameter. Some cord edema is present in 10% of deliveries, and it can be associated with a variety of fetal pathologic conditions including abruption, diabetes, intrauterine demise, prematurity, and cesarean delivery, although it is usually an incidental finding. Coulter and colleagues[511] found that cord edema was associated with idiopathic respiratory distress syndrome and transient tachypnea in the newborn, but not with fetal distress. Increased hydrostatic and lower osmotic fetal intravascular pressures and increased water content of the fetus and placenta are considered as predisposing factors for cord edema[511]. Rarely, the diagnosis has been made prior to delivery[512].

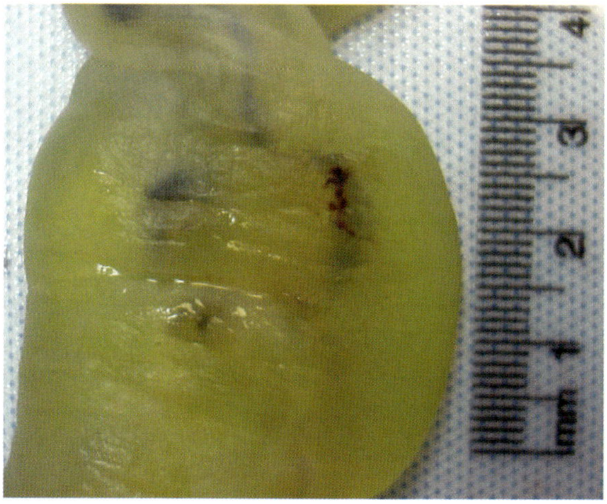

Figure 82 Cord edema

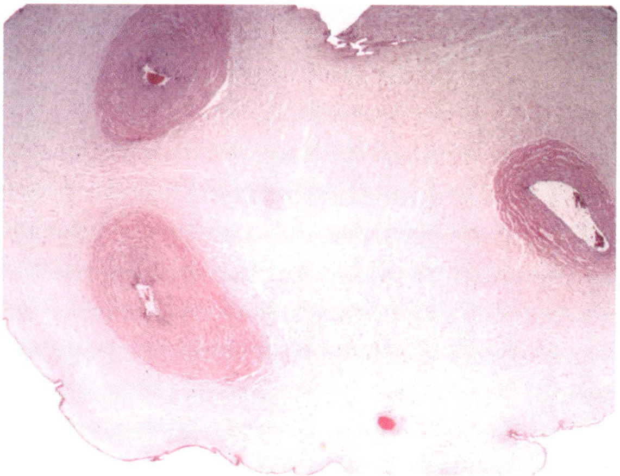

Figure 83 The umbilical cord section shows a small circular structure lined by epithelium to the right and center of the umbilical arteries, the urachal remnant (see also Figure 85). The vitelline vessel remnant is the peripheral lower aspect of the cord

EMBRYONIC REMNANTS OF THE UMBILICAL CORD

Three types of embryonic remnants may be seen on histologic examination: two are visible in Figure 83, the urachal remnant and the vitelline vessel remnant. The third, the omphalomesenteric remnant, is shown in Figure 84.

(1) Omphalomesenteric (vitelline) duct remnants consist of tubular structures < 1 mm in diameter lined by a cuboidal to columnar epithelium. At the third week of development the omphalomesenteric duct, also known as the extraembryonic yolk sac and the vitelline duct, is an outpouching of the primitive endodermal tube (gut). At this time it becomes supplied with embryonic vessels, and with folding of the embryo, during the third and fourth weeks, it and its vessel come to lay *alongside* the umbilical vessels. Eventually, the cord vessels and the neighboring omphalomesenteric duct become surrounded by Wharton's jelly and the omphalomesenteric duct becomes incorporated within the cord jelly and enclosed within the amnion of the cord. The structure normally involutes, but it can be seen as a tubular remnant with a thin muscle cuff lined by mucin-secreting cells[4]. Because the omphalomesenteric duct is originally peripheral to the cord vessels, its remnant is peripherally located on cross-sections of the cord (Figure 84).

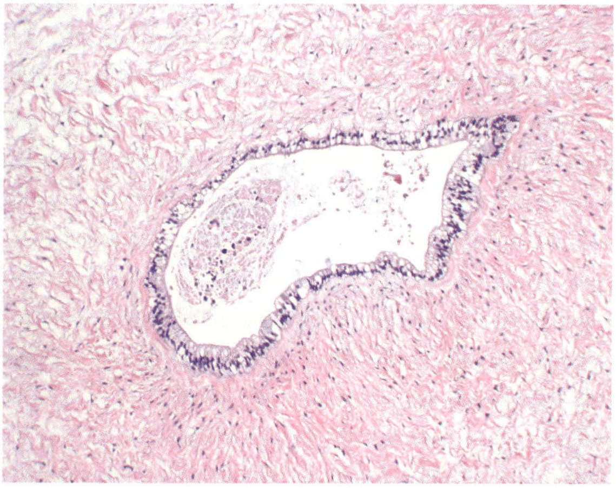

Figure 84 High-power photomicrograph of omphalomesenteric (vitelline) duct remnant showing mucinous epithelium

(2) Urachal (or allantoic duct, the allantois being the very early embryonic structure) remnant consists of clusters of epithelial cells or microcystic structures lined by a flattened, mucinous, or transitional epithelium. Because the urachus is attached to the dome of the bladder and

because the two umbilical arteries lie on either side of the urinary bladder, within the fetus, cross-sections of the umbilical cord will reveal preservation of this anatomic relationship; the urachal remnant is characteristically located between the two umbilical arteries (Figures 83 and 85) on histologic sections of the cord. Urachal remnants can occur in association with persistent patent urachus, a rare anomaly. In this anomaly, the cord is turgid and swollen at birth, and, subsequently, urine drains from the umbilicus, after the cord stump falls away.

Omphalomesenteric and urachal remnants may dilate and form cysts within the cord (see below).

(3) Vitelline vessel remnants are thin-walled capillary-like vascular structures that supplied the omphalomesenteric duct described above. Grossly they can be seen as a delicate thin vessel running in parallel with the umbilical vessels and are most easily identified at the fetal end of the cord. Microscopically, a single capillary-like vessel or a focal angioma-like cluster may be seen (Figure 83).

The overall incidence of these remnants was 23.1% in one series[513]. No complications or anomalies occur in the overwhelming majority of cases, although a case of acid-secreting gastric cells in an omphalomesenteric remnant leading to cord perforation, hemorrhage, and fetal death has been reported[514].

CYSTS OF THE UMBILICAL CORD

Cystic lesions may be true epithelial-lined cysts, pseudocysts due to segmental edema or degeneration of Wharton's jelly, or neoplastic (see below). Epithelial cysts arise from cystic dilatation of omphalomesenteric or allantoic remnants, or from amniotic epithelial inclusions, and are usually small and of no clinical significance. Large cysts may cause compression of cord vessels[513,515].

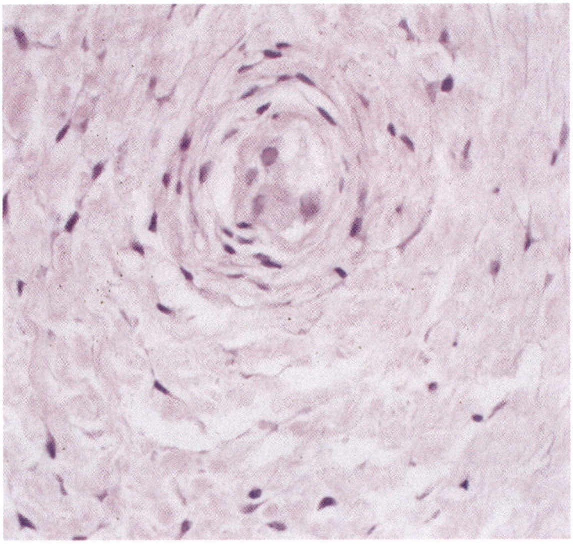

Figure 85 Urachal remnant

TUMORS OF THE UMBILICAL CORD

Tumors of the cord are rare, and are usually hemangiomas. Teratomas occur even more uncommonly. Hemangiomas are more common at the placental end of the cord[4], and are usually of no clinical significance, but large ones have been associated with intrauterine demise[516]. Angiomyxomas have also been described[517].

PROLAPSE OF THE UMBILICAL CORD

Cord prolapse is associated with increased perinatal morbidity and mortality. The pathologist may note thrombosis of vessels in such cases, but cord prolapse remains a clinical diagnosis. The risk of cord prolapse is increased with long cords, multiparity, rupture of membranes with an unengaged presenting part, prematurity, and malpresentation. In one study, cord prolapse was associated with obstetrical interventions in 47% of cases[518]. The presenting part can then come down and compress the prolapsed cord. Prolapsed cord is an obstetrical emergency[519].

ENTANGLEMENT OF THE UMBILICAL CORD

Entanglement of the cords is a risk in monoamniotic twin pregnancies, and may occur in singletons with excessively long cords. Tight entanglements may leave indentations on the fetal part entrapped, and may compromise flow through the cord. The cord may also be strangled by amniotic bands[520].

UMBILICAL VASCULITIS AND FUNISITIS

These lesions are described in the sections on chorioamnionitis (Chapter 12).

12

Lesions of the membranes

SQUAMOUS METAPLASIA

Squamous metaplasia of the membranes is a frequently seen phenomenon of no clinicopathologic significance. It is characteristically distributed on the amnion around the cord insertion site and appears as slightly elevated, gray-white plaques, which are usually only a few millimeters in diameter (Figure 86a). Since the plaques represent sites of amniotic epithelial metaplasia, and are not deposits, they cannot be easily removed from the amniotic surface by scraping. This resistance to removal and the peri-insertional distribution are helpful features in distinguishing squamous metaplasia from amnion nodosum, described below. Histologically, the plaques are seen as sites of change in the monolayer of amniotic cuboidal epithelium to a multilayered keratinizing squamous epithelium (Figure 86b). Their location and appearance are compatible with sites of reactive change, due to traction and associated displacement of the amnion from the chorion, at the cord insertion site, that likely occur with fetal movement.

AMNION NODOSUM

Amnion nodosum is seen in cases of severe and longstanding oligohydramnios, and, as such, it is always a

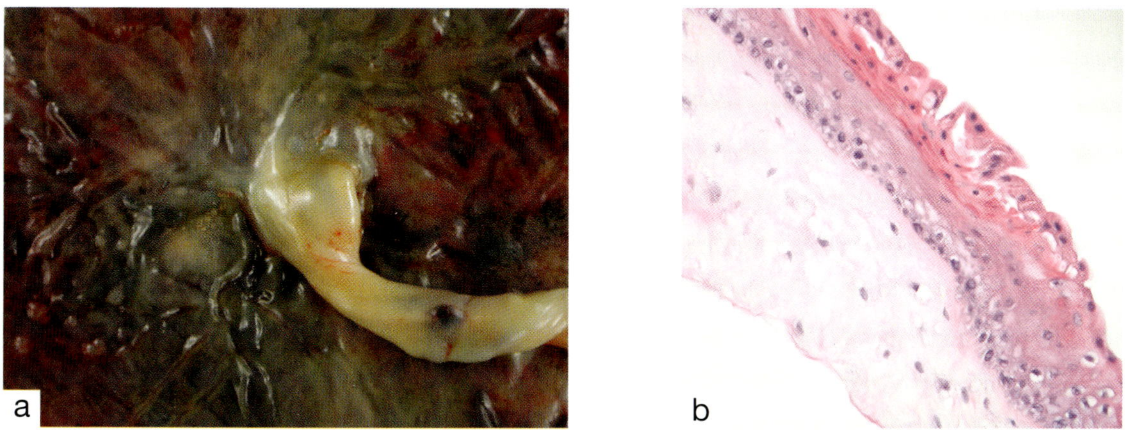

Figure 86 Squamous metaplasia of the amnion. (a) Gross findings: 1–2-mm, tan nodules are present around the cord insertion site. Meconium staining is also present in this case. (b) Histology of squamous metaplasia

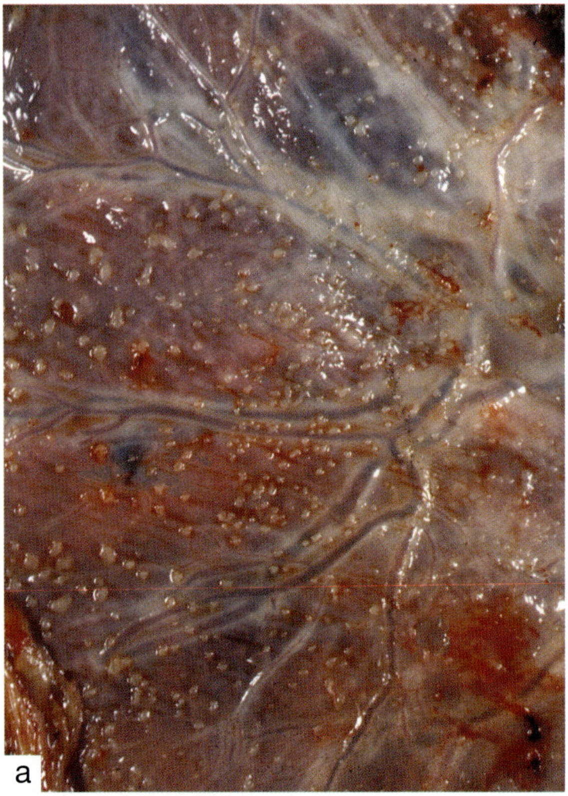

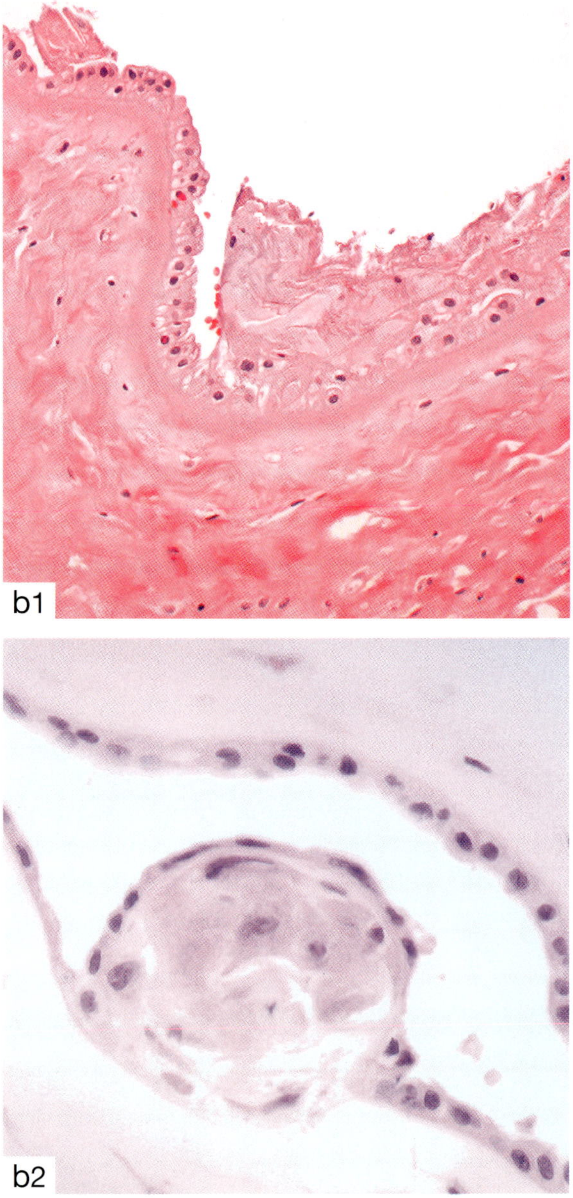

Figure 87 Amnion nodusum. (a) Amnion nodosum diffusely studs the amniotic surface, as tiny yellow-white nodules. (b-1) Microscopically, they are foci of compacted deposits of shed vernix and sebaceous debris. (b-2) The aggregates may become covered over with amniotic epithelium, and seen as clumps of keratinized cellular debris on the membrane roll or fetal surface

pathologic lesion. It is an important marker of fetal genitourinary anomalies and associated pulmonary hypoplasia, and may also be seen in cases of oligohydramnios due to premature membrane rupture and chronic amniorrhea. Amnion nodosum consists of small, yellowish-white nodules (1–5 mm) that are most easily detected on an oblique view of the amnion of the chorionic plate (Figure 87a), but they may also be seen on the amnion of the free membranes and, very rarely, of the umbilical cord. They are readily scraped from and diffusely distributed over the fetal surface, in contrast to the incidental foci of squamous metaplasia. Their gross characteristics reflect their histology: the lesions are composed of deposits of vernix caseosa (an admixture of amorphous, fibrillar, eosinophilic sebum, fetal skin squames, and/or lanugo hairs), compressed and affixed to the fetal surface (Figure 87b-1). In addition, the lesions may demonstrate a covering of regenerated amniotic epithelium (Figure 87b-2). Because of their composition of keratinizing epithelium and skin adnexal structures, placentas from gestations of 26 weeks or less rarely show amnion nodosum, despite an accompanying history of marked oligohydramnios. The pathogenesis of amnion nodosum is unclear, but deficient amniotic fluid volume is generally believed to result in deprivation of nutrients and oxygen that leads to necrosis of and defects in the amniotic epithelium[4]. Presumably, the sites of denudation and secondary exposure of underlying chorionic collagen permit abnormal adherence of 'precipitates' of solid cellular and proteinaceous elements present in abnormally high concentrations, due to the scant amount of amniotic liquor.

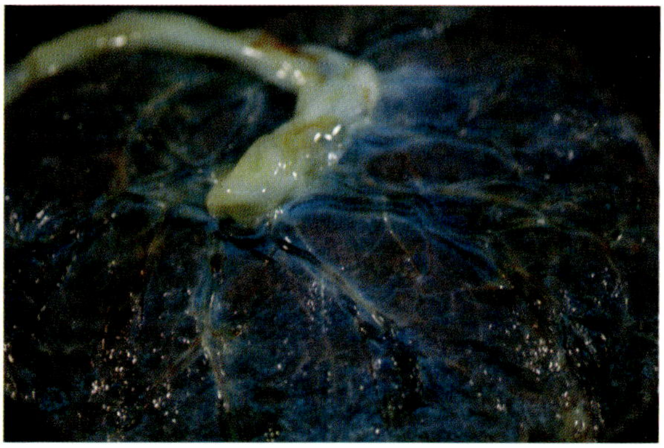

Figure 88 An amniotic web has tethered the umbilical cord to the surface of the placenta

AMNIOTIC CYSTS, RESTS, AND POLYPS

These lesions are rare. Cysts may arise from localized edema (pseudocysts), amniotic epithelial inclusions, or rests of squamous epithelium under the surface epithelium. Cartilaginous or bony rests may rarely occur. Amniotic polyps, composed of hyperplastic epithelium, are of unknown significance.

AMNIOTIC WEB

An amniotic web ('chorda') extends from the fetal surface of the placenta to the cord[521], where it may potentially tether (Figure 88) the cord and/or interfere with circulation in the cord or fetal movement, or result in vascular trauma due to traction.

AMNIOTIC BAND SYNDROME/ AMNIOTIC DISRUPTION SEQUENCE

Amniotic band syndrome (ABS) is characterized by the presence of strands of amnion that are entangled with the umbilical cord and/or fetal parts. These bands are associated with features of strangulation, including cord strangulation with fetal death[520] and/or amputations. In most cases, the findings and the asymmetric distribution of the defects are consistent with sequelae of rupture of the amniotic sac[4,522]. As stated in Chapter 2, the amniotic sac enlarges during the first trimester, as fluid (a transudate of maternal plasma that crosses the chorionic plate and fetal plasma that passes through the nonkeratinized fetal skin) accumulates within it, until, at about 12 weeks of gestation, the amnion apposes the chorion[522]. By prenatal ultrasonographic findings, attachment to the chorion is fully developed by about 17 weeks[523]. With amniotic rupture and its detachment from the chorion, portions of the fetus come to lie within the chorionic cavity, and the shriveled, rolled remnants of amnion become hazards to the fetus. The most common sequelae are amputations of the fingers, likely reflecting their greater vulnerability due to their more active movement[4] (Figure 89 a–c).

Typically, amniotic bands involve constrictions of the cord or asymmetric constrictions or amputations of extremities, and the fetus/infant is otherwise normally formed[4]. Some investigators state that amniotic bands may occur before 12–17 weeks of gestation[523]. However, in some rare cases, broad amniotic *sheets* are seen that are *contiguous* with the fetal skull and/or the fetal abdominoperitoneal sac in cases of limb–body wall complex (LBWC) (limb defects, abdominoschisis, kyphoscoliosis, with or without facial clefting, exencephaly or encephalocele)[4,522,524,525] (Figure 90). While some have proposed that more severe cases of ABS represent very early amnion rupture, there is mounting evidence

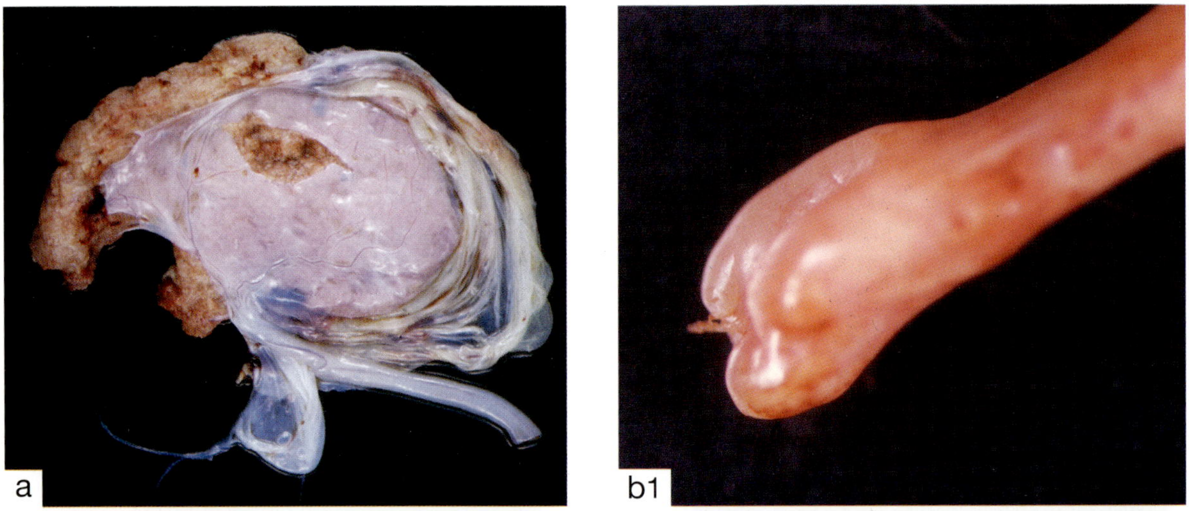

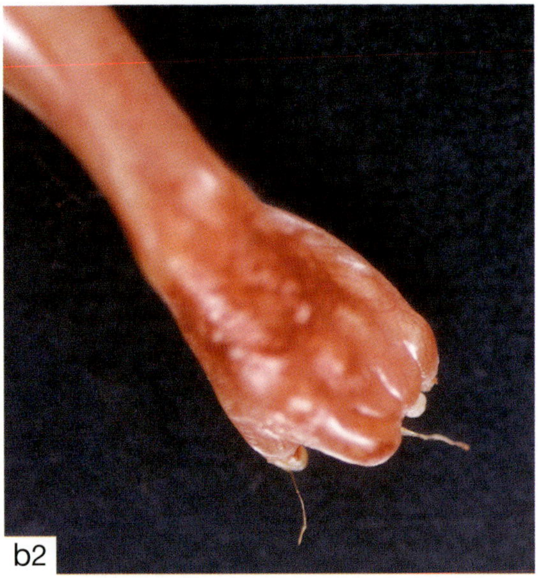

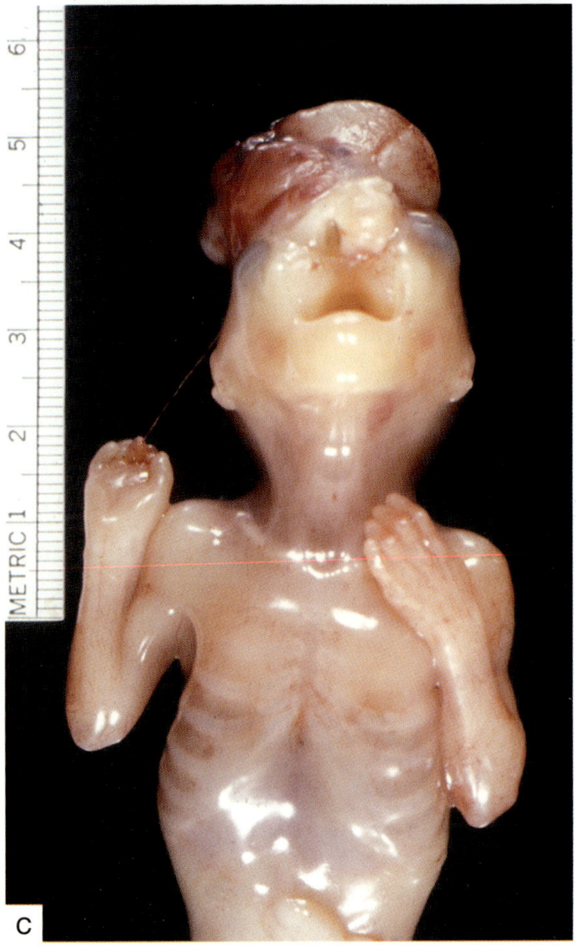

Figure 89 Amniotic band. (a) Delicate amniotic bands were seen around the umbilical cord and as free strands from the chorionic plate. The spontaneously aborted 18-week fetus had bilateral but asymmetric amputations of the fingers and toes. The more severely affected right and the left hands, with strands of the band material, are shown in (b-1) and (b-2), respectively. (c) This previable fetus has a delicate hair-like band from the fingers of the right hand to exposed brain and disrupted skin with central clefting and deformation of the face and skull. A thicker strip of band material is seen crossing the face over the right nasolabial cleft and entangled with band material at the top of the head. A small amount was also present in the oropharyngeal space. The remainder of the fetus was completely normal and surprisingly intact, except for a right toe amputation. (d) Placenta with saccular remains of disrupted amnion surrounding the umbilical cord insertion site, and strands of amniotic bands visible on the right, and also, one on the left center. (e) The free membranes of this placenta also show residual amniotic bands

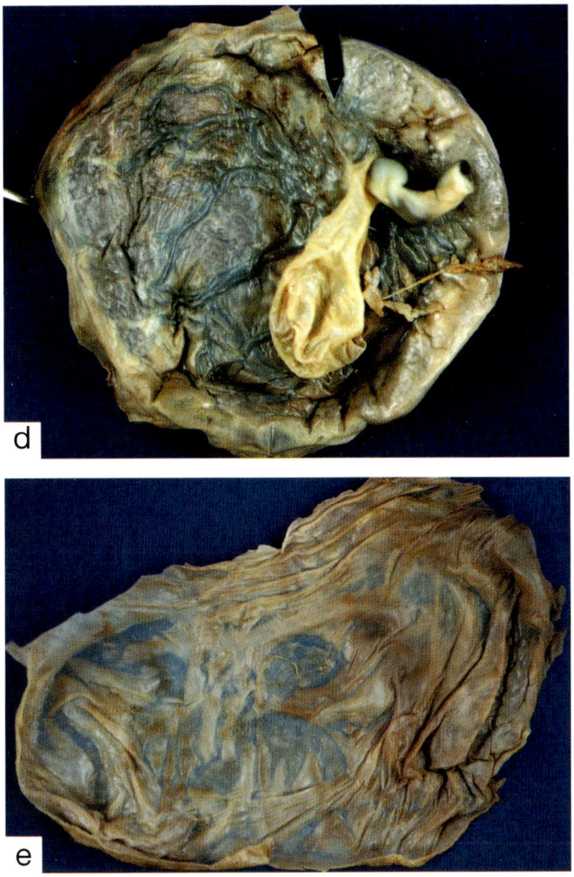

Figure 89 *Continued*

that anomalous complexes with amniotic sheets and/or limb–body complex are due to more complex, and different pathogenetic mechanisms[4], such as epiblast damage to the amnion and embryo[526] and/or malfunction of the ectodermal placodes involving the early embryonic folding process[525]. We concur that amniotic bands should be distinguished from amniotic sheets, even though they both almost always exhibit a sporadic occurrence[4]. In addition to the proposed differences in pathogenesis, they also have very different prognoses; the defects seen with amniotic sheets are associated with severe morbidity and very high mortality (LBWC is lethal)[522].

The proposed pathogenesis for the formation of amniotic bands has led to the use of the alternative term, amniotic disruption sequence (ADS). The notion that amniotic bands adhere to areas of fetal skin, and may be swallowed by the fetus and be associated with facial clefts or other defects (Figure 89c), has led to the use of an additional acronym, ADAM (amniotic deformities, adhesions, mutilations) complex. However, not all investigators concur that amniotic rupture leads to fluid loss from fluid transfer by the chorion or that ensuing oligohydramnios leads to abrasions[4], as was proposed by Lockwood and colleagues[526]. However, the cause of rupture of the amnion remains uncertain. Trauma during pregnancy[523] and hereditary collagen defects occurring in metabolic disorders such as osteogenesis imperfecta or Ehlers–Danlos syndrome (characterized by abnormalities of collagen, fibronectin, etc.)[527] have been implicated in some cases, but bands are not seen in all cases of these conditions and these risks do not explain the overall sporadic occurrence of ABS.

The placenta should be examined in all cases of suspected ABS. In cases of spontaneous abortion or pregnancy termination, both the placenta and the fetus should be submitted to the pathologist. The placenta in ABS shows separation of the amnion from the chorion. The chorionic plate may be devoid of amnion, and relatively opacified-appearing due to macrophage infiltrate, but delicate, shredded-appearing or short amniotic remnants may also remain at the margin or the cord insertion site. In some cases, a remnant saccular structure may be detectable at the cord insertion site, since the amnion is normally firmly attached to the chorion at this location[4] (Figure 89d). Careful examination, including a search of the amniotic surface following submersion of the specimen in water, may be required to identify these remnants. In cases of stillbirth or neonatal death, infant features such as asymmetry of missing parts, constriction grooves on the skin with edema distal to the grooves, fenestrated syndactyly, and demonstration of amniotic bands attached to or encircling fetal parts enable the diagnosis of ABS. Multiple, thin amniotic bands (in the absence of a sheet) may surround several fetal parts, and may represent more than one disruption or fragmentation of a band. The amniotic nature of the bands should be confirmed by histologic examination; microscopic examination reveals connective tissue lined by amniotic epithelium. Inflammatory or degenerative changes are rarely identified.

In cases of suspected ABS, in which a band cannot be identified on the chorionic plate surface, examination of the free membranes may reveal a large area of amniotic necrosis and vernix caseosa in the decidua capsularis[4] or the presence of residual bands (Figure 89e). Apparent amniotic bands may also be seen on ultrasonography in some pregnancies, without detectable amniotic bands on placental examination at delivery. This potential pitfall in the sonographic diagnosis may result from the presence of decidual bands adherent to previously damaged endometrium (previous abortion, myomectomy, infection, etc.). More detailed studies are necessary to elucidate the precise nature of this condition[4,528].

EXTRAMEMBRANOUS PREGNANCY

If the amnion and chorion rupture during pregnancy with prolonged leakage, the fetus may develop out-

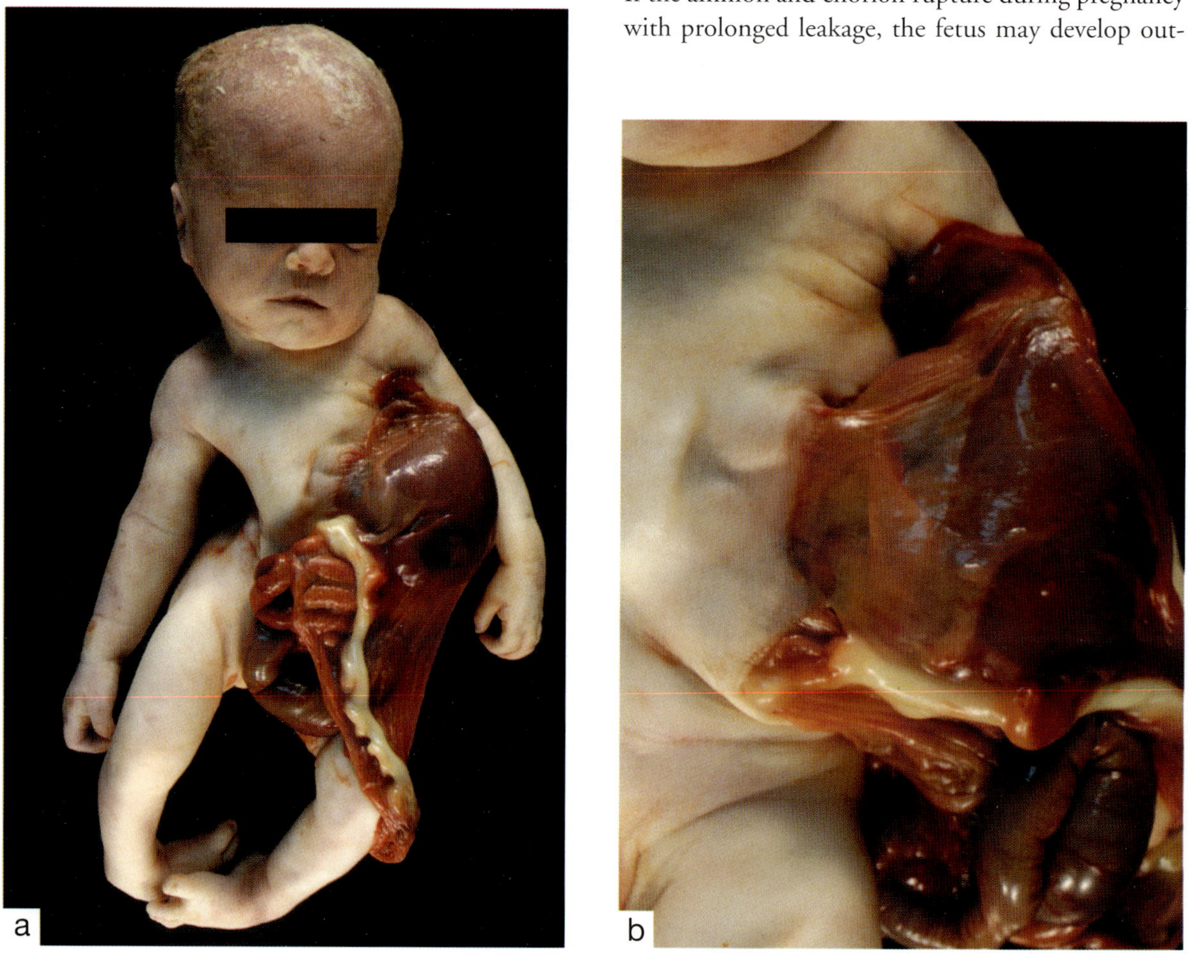

Figure 90 (a) Example of limb–body wall complex. This 38-week gestation infant has a severe thoracoabdominal defect such that the lateral abdominal wall skin is continuous with the amnion of the amniotic sac, there is diminution to absence of the lateral and central thoracoabdominal wall musculature, and the peritoneal sac rests directly on the chorionic surface of the fetal plate of the placenta. The umbilical arteries coursed as separate vessels on either side of the short, broad saccular structure formed by fusion of the amnion with the peritoneum. The right was joined by the umbilical vein, to form a cord-like structure with multiple varices. The infant has multiple anomalies including severe kyphoscoliosis and vertebral defects. Birth resulted in immediate exsanguination. (b) This photograph shows a close-up of the amnioperitoneal membrane, the ectopia of the heart in the pericardium, and the formation of a right-sided aspect of an umbilical cord ensheathed in the fused membranes

side the membranous sac. The remaining sac is small, and the placenta is always circumvallate. These pregnancies usually deliver preterm. Abruption is common. The infant may show the manifestations of oligohydramnios, namely Potter's facies, limb deformities, and pulmonary hypoplasia[529].

EXTRA-AMNIOTIC PREGNANCY

If the amnion ruptures without formation of bands, the fetus may develop within the intact chorion. Remnants of the amnion may be seen as a thickening of the membranes around the cord.

MECONIUM STAINING OF THE MEMBRANES

The fetus may pass meconium during or remote from labor. The obstetrician will observe recent meconium as a dark pea-green, either thick or thin within the amniotic fluid, or as staining of the placenta (Figure 91a) or on the infant's perineum, nails, or skin creases. Old meconium is paler in color. Meconium is usually not passed before 30 weeks of gestation, but this can occur earlier. While traditionally viewed as a sign of fetal distress, meconium may be passed in the absence of distress, and distressed babies may not pass meconium. Passage of meconium becomes more frequent after 40 weeks of gestational age. Occasionally, the pathologist can detect meconium pigment in vernix debris on the amniotic surface histologically. However, more commonly, meconium is detectable upon its uptake by chorionic, vacuolated macrophages as finely granular, golden brown, cytoplasmic pigment (Figure 91b and c). Membrane exposure of greater duration can lead to meconium staining of decidual cells of the capsularis. Meconium can cause vasoconstriction of the umbilical cord and chorionic plate fetal vessels, and even necrosis of the muscular wall of these vessels (Figure 91c), and hence produce significant fetal compromise[530–532]. It has been demonstrated[533] that the wall of chorionic plate vessels that face the amniotic cavity, but not the portion facing the villi, shows significantly increased apoptosis, in cases of meconium-associated vascular necrosis.

The timing of the passage of meconium and penetration through the membranes is a subject that comes up in the legal arena, but is not reliably assessed in the individual case. In addition, meconium may be passed more than once. In one study[534], gross staining occurred at 1 h, and meconium macrophages were present in the amnion after 1 h, and in the chorion by 3 h. However, this was an *in vitro* study, and transmembrane passage may occur after birth if the placenta is not refrigerated or fixed[4].

Pathologic features of meconium staining Grossly, the meconium-stained placenta shows various shades of green to green-brown staining of the fetal surface and membranes (Figure 91a). Edema of the amnion is a consistent feature of meconium staining. The amnion, when exposed to meconium, undergoes reactive changes. Pseudostratification, epithelial disorganization, cuboidal to columnar change, and cytoplasmic vacuolation may be observed (Figure 91d). Alternatively, there may be denudation of the amniotic epithelium. As stated above, pigment-laden macrophages may be seen (Figure 91b). However, it has been shown that exposure of the placental slides to fluorescent lighting markedly diminishes the intensity of the meconium pigment. Hence, protecting the placental slides from excessive light is helpful in retaining the histopathological finding[535]. Yellow-brown discoloration of amniotic debris on the fetal surface of the membranes may also be seen. Meconium containing macrophages may be found in the absence of greenish discoloration of the membranes on gross examination. A diligent and careful search may be necessary for detection of the macrophages.

There are several other findings that may be confused with meconium. The gross appearance of severe chorioamnionitis, with its green-yellow color, may be mistaken for meconium. Meconium is odorless, while there may be an odor with chorioamnionitis, and the histology will clarify the distinction. Pigmented macrophages seen in the membranes may actually contain iron stain-positive hemosiderin, while meconium will be iron stain-negative. The granules of hemosiderin are coarser, golden-brown, and refractile, while meconium produces a less coarse, more diffuse staining, and is more red-brown. Significant maternal hyperbilirubinemia can also result in gross golden-yellow discoloration of the membranes. Meconium does not stain with routine cytochemical stains for bile.

ACUTE CHORIOAMNIONITIS

Acute chorioamnionitis (ACA) may be defined in histologic, clinical, or microbiologic terms. Histologically, ACA consists of an acute inflammatory infiltrate in any of the following: the free membranes, chorionic plate, subchorionic space, vessels of the chorionic plate or umbilical cord, or the Wharton's jelly of the cord. Inflammatory changes may be absent in individual sections of one or more of these structures. Therefore, sections from all of these structures should be routinely assessed for evidence of ACA. The inflammatory changes are more consistently found in the sections that include the site of rupture of the membranes and the undersurface of the chorionic plate[536]. Clinically, ACA is characterized by fever ($\leq 38°C$), leukocytosis, uterine tenderness in the mother, and turbid or foul-smelling amniotic fluid. In many cases, only fever may be present. The other features are present only in severe cases. In those cases where there are no maternal signs, and ACA is diagnosed histologically, the lesion is considered 'silent' ACA. In group B streptococcal infection, cultures from the maternal genital tract and the neonate may be positive in the absence of demonstrable histologic chorioamnionitis[537], and may be considered as ACA in microbiologic terms.

The inflammatory cells seen in the membranes, chorionic plate, and subchorionic space are of maternal origin, and consist predominantly of polymorphonuclear leukocytes (PMNs). The PMNs seen in the cord or chorionic plate vessels are of fetal origin, and may be seen migrating from inside the vessel out, often polarized towards the source of infection in the amniotic sac. The finding of inflammation in the fetal vessels signifies that the fetus has mounted an immune response, and studies suggest that this response and subsequent release of cytokines causing damage to or spasm of large placental blood vessels may be responsible for cases of cerebral palsy, particularly in the preterm neonate[538].

Etiology A variety of bacterial organisms present in the maternal genital tract may lead to ACA. Group B *Streptococcus* (GBS), *Escherichia coli*, and *Staphylococcus*, *Pseudomonas*, *Proteus*, and *Klebsiella* spp. are among the common causes of ACA. Anaerobic organisms, such as *Clostridium perfringens* and *Fusobacterium*, and fastidious organisms, particularly *Mycoplasma hominis* and *Ureaplasma urealyticum*, have also been recognized as important causes of ACA. Of note is that when culture techniques are expanded, *M. hominis* and *U. urealyticum*, together with *Fusobacterium* species, are the most common organisms identified in ascending intrauterine infections[539], and *U. urealyticum* is a leading partner with *E. coli* and group B streptococci as major causes of stillbirth in developing countries[280]. *Chlamydia trachomatis*, which causes acute cervicitis, has been implicated as a cause of premature rupture of the membranes and chorioamnionitis. A rat model of chlamydial chorioamnionitis has been described; however, there is no definite evidence of chlamydial chorioamnionitis in humans, and it has not been isolated from the placenta. Among fungi, *Candida* is the most important, and may produce chorioamnionitis and/or funisitis. Viruses generally produce villitis (see section on villitides in Chapter 10), rather than chorioamnionitis, as do infections with *Listeria* and syphilis. An under-recognized cause of chorioamnionitis is *Fusobacterium*[532], which is difficult to see on routine hematoxylin–eosin stained sections, and is better demonstrated with the Warthin–Starry stain (Figure 92).

Cultures to identify the pathogenic organism are best taken in the delivery room. To obtain cultures, the amnion should be peeled away, and cultures taken between the amnion and chorion. In addition to aerobic and candidal cultures, anaerobic cultures should be obtained as well. Culture for *Mycoplasma*, if the pathology department has appropriate transport media and the means to culture these organisms, is also recommended. If these guidelines are not followed, negative cultures may be obtained in 50% of cases. Because of the negative results on routinely processed cultures and lack of clinical manifestations in the mother and fetus, in such a high proportion of cases with histologic ACA, some investigators have suggested that non-infectious factors such as the maternal immunological reaction to fetal tissue, gastric juice, amniotic debris, meconium, pH changes, and hypertonicity of the amniotic fluid may be the cause(s) of ACA. Lauweryns and colleagues[540] failed to produce any inflammatory reaction in the membranes (or fetal lungs) when amniotic debris, meconium, gastric juice, and acidified amniotic fluid were injected into the amniotic sac of pregnant rabbits. They concluded that ACA is always infectious in origin. Furthermore, as indicated above, the high proportion of negative results of cultures is likely related to the lack of use of proper methodology for culture

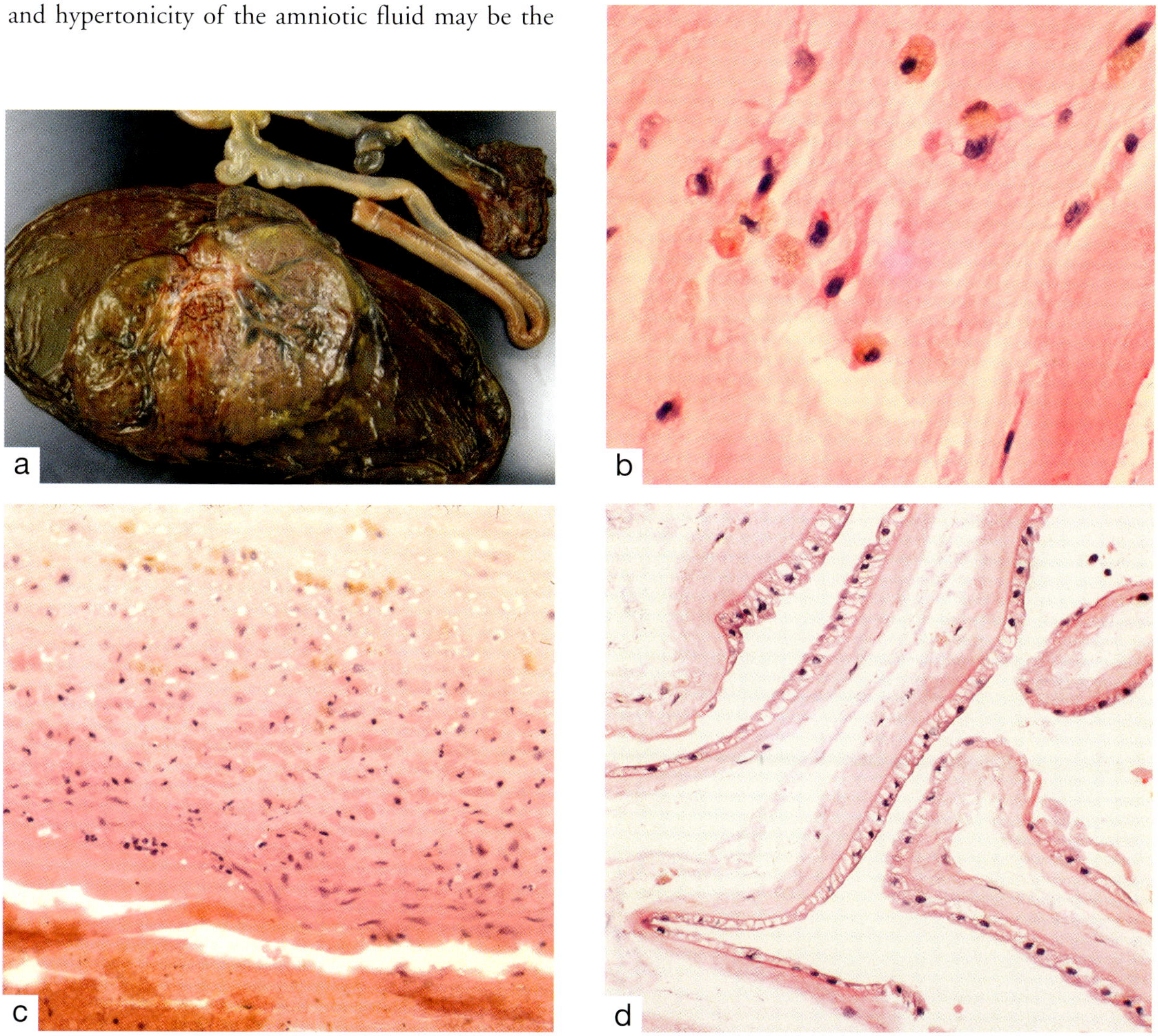

Figure 91 Meconium staining. (a) Dark green-brown meconium staining is evident on the fetal surface, the free membranes, and the cord. (b) Brown, finely granular, pigment is seen within chorionic macrophages. (c) Brownish meconium-laden macrophages are seen in a region of degeneration of vascular smooth muscle. (d) The amniotic epithelium may slough and/or the cells may become vacuolated and taller, when exposed to meconium, as shown here

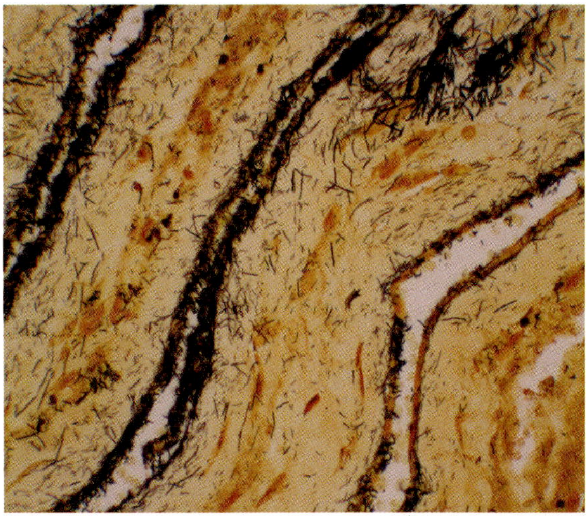

Figure 92 Fusobacterium. The filamentous organisms are demonstrated by Warthin–Starry stain on sections of membrane roll

of fastidious organisms, and the absence of clinical manifestations may be due to low virulence of the infecting organisms.

ACA is usually due to an ascending infection, in contrast to villitis, which largely represents hematogenous transmission of pathogens from the mother to the fetus. Anything that facilitates cervical entry of organisms into the gestational sac, such as cervical incompetence and vaginal examination or instrumentation, can increase the likelihood of developing ACA, but many organisms can penetrate intact membranes. Loss or diminution of bactericidal factors (lysozyme, immunoglobulins, etc.) in the amniotic fluid due to prematurity, presence of meconium, or unknown reasons may contribute to the occurrence of ACA[541,542].

Since the membranes covering the cervical os are those first exposed to infecting organisms, the inflammatory infiltrate on microscopic examination is generally most evident at the site of membrane rupture (which should be at the center of the membrane roll taken for histologic section). A slight infiltrate of neutrophils at the rupture site may be reactive and due to trauma from fetal head contact and membrane rupture, rather than representing an inflammatory response to an ascending infection. Inflammation limited to the point of rupture should be interpreted with caution, particularly in a stillbirth, where this may be a postmortem change.

As noted above, the neutrophilic infiltration in the free membranes and the initial infiltrate of the chorionic plate represent a maternal response (from the maternal blood vessels in the decidua vera and blood of the maternal space supplied by vessels in the decidua basalis, respectively). In both the free membranes and the chorionic plate, neutrophils first infiltrate the subchorion and then the chorion, to which they may be confined in many cases. Of note is that in dichorionic diamniotic twin placentas, ACA may be confined to the membranes of twin A's (the presenting twin) placenta, with no ACA seen in the membranes of the placenta of twin B. (However, ACA of the placenta of twin B is not seen in the absence of ACA of that of twin A.) Acute inflammation of the chorionic plate is seen first as maternal neutrophils, originating from the intervillous space, forming clusters or a linear aggregation along the undersurface of the chorionic plate. Subsequent migration into and up through the chorion also involves the amnion, as the PMNs respond to bacteria, bacterial byproducts, and other chemoattractants in the amniotic fluid.

The umbilical cord is also exposed to the organisms in the amniotic fluid, and there is a *fetal* neutrophilic response, most commonly first originating from the umbilical vein, and later, from one, and then both, of the arteries (umbilical vasculitis); the inflammation may subsequently extend out into Wharton's jelly (funisitis). Umbilical vasculitis and funisitis are usually eccentric since the inflammatory response is directed towards the organisms in the amniotic cavity.

The fetal response in the umbilical cord may also be followed/accompanied by ACA of the chorionic plate in which a fetal neutrophilic response can be seen originating in the blood vessels of the chorionic plate; this egress of neutrophils into and through the vessel wall is referred to as 'chorionic vasculitis', and exhibits polarity; it is oriented toward the amniotic surface and fluid. This vasculitis also does not extend beyond the chorionic plate into the stem or chorionic villous vessels. However, focal acute villitis may occur if there is fetal septicemia; presumably, in fetal septicemia, organisms gain access to the fetal blood via intrauterine aspiration of infected amniotic fluid. Amniotic neutrophils and organisms may enter developing lung and stomach lumina with normal fetal breathing and swallowing movements, and evidence of such intrauterine aspiration/ingestion can include the presence of neutrophils in the lumina of alveoli and/or of the gastrointestinal tract of the fetus. The neutrophils seen in the fetal airspaces have been largely regarded as being maternal in origin, but recent literature has suggested that they may be of fetal (lung microvascular) origin. Scott and colleagues[543] showed that 70–80% of neutrophils in airspaces of five male fetuses were found to contain the Y chromosome, consistent with fetal origin. Gastric samples were not evaluated in this study, however, so it is possible that the aspirated neutrophils containing the Y chromosome may also have included PMNs from the amniotic fluid that migrated out of fetal plate or cord vessels.

Pathology Grossly, the membranes may appear opaque and yellow or yellow-green (Figure 93a), although there may be no grossly recognizable feature. Histologic ACA may not be present in all placental sections, so it is important to take an adequate number of sections. Inclusion of the point of rupture in the membrane roll, and sections incorporating the subchorionic space, will maximize the chances of finding the inflammatory cells.

The neutrophilic response in ACA may vary from minimal and focal to severe and diffuse. It is worth re-emphasizing that, in GBS infection, there may an absence or paucity of inflammatory response[537]. Conversely, the nuclei of the cells of the chorion may show pyknosis, which may be mistaken for a neutrophilic infiltrate. In addition, the subchorionic fibrinoid may passively 'entrap' an occasional PMN from the maternal space (non-specifically chemotaxed by the presence of fibrinoid material) and scattered, sparse numbers of neutrophils in the subchorion should not be overinterpreted as subchorionitis.

ACA may be graded in the chorionic plate according to the criteria of Blanc[544] (Figure 94); stage I, acute subchorionic intervillositis (Figure 93b); stage II, acute chorionitis; stage III, acute chorioamnionitis (Figure 93c). A more recently proposed nomenclature is shown in Table 11[545]. As noted above, acute chorioamnionitis can also be considered in terms of maternal and fetal response, particularly in light of recent evidence of the significance of the fetal inflammatory response (cited previously and below). The fetal response is shown in Figure 93d (chorionic vasculitis) and 93e (umbilical vasculitis and funisitis). Fetal plate vascular thrombosis (Figure 93f) and/or mural necrosis may also be seen and may be involved in the pathologic mechanisms of adverse neurologic sequelae in the infant[546].

Clinical significance of ACA ACA has been linked to premature labor, placental abruption, fetal/neonatal sepsis, and neonatal respiratory distress syndrome, chronic lung disease, intraventricular hemorrhage, periventricular leukomalacia, and later findings of cerebral palsy. In addition, ACA is detected in 40–60% of placentas from very-low-birth-weight infants[29]. Despite the severe perinatal morbidity with ACA, associated maternal sepsis is rare, and ACA and maternal fever have been linked to the use of epidural analgesia in labor, possibly due to prolonged labor[547]. Finally, it needs to be re-emphasized that ACA, although it is associated with prolonged rupture of the membranes, can also be the cause of premature rupture of the membranes.

The most important and most frequent complication of ACA appears to be the initiation of premature labor. Of note is that one-quarter to one-third of preterm deliveries are attributed to ascending intrauterine infection[548,549]. Phospholipases from the bacteria and neutrophils of ACA cause the release of prostaglandins from the membranes[536]. Uterine contractions and dilatation of the cervix due to prostaglandin release herald the onset of premature labor. Collagenases and elastases of neutrophilic origin produce rupture of the membranes. Premature labor culminates in delivery of a premature infant, with all the sequelae of prematurity, who may in

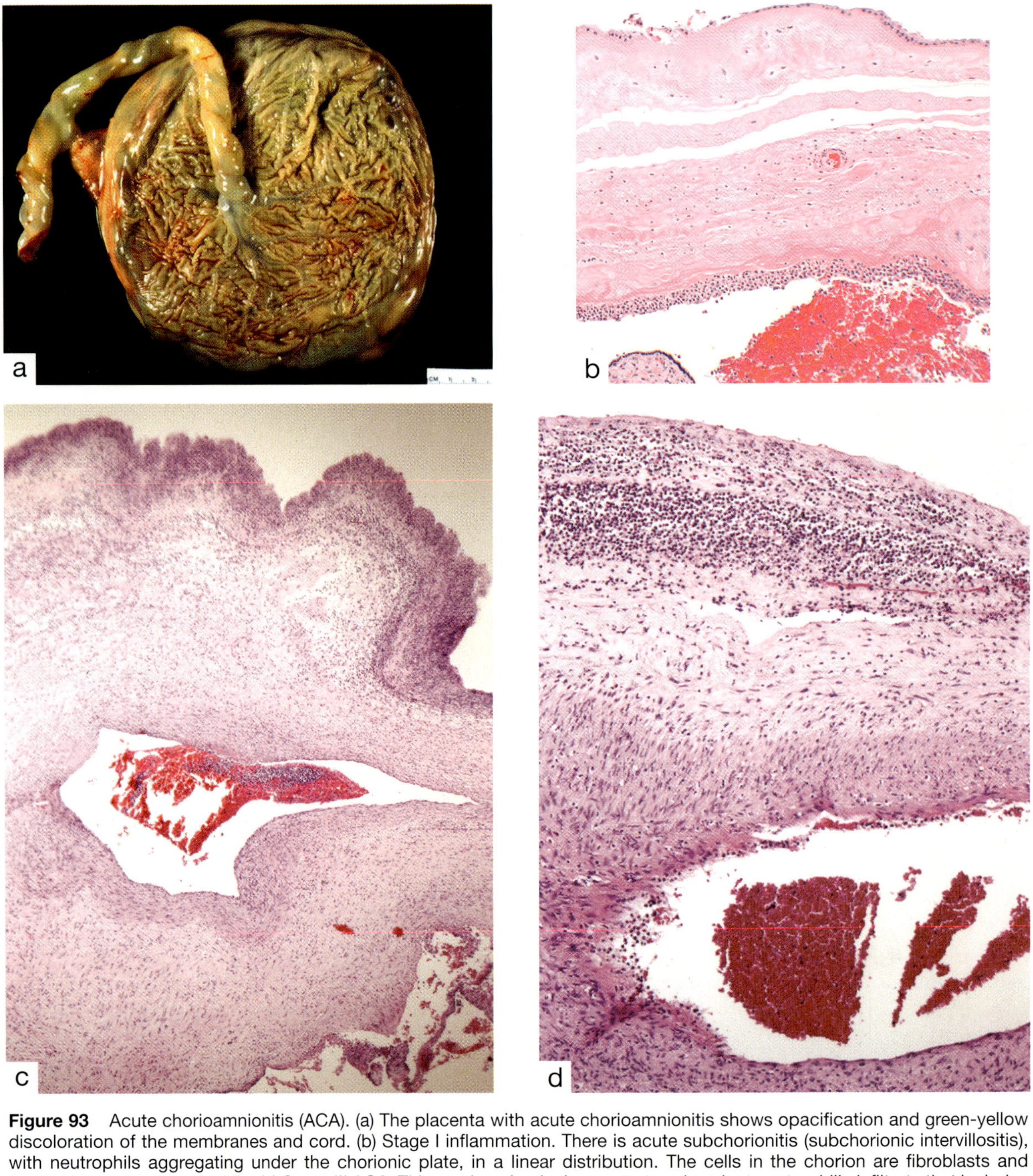

Figure 93 Acute chorioamnionitis (ACA). (a) The placenta with acute chorioamnionitis shows opacification and green-yellow discoloration of the membranes and cord. (b) Stage I inflammation. There is acute subchorionitis (subchorionic intervillositis), with neutrophils aggregating under the chorionic plate, in a linear distribution. The cells in the chorion are fibroblasts and macrophages, not neutrophils. (c) Stage III ACA. This section clearly demonstrates abundant neutrophilic infiltrate that includes involvement of the chorionic plate (fulfilling stage II) and the amniotic epithelium (and therefore, also stage III). (d) Acute chorionic vasculitis. The neutrophils are of fetal origin, evidenced by their margination within the vascular lumen of the fetal plate and their migration into the subamniotic chorion and amnion. Their migration exhibits polarity toward the amniotic sac. (e) Acute umbilical arteritis–like chorionic vasculitis; this fetal response is manifested as migration of the inflammatory cells from the vascular lumen outward, through Wharton's jelly (funisitis) toward the amniotic surface of the cord. (f) Acute thrombosis is also present with this chorionic plate vasculitis

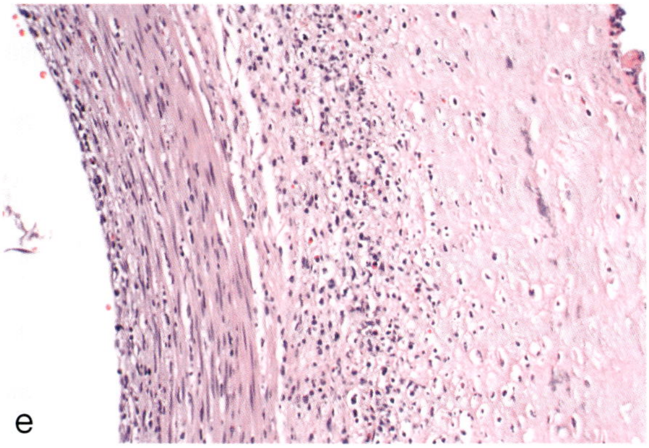

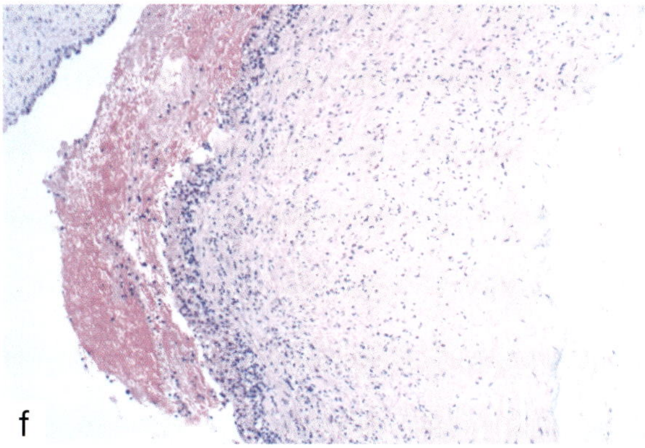

Figure 93 *Continued*

addition have pneumonitis. In a prospective, case-controlled study, Hillier and colleagues[549] found that infection of the chorioamnion is strongly related to histologic chorioamnionitis, and may be related to premature birth. The organisms that were most frequently isolated included *Ureaplasma urealyticum* and *Gardnerella*. However, *C. trachomatis*, *Neisseria gonorrhoeae*, *Trichomonas vaginalis*, GBS, *M. hominis*, and *Bacteroides* species have also been implicated as being associated with prematurity[3,4,549].

As indicated above, the fetus may develop intrauterine pneumonitis secondary to aspiration of infected amniotic fluid, or as a fetal response, or both, as well as septicemia, with subsequent potential for intrauterine death, or neonatal morbidity or mortality. Infected amniotic fluid is also swallowed into the gastrointestinal tract and gains access to the middle ears due to passage through the eustachian tube[148].

Recent literature has focused on the significance of the clinical condition of fetal inflammatory responsc syndrome (FIRS)[548] due to the release of cytokines, and their roles in initiating fetal organ damage, in cases of ACA. As noted above, the *histologic* evidence of a fetal inflammatory response is seen in fetal vessels as acute umbilical vasculitis and funisitis, and in the chorionic plate as acute chorionic vasculitis, and numerous studies have linked the histopathologic findings in ACA with elevated amniotic fluid and fetal/neonatal blood cytokine levels. Pacora and colleagues[550] found that increased fetal plasma interleukin 6 (IL-6) levels were associated with inflammation of the membranes and cord, and that significantly higher levels were associated with the presence of funisitis, and/or chorionic vasculitis, strongly suggesting that these histolopathologic vascular findings are evidence of a fetal inflammatory response. In addition, Mittendorf and associates[551] found funisitis to be a more specific predictor of high IL-6 levels and of neurologic impairment, and Yoon and co-workers[552] found elevated IL-6 associated with bronchopulmonary dysplasia. Recently, a subset of chorioamnionitis (and funisitis), termed subacute chorioamnionitis[245,553,554], whose histopathology is compatible with prolonged inflammation of the chorionic plate and which is associated with a variety of fetal blood proinflammatory cytokines, has been associated with a particular risk for chronic lung disease of the so-called 'dry lung' type[553,554], especially when seen in combination with amniotic necrosis[554]. The inflammatory infiltrate in subacute chorioamnionitis includes eosinophils, but the pathology of this form is distinct from the histologically focal and very rare eosinophilic and T-lymphocytic CD3+ cell chorionic inflammation identified by Fraser and Wright, in which the inflammatory cells radiate *away* from the amniotic cavity[555].

The largest emphasis of investigations of the relationship of ACA and elevations of inflammatory mediators as risk factors for infant morbidity has been focused on their linkage to cerebral palsy (CP). A full discussion of intrauterine infection as a risk for CP is beyond the scope of this manual. However, some have linked proinflammatory cytokines with

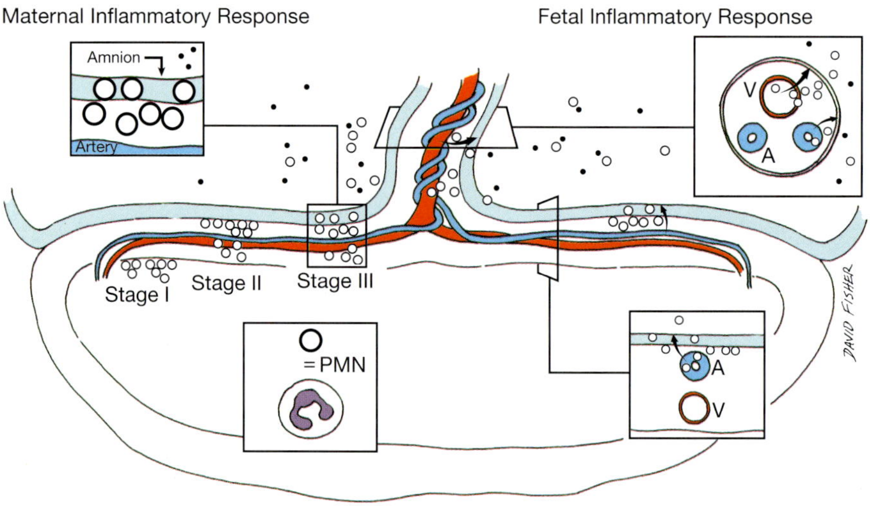

Figure 94 Acute chorioamnionitis: The left side of the diagram shows the stages of acute chorioamnionitis, the right, the fetal response, in ascending intrauterine infection. The open circles (o) represent neutrophils, the solid dots (•), bacteria. Maternal neutrophils aggregate in the subchorionic intervillous space (stage I), migrate into the chorion (stage II), and then into the amnion (stage III). Fetal neutrophils migrate from the umbilical vein out into Wharton's jelly, and into the amnion; an inflammatory response from an umbilical artery usually follows the venous one. Fetal response in the chorionic plate is first manifest in the arteries. The arteries show neutrophilic margination along the endothelial surface closest to the amniotic cavity, then a neutrophilic egress across the vascular smooth muscle, followed by a migration into the subamniotic chorion, and then an infiltration of the amnion. PMN, polymorphonuclear cells; A, artery; V, vein

CP in the very-low-birth-weight and/or premature infant[538,552], and others have not found intrauterine infection to be an independent risk factor for CP, when prematurity and low birth weight were factored[556]. Research into the relationship between ACA, FIRS, and CP and other long-term childhood disabilities and illnesses, including asthma[557] and autism[558–560], and other disorders, is currently in progress. Antenatal cytokines seem to exert direct and immediate deleterious effects on fetal tissues and their development, but these mediators may also initiate a self-perpetuating inflammatory response in the fetus. This ongoing response may participate in or predispose the infant to the development of neurologic and organ damage during infancy, and the risks may be exacerbated with superimposed infections by common viral diseases during childhood[558,561,562].

Investigations into the perinatal transmission of HIV have led to decreased transmission rates with appropriate antiviral therapy of the mother and the newborn infant. Studies have sought to evaluate the placental factors associated with perinatal transmission in these pregnancies. Although many of the placentas of women who are HIV-positive are normal, the presence of ACA has been suggested as facilitating peripartum transmission of the virus[384] (see section on 'Villitis' in Chapter 10).

CHRONIC CHORIOAMNIONITIS

Chronic chorioamnionitis (CCA), defined as infiltration of the membranes, chorionic plate, and/or umbilical cord by mature lymphocytes, with or without plasma cells, histiocytes, and large lymphocytes and immunoblasts[249], is rare (Figure 95). Most cases are of unknown origin, and are often associated with a chronic lymphohistiocytic villitis (see section on 'Villitides' in Chapter 10); however, some may occur

Table 11 Placenta reaction patterns related to amniotic fluid infection: nomenclature and definitions. Modified from reference 545, with permission

Diagnostic categories	*Suggested diagnostic terminology*	*Definitions*
Maternal inflammatory response		
Stage		
1 early	acute subchorionitis or chorionitis	PMN in subchorionic fibrin and/or membrane trophoblast
2 intermediate	acute chorioamnionitis	diffuse-patchy PMN in fibrous chorion and/or amnion
3 advanced	necrotizing chorioamnionitis	PMN karyorrhexis, amniocyte necrosis, and/or amnion basement membrane thickening/hypereosinophilia
Grade		
1 mild–moderate	no special terminology required	not severe as defined below
2 severe	severe acute chorioamnionitis or with subchorionic microabscesses	confluent PMN (aggregates of $\geq 10 \times 20$ cells) between chorion and deciduas; ≥ 3 isolated foci or continuous band
other	chronic (or subacute) chorioamnionitis	subamniotic mononuclear cell infiltrate with occasional PMN (meconium and hemosiderin-laden macrophages excluded)
Fetal inflammatory response		
Stage		
1 early	with chorionic vasculitis or umbilical phlebitis	intramural PMN – chorionic vessels and/or umbilical vein
2 intermediate	with umbilical vasculitis (one or two arteries ± vein) or umbilical panvasculitis (all vessels)	intramural PMN – umbilical artery or arteries (± umbilical vein)
3 advanced	with (subacute) necrotizing funisitis or with concentric umbilical perivasculitis	PMN ± associated debris in concentric bands/rings/halos around one or more umbilical vessels
Grade		
1 mild–moderate	no special terminology required	not severe as defined below
2 severe	with a severe fetal inflammatory response or with intense chorionic (umbilical) vasculitis	near confluent intramural PMN – chorionic and/or umbilical vessels with attenuation/degeneration of VSMC
other	with associated fetal vessel thrombi	recent thrombosis associated with intramural PMN
Other specific features	peripheral funisitis	focal aggregates of PMN at the umbilical cord surface
	acute villitis	PMN in villous stroma (or between trophoblast and stroma)
	acute intervillositis with intervillous abscesses	patchy-diffuse PMN in intervillous space
	decidual plasma cells	unequivocal plasma cells in decidua basalis or capsularis

PMN, polymorphonuclear cells; VSMC, vascular smooth muscle cells

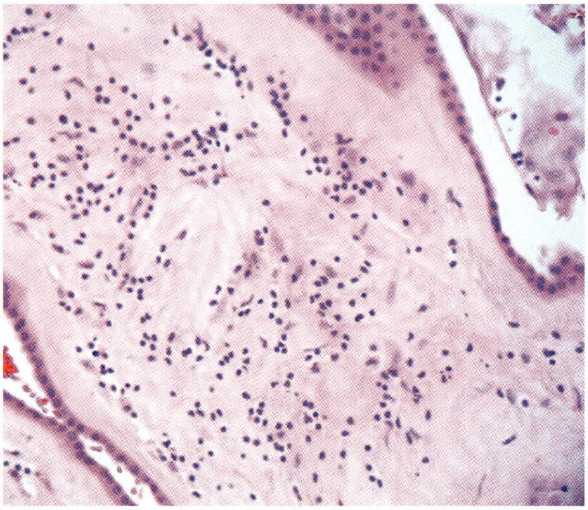

Figure 95 Chronic chorioamnionitis in which the infiltrate is generally lymphohistiocytic and patchy

in the absence of villitis, or in association with chronic or subacute necrotizing funisitis[563,564]. In a series of 31 cases of chronic chorioamnionitis, Jacques and Qureshi[353] found that 71% had associated villitis of unknown etiology. A tendency towards low birth weight may relate to the association with villitis[249]. Some cases may be due to herpes simplex, toxoplasmosis, or syphilis.

FUNISITIS

Acute funisitis is most often seen in association with ACA. The neutrophils may be seen migrating out of the fetal vessels into Wharton's jelly (Figure 96a). *Candida* may be a cause of isolated acute funisitis, although many of these cases have associated ACA, and a small percentage of cases have evidence of congenital candidiasis[406]. Characteristically, in candidal funisitis, multiple tiny white-yellow nodules are seen on the surface of the cord (Figure 96b-1), which are foci of subamniotic microabscess formation by hematoxylin–eosin stain (Figure 96b-2). The organisms may be identified with fungal stains such as Gomori methenamine silver (Figure 96b-3 and b-4). Syphilis may be associated with necrotizing

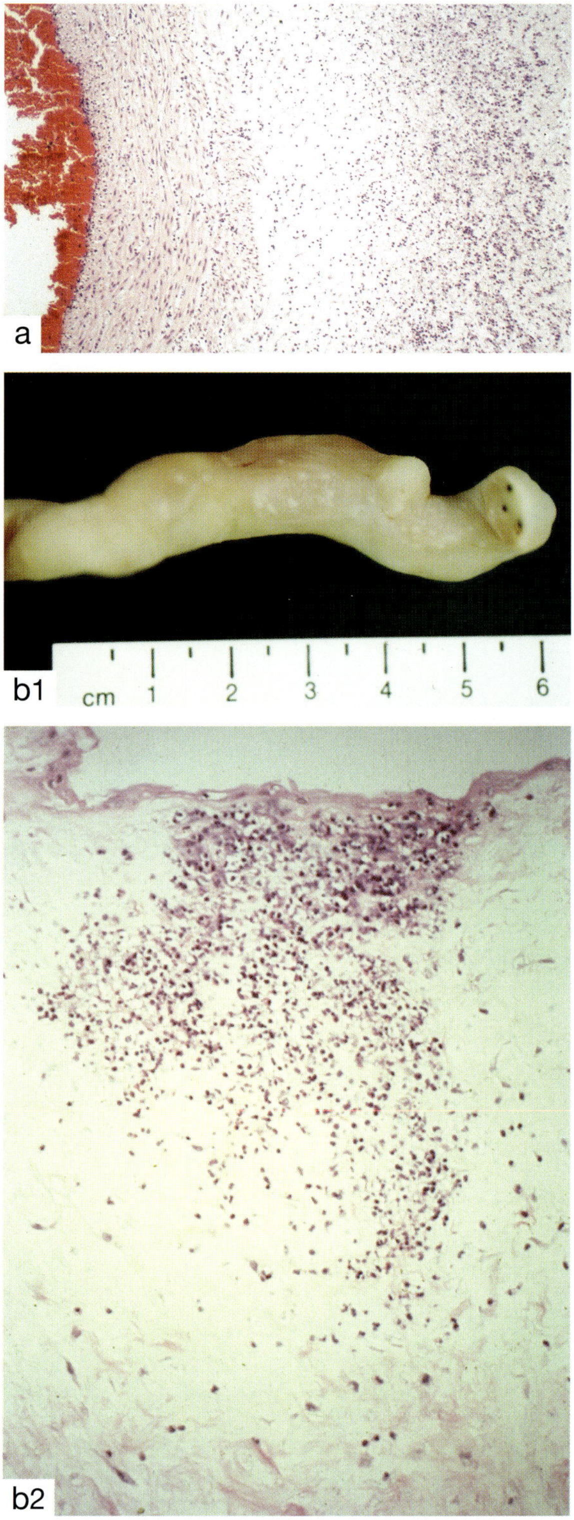

Figure 96 *See opposite for legend*

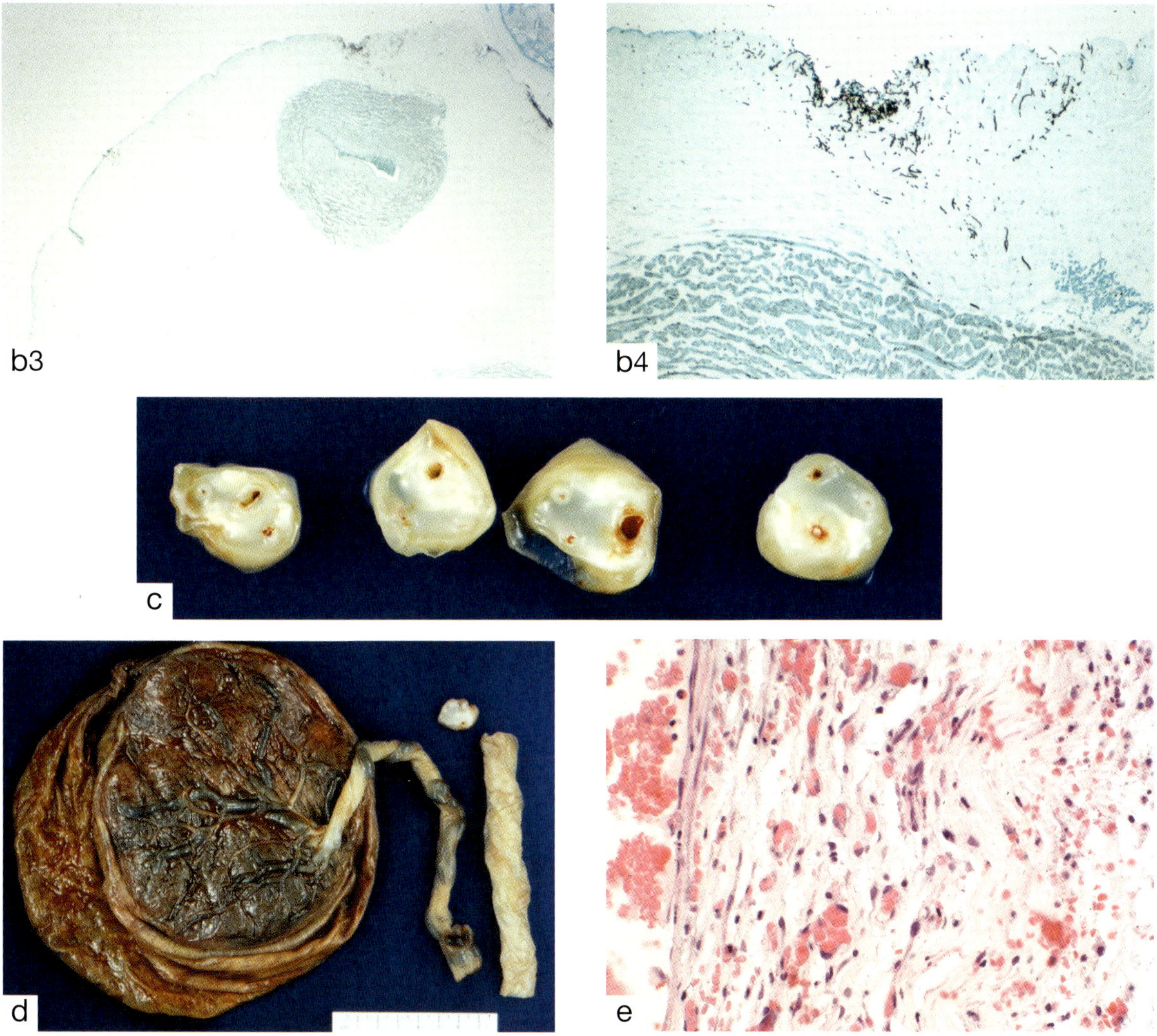

Figure 96 Necrotizing funisitis. (a) Neutrophils migrate out into Wharton's jelly toward the amniotic surface. The inflammatory waves encounter invading organisms and their interactions produce arcs of inflammatory debris in Wharton's jelly, near the amniotic surface. These may calcify (see Figures 77 and 96c). (b-1) Necrotizing funisitis due to *Candida* funisitis. *Candida* funisitis is seen as punctate, 1–2-mm, yellow-white nodules on the cord. They generally track the coils of the cord vessels and are first noted along the perimeter of the umbilical vein. A hand lens and tangential lighting are helpful in detecting their presence. A false knot is present on the left. (b-2) Hematoxylin–eosin stained section of subamniotic microabscess typical of candidal funisitis. The lesion is highly characteristic, but not specific for the organism. (b-3) *Candida* psuedohyphae revealed with Gomori methenamine silver stain in subamniotic foci in this low-power photomicrograph of an umbilical cord with subamniotic microabscesses. (b-4) High-power photomicrograph of the pseudophyphae in the upper lesion in (b-3) (×400). (c) Several cut surfaces of umbilical cord are shown. They demonstrate arc-like, white to yellow-white deposits in Wharton's jelly in the spaces between the amniotic surfaces of the cord segments and the vessels within. The cords are edematous and the vessels are somewhat thickened as well. (d) Sclerosing necrotizing funisitis. Placenta and cord segments from a case of a live-born 35-week gestation age infant with marked growth restriction due to chronic *Candida albicans* infection. Note that the umbilical cord is alternately thin and sclerotic, to thicker, white-yellow and wrinkled. The thicker segment was also rigid due to sclerosis and calcification. Note the white punctate subamniotic region lesions on the cord cross-section. (e) Reactive neovascularization in the wall of the umbilical vein in necrotizing funisitis (due to *Toxoplasma gondii*, cysts not included in image)

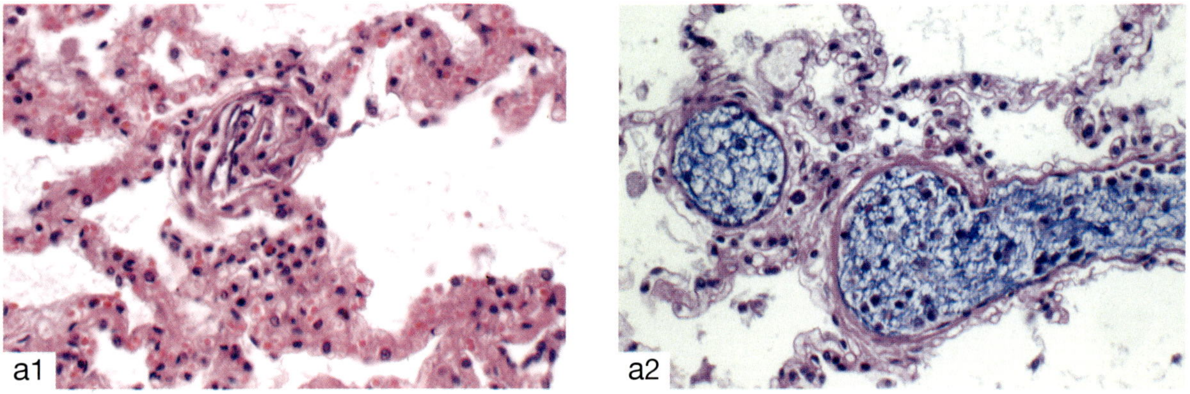

Figure 97 Amniotic fluid embolism. (a-1) Hematoxylin–eosin section showing squames in pulmonary arteriole. (a-2) Alcian blue stain for neutral mucin shows abundant positive material in pulmonary arterioles in this section of lung

funisitis[565] or it may be polymicrobial[353]. Necrotizing funisitis is grossly characterized by whitish-yellow, firm to gritty, perivascular arcs of material deposited between the vessels and the cord surface (Figure 96c), that microscopically consists of an admixture of inflammatory cells, necrotic debris, and/or calcium (Figures 96a and 77).

Subacute necrotizing funisitis has been associated with high rates of perinatal infection and death[564]. Subacute funisitis is characterized by a mixed acute and chronic inflammatory infiltrate. Sclerosing funisitis is characterized by a rigid cord, in which sclerosis and an inflammatory exudate are seen around the umbilical cord vessels (Figure 96d). The etiology remains undetermined in many cases. Rarely, cases of chronic funisitis, characterized by lymphoplasmacytic infiltrate, coagulative necrosis of the vascular media with calcification, and association with chronic chorioamnionitis and funisitis, may be related to viral infections[563]. Navarro and Blanc identified pox virus and herpes simplex virus each in one case[563]. Chronic changes can also include reactive neovascularization within the thickened walls of damaged vessels, such as in *Toxoplasma* infection (Figure 96e).

Genest and colleagues[566] have described a lesion that they term umbilical cord 'pseudovasculitis', seen in second-trimester fetal deaths, where autolytic changes in the nuclei of smooth muscle cells of the umbilical vasculature mimic a neutrophilic infiltrate.

AMNIOTIC FLUID EMBOLISM

In this condition, amniotic fluid and its particulate elements (fetal squames and hair, gastrointestinal mucin and cellular debris, sebaceous fat, and possibly meconium) gain access to the maternal circulation through breaches in the barrier between maternal blood and amniotic cavity. Access of at least squamous elements may not always be pathologic, since squames have been identified in the pulmonary blood of pregnant women subject to pulmonary arterial catheterization or invasive hemodynamic monitoring studies in the peripartum period[567,568]. However, in about 1 in 20 000 deliveries, amniotic fluid embolism (AFE) manifests as a catastrophic event with maternal hypoxia, hypotension, and consumptive coagulopathy, during or following precipitous or difficult labor, cesarean section delivery, delivery complicated by placenta previa or accreta, or in association with elective termination during the second trimester. The manifestations of AFE are not fully explainable as sequelae of sudden pulmonary arterial obstruction due to embolization, and more closely resemble anaphylaxis- or sepsis-like reactions, in which pathologic cascades are initiated by proinflammatory mediators and chemokines. Of note, endothelin-1 expression by fetal squames recovered from maternal lung vessels from fatal cases of AFE has been identified[569]. Other mediators will likely also be identified, and may include TNF, released upon bile-induced endothelial injury, or potentially even cytokines, such as IL-6, that are present in the amniotic liquor, due to an ascending amniotic fluid infection.

In fatal cases, pathologic documentation at autopsy requires demonstration of squames and mucin (by Alcian blue or mucicarmine stain) in the lumina of branches of pulmonary arteries (Figure 97a). Lipid demonstration (in the absence of evidence of bone marrow elements) on frozen section is also helpful. Of these, we favor Alcian blue, since with pH variation, it can be used to demonstrate the presence of neutral mucins. If such methods fail to demonstrate the presence of amniotic fluid particulates, in cases of clinically suspected AFE, then immunohistochemical stains for fetal isoantigen A and mucin-type glycoprotein[570] should be considered. Placental examination is not helpful in the diagnosis. Amniotic debris dissecting between amnion and chorion, in the absence of chorionic reaction, seen in some placentas is considered to be incidental and unrelated to AFE[571].

TUMORS OF THE PLACENTAL MEMBRANES

Placental teratomas, described above, lie between the amnion and the chorion on the fetal surface or at the placental margin. Therefore, these tumors can be considered to arise primarily in the membranes. The two reports of intramembranous leiomyomas, by Misselevich and colleagues[464] and Tarim and associates[465], have also been previously addressed in Chapter 10. A localized thickening in the membranes related to a vanished twin may be mistaken for a tumor (see section on 'Types of placentas in twin pregnancy' in Chapter 15).

13

Abnormalities of the decidua

TERMINOLOGY

Decidua basalis (DB) is the decidua at the maternal surface of the placental disk, decidua capsularis (DC) is the decidua attached to the free membranes of the protruding embryo, and decidua parietalis (DP) or decidua vera is the decidua lining the uterine cavity. The DC fuses with the DP at about 17 weeks' gestation when the membranes come into contact with the uterine wall, largely obliterating the uterine cavity.

DECIDUITIS

Chronic deciduitis, defined as increased lymphocytes and the presence of plasma cells in the decidua, is a poorly defined entity, which has been postulated to correlate with TORCH infections (toxoplasmosis, other infections, rubella, cytomegalovirus infection, herpes simplex), abnormal maternal immune status, or pelvic inflammatory disease[15]. However, it is likely that these conditions are absent in the majority of observed cases. The lesion has been associated with IUGR. Chronic deciduitis may accompany specific villitides and VUE. Mild acute inflammatory infiltrates of the decidua are common and not pathological. Keski-Nisula and colleagues[572] found a high frequency of decidual low-grade inflammation in clinically non-infected gestations after labor ensued. Widespread severe acute deciduitis, often associated with necrosis of the decidua, is associated with ACA.

DECIDUAL VASCULOPATHY

Decidual vasculopathy is most often seen in preeclampsia, but may be seen in other maternal conditions such as systemic lupus erythematosus or antiphospholipid syndrome (see Chapter 14), and there is an increased incidence of vascular as well as thrombotic placental changes in the placentas of women with autoantibodies[573]. The earliest changes appreciable are absence of the usual physiologic remodeling of maternal decidual arterioles, with persistence of endothelium instead of the usual replacement by invading intermediate trophoblast. More advanced changes include mural hyalinization with eosinophilic material accumulating in the vessel wall, and atherosis with foamy macrophages. Other changes include fibrinoid necrosis and thrombosis (Figure 98).

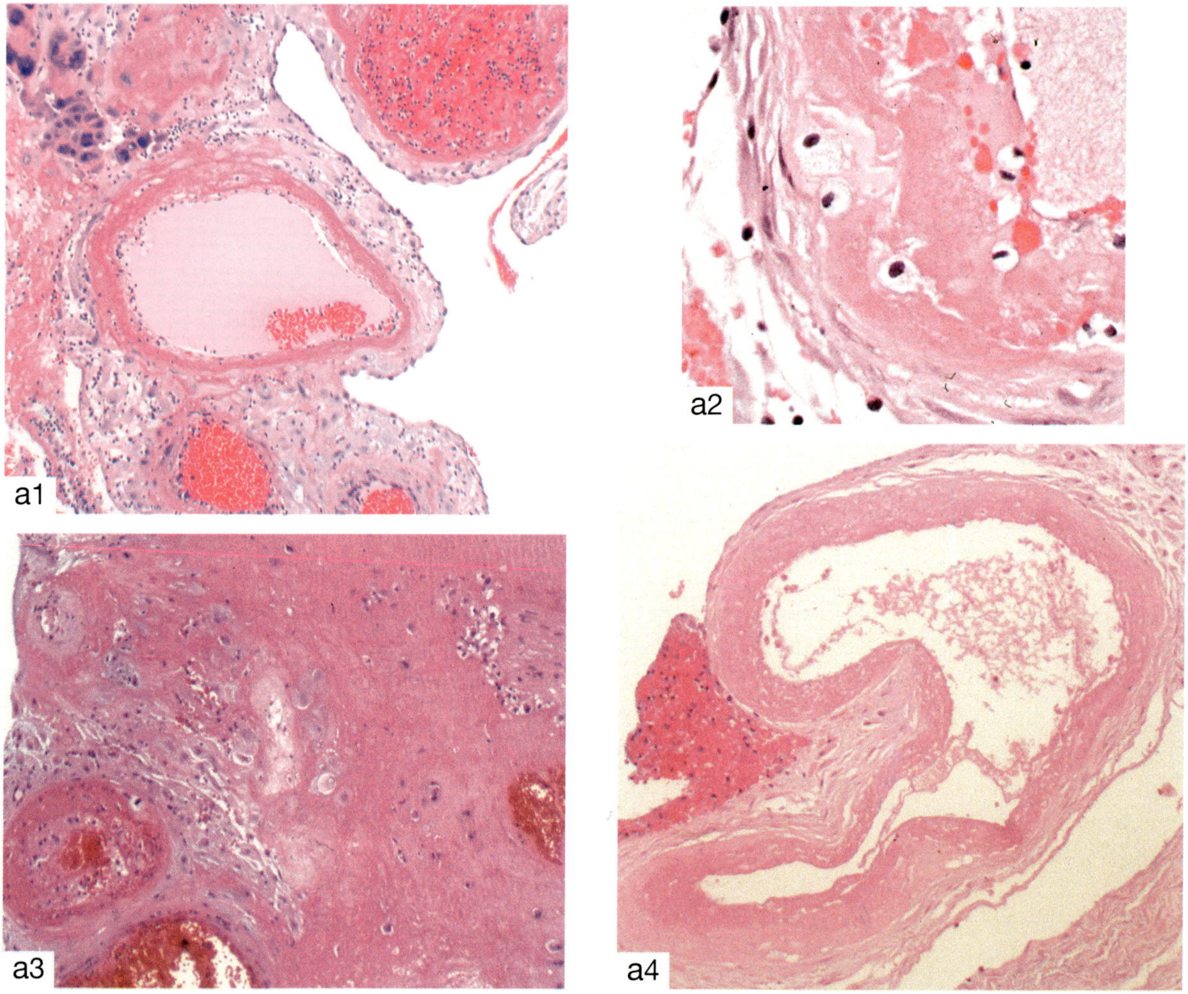

Figure 98 Decidual vasculopathy. (a-1) Decidual vasculopathy, with mural hyalinization and atherosis, with foamy macrophages in the arteriolar wall. (a-2) Higher magnification reveals the foamy cytoplasm of the intramural macrophages and lipid-laden smooth muscle cells of atherosis. (a-3) The top two arteriolar decidual vessels in this section show thick walls, small lumina, and the lower one also shows atherosis. (a-4) An example of fibrinoid necrosis

14

Lesions of the placenta associated with pathologic maternal clinical presentations and/or underlying maternal disorders

PRE-ECLAMPSIA

Pre-eclampsia (Table 12) is defined as pregnancy-induced hypertension with proteinuria. Hypertension in pregnancy is defined as a systolic pressure of ≥ 140 mmHg, and/or a diastolic pressure of ≥ 90 mmHg in pregnancies over 20 weeks in previously normotensive women. Proteinuria is defined as 0.3 g or more of protein in a 24-h urine collection. Severe pre-eclampsia is classified when at least one of the following is present: a blood pressure of ≥ 160 mmHg systolic and/or ≥ 110 mmHg diastolic on two separate occasions 6 h or more apart on bedrest; ≥ 5 g of protein in a 24-h collection (or two separate spot readings of 3+ over 4 h apart); oliguria (< 500 ml in 24 h); cerebral or visual disturbances; pulmonary edema or cyanosis; epigastric or right upper quadrant pain; impaired hepatic function; thrombocytopenia; or fetal growth restriction[574]. Edema is often associated with pre-eclampsia. A variety of terms may be applied to this condition, including pre-eclampsia, toxemia, and pregnancy-induced hypertension (PIH). If new-onset grand mal seizures have occurred, the diagnosis is eclampsia. The HELLP syndrome (hemolysis, elevated liver enzymes, low platelets) is a severe form of pre-eclampsia. Proteinuria may be absent in HELLP syndrome.

Gross features Placentas from pre-eclamptic pregnancies may be of reduced weight, or may be within normal limits. Infarcts involving more than 5% of the placenta are commonly seen, and in severe pre-eclampsia, more than 50% of the placenta may be infarcted. Retroplacental hematoma (with or without a clinical history of abruption) may be present.

Histologic features Increased syncytial knots (see Figure 39a-1), stromal fibrosis, prominent and cytotrophoblastic hyperplasia (cytotrophoblast present in > 20–40% of villi at term), and excessive fibrinoid necrosis may also be seen in the villi (see Chapter 9). PAS stain and thin sections of plastic embedded material may enhance detection of cytotrophoblastic hyperplasia, but these special steps are not generally taken in routine practice. Hypoplasia of the distal villous tree with reduced vascularity with increased knots (see Figure 45), and/or fibromuscular hyperplasia and obliterative endarteritis of the fetal stem arteries, may be present. Increased apoptosis has been reported in placentas, and in their respective sites of implantation in the uterus, from gestations complicated by pre-eclampsia[111,575], but this feature cannot be readily assessed in practice. The basic and most consistently seen (although not pathognomonic) lesion is acute atherosis in the basal arteries of the decidua basalis and the spiral arteries of the decidua parietalis, characterized by fibrinoid necrosis and lipid-laden macrophages in the vessel wall, with perivascular lymphocytic infiltration (Figure 98). Occlusive thrombosis may also occur in these maternal arteries, particularly associated with

Table 12 Salient features of the placenta associated with pathologic maternal clinical presentations and/or underlying maternal disorders

Disorder	*Gross*	*Microscopic*	*Comment*
Pre-eclampsia	low weight, infarcts, retroplacental hematoma	villi – distal villous hypoplasia, cytotrophoblast hyperplasia, thickened trophoblast basement membrane; maternal arteries – acute atherosis, thrombosis	changes may be absent or require extra sampling of maternal arteries; severe cases and HELLP syndrome tend to show more severe changes
Maternal hypertension	low weight, infarcts, retroplacental hematoma	villi – same as above, less prominent syncytial knots; maternal arteries – intimal hyperplasia, medial thickening	may see atherosis if there is superimposed pre-eclampsia
Maternal diabetes	increased or decreased weight, pallor, single umbilical artery	edema, variable maturation, obliterative endarteritis, fetal artery thrombosis	may see no change, particularly in gestational diabetes; may see vascular changes of superimposed pre-eclampsia or hypertension
Abortion	torsion, stricture, true knot of cord, massive subchorial thrombosis, molar change, maternal floor infarction	stromal fibrosis, hydropic change, decreased/absent fetal vessels in villi, hypoplastic villi, trophoblast hyperplasia in moles	circumferential trophoblast hyperplasia best distinguishing histologic feature between moles and missed abortions
Premature labor and delivery	variable by etiology	variable by etiology	placenta may be normal for gestational age
Postmaturity	heavy placenta, infarcts, calcifications (similar to term gestation), meconium more frequent than term	villi – stromal fibrosis, prominent syncytiotrophoblast, thickened trophoblastic basement membrane, obliterative endarteritis of fetal stem vessels, variable vascularity	clinical gestational age may have been inaccurate
Polyhydramnios	fetal malformations, e.g. esophageal atresia, twin–twin transfusion syndrome, maternal diabetes, chorangioma	none	findings relate to underlying condition
Oligohydramnios	postmaturity, fetal urinary tract abnormality (obstructive, anomalous), chronic fluid leakage; amnion nodosum seen in severe cases	amnion nodosum	chorioamnionitis may be seen in chronic fluid leakage

Continued

Table 12 *Continued*

Disorder	*Gross*	*Microscopic*	*Comment*
Premature, preterm, and/or prolonged rupture of membranes	increased incidence of retroplacental hematoma	acute chorioamnionitis	cultures are useful
Maternal fever	opacification of membranes in some cases of chorioamnionitis	chorioamnionitis, villitis, funisitis, depending on causative organism	may see no changes in placenta
Maternal substance abuse	low weight, retroplacental hematoma, premature rupture of membranes, meconium	chorioamnionitis, villitis, hypovascularity of villi, stromal fibrosis	may see no changes; cocaine may cause acute abruption
Abruptio placentae	retroplacental hematoma with compression of parenchyma, possibly associated with infarction	may see lesions of pre-eclampsia and hypertension	in the majority of cases, no retroplacental hematoma is seen, particularly if the blood has escaped through vaginal bleeding; in such cases, localized crater-like depression without blood clot can be considered as evidence of retroplacental hematoma
Systemic lupus erythematosus (SLE)	infarcts, retroplacental hematoma	premature aging of villi, atherosis, obliterative fetal vessels	atherosis may be seen in lupus anticoagulant in the absence of SLE, and in SLE with superimposed pre-eclampsia

HELLP, hemolysis, elevated liver enzymes, low platelets

infarcts. Careful examination of the arteries in the decidua of the membrane roll and along the maternal surface is essential to recognize the lesion, and extra sections to ensure adequate sampling of the maternal arteries may be considered. The membrane roll is particularly useful. In cases of mild pre-eclampsia, and if sampling is inadequate, there may be no abnormalities appreciated in placental sections. It is also possible that the clinical diagnosis of pre-eclampsia may have been incorrect. If insufficient arteries are present to assess, a comment can be made on the report. A shave section of the basal plate is helpful if the other sections do not demonstrate the lesion.

Pathogenesis The villous lesions are associated with ischemia, due to what is thought to be abnormal implantation without normal physiologic remodeling of maternal arteries in early pregnancy. Normally, there is trophoblastic infiltration of maternal arteries, converting them into dilated, non-contractile channels. In pre-eclampsia, narrow undilated segments of maternal arteries persist throughout pregnancy, leading to ischemia as pregnancy progresses. The vascular changes (atherosis) compound the ischemia, leading to further compromise of the villi. Occlusive thrombi in these vessels cause villous infarctions, as do retroplacental hematomas, which are secondary to rupture of these abnormal maternal arteries. Villous changes correspond to ischemia. The pathogenesis of acute atherosis is not known. An immunopathologic basis has been postulated, as there is IgM, and complement deposition in these vessels[192].

Comment In some cases, particularly those with mild toxemia, the placenta may not show any recognizable gross and microscopic lesions. This may be partly due to the absence of maternal arteries in the sections (including the extra ones) taken for histologic assessment. The most characteristic primary histologic lesion is acute atherosis of maternal arteries, although this finding, a manifestation of endothelial injury (see Chapter 9) is not pathognomonic for pre-eclampsia. A granulomatous reaction around decidual arteries may be seen on rare occasions. Prominent and excessive numbers of syncytial knots have been emphasized as a characteristic finding[4]. Some investigators have observed acute atherosis in hypertension, systemic lupus erythematosus (SLE), diabetes, and IUGR[576,577]. The other histologic features, such as cytotrophoblastic hyperplasia and trophoblastic membrane thickening, are difficult to demonstrate consistently.

If maternal arteries are present in sections of decidua, acute atherosis is readily recognizable. Sections from the margin of the placenta, along with the attached membranes, tend to show maternal arteries more frequently than sections from the maternal surface. However, in some cases, the absence of maternal arteries or of an adequate amount of decidua, even in additional sections of the placenta and membranes, makes assessment of maternal vascular changes associated with pre-eclampsia impossible. A shave section of the basal plate is helpful if the other sections do not demonstrate the lesion. A comment to that effect should be added in the surgical pathology report. In occasional cases diagnosed clinically as pre-eclampsia, no maternal vascular lesions may be seen. It is possible that the clinical diagnosis may have been inappropriate. Conversely, acute atherosis may be seen rarely in the absence of overt clinical features of pre-eclampsia. It is possible that in such cases the disease process of pre-eclampsia is present in a subclinical form.

In the HELLP syndrome, characterized by hemolysis, elevated liver enzymes, and low platelets, and more commonly seen in Caucasian women[578], the placental pathologic lesions are similar to those in pre-eclampsia. (The HELLP syndrome is considered to be a severe variant of pre-eclampsia.) The lesions may be more severe, and the incidence of thrombosis of maternal arteries may be more frequent. A systematic description of placental findings in the HELLP syndrome is lacking in the literature.

MATERNAL HYPERTENSION

Maternal vasculopathy, and in some cases, chronic villitis of unknown etiology have been reported in maternal hypertension[579] (Table 12). The maternal vasculopathy is characterized by medial thickening and intimal hyperplasia. The fibrinoid necrosis of villi and obliterative endarteritis of villi seen in pre-eclampsia are absent or less marked.

MATERNAL DIABETES

Introduction Diabetes in pregnancy (Table 12) is classified according to the White classification[580] (Table 13). Pregnancies associated with gestational diabetes without maternal vascular disease are associated with large placentas, while more severely diabetic women have small placentas associated with growth-restricted infants.

Pathology Grossly, the placentas may be pale, and there is an increased incidence of single umbilical artery. Microscopically, the villi may be immature, with larger terminal villi, edema, and increased numbers of residual cytotrophoblast and Hofbauer cells[581]. Accelerated maturation may also be seen. Diabetes is also associated with fetal arterial thrombosis[4], stromal fibrosis, prominent syncytial knots, thickened trophoblastic basement membrane, variable vascularity (normal, hypovascularity, or chorangiosis), and excessive fibrinoid necrosis. The fetal stem arteries show thrombosis in about 10% of cases, compared with 4.5% of normal placentas, and 25% show obliterative endarteritis, compared with 10% of normal placentas. Maternal vascular changes are seen only if there is superimposed pre-eclampsia.

Table 13 Classification of diabetes in pregnancy[580]

Class	*Criteria*	*Vascular disease*
A_1	gestational, diet controlled	no
A_2	gestational, insulin required	no
B	onset after age 20 with < 10 years' duration	no
C	onset before age 20 or 10–19 years' duration	no
D	onset before age 10 or > 20 years' duration	retina
F	any age/duration, with nephropathy	kidneys
R	any age/duration, with proliferative retinopathy	retina
H	any age/duration, with atherosclerotic heart disease	heart disease
T	any age/duration, with renal transplant	

Pathogenesis The pathogenesis of the placental lesions associated with maternal diabetes is unclear. The maternal arteries are not narrowed in uncomplicated diabetes, mitigating against ischemia. Immunologic factors and abnormal internal metabolic environment have been postulated.

Comment The histopathology of maternal diabetes more frequently shows chorionic villous dyssynchrony and variability. Diabetic hyperglycemia characteristically results in fetal hyperglycemia, hyperinsulinemia, and increased insulin growth factor production that result in increased fetoplacental growth, metabolic rate, and oxygen demands[582]. Typically, the villi of a placenta from an insulin-dependent diabetic gestation are relatively enlarged and irregularly shaped, and, despite their size, may show numerous capillary outlines along with increased numbers of cytotrophoblast cells, hypercellular fibroblastic stroma, and decreased VSM (increased fetomaternal diffusional distances) (see section on 'Chorangiosis' in Chapter 9). Thus, their morphology does not conform to any normally occurring stage of villous development (see Figure 41). Chorionic villous dysmorphogenesis of diabetes likely reflects a complex, deleterious interplay of fetal and maternal responses to elevations in maternal glucose levels, which, in turn, alter the availability, clearance, and function of factors necessary for proper villous maturation and the formation of VSM. The affected mediating factors include fetoplacental levels of glucose and oxygen, insulin-like growth factors I and II, and their binding proteins[583]. Results of recent studies lend support to the hypothesis that the placenta-to-placenta variations in diabetic histopathology are at least partially explained by differences in patients' glucose control. Mayhew[584] found that placental villi showed increased longitudinal angiogenesis, but no accompanying microvascular remodeling, in well-controlled pre-gestational diabetes, whereas, Jirkovska and colleagues[585] found abnormal increases in both longitudinal and branching capillarization, in placentas from variably controlled patients. The degree of reduction of VSM in a given case may also reflect the complicating effect of hypoxia due to maternal vascular disease.

There are no consistent or pathognomonic histologic findings in diabetic placentas, and many may appear normal. Detailed morphometric studies of histologic and ultrastructural features of placentas in diabetic and non-diabetic normal women have revealed few statistically significant differences[586,587]. Histologic features do not correspond to disease severity, although lesions are more consistently present in pre-existing diabetes than in gestational diabetes. Figure 99 shows examples of the placental histopathology associated with maternal diabetes.

ABORTION (SPONTANEOUS OR MISSED)

Gross findings Grossly, torsion, stricture, and true knots of the cord may be seen (Table 12). Other findings include massive subchorial hemorrhage (Breus' mole), molar change, and maternal floor infarction.

Histologic findings Placentas from spontaneous or missed abortions may be histologically unremarkable,

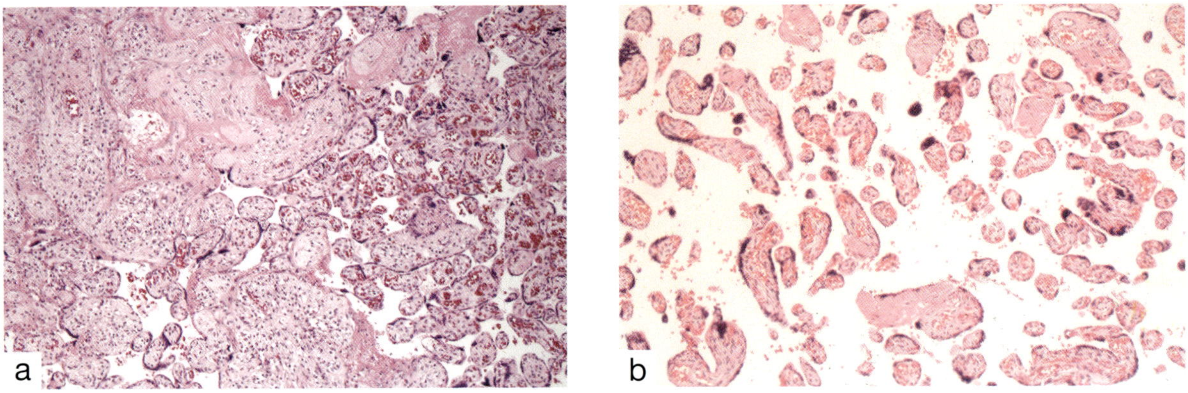

Figure 99 Diabetes mellitus. (a) Chorionic villi are dysmature, but also, coincidental villitis of unknown eitiology is present. (b) This gestation was complicated by maternal class C diabetes mellitus, and villi show distal villous hypoplasia (see Figure 45)

or show a variety of villous changes including hypoplastic villi, fetal vascular obliteration, stromal fibrosis, and prominent syncytio- and cytotrophoblast. Missed abortions in particular may show hydropic change, with loss of fetal vasculature in the villi, which must be distinguished from hydatidiform mole. The circumferential trophoblastic proliferation of moles is not present in missed abortions, and the physiologic polar trophoblast proliferation of normal pregnancy ('polar capping') should not be mistaken for molar change.

Missed abortion versus hydatidiform mole Placentas from missed abortions are particularly difficult at times to distinguish from partial hydatidiform moles, and ploidy analysis by flow cytometry may be helpful in the distinction. It should be noted that while partial moles are usually triploid, not all triploid gestations are partial moles. Placentas with chromosomal anomalies, from spontaneous abortions, may show irregular outlines with villous scalloping and trophoblast inclusions. This is particularly true of triploid gestations that are not partial moles, i.e. are due to digyny versus diandry. These gestations lack the trophoblast proliferation of molar pregnancies[588]. In addition, complete hydatidiform moles, which are diploid, tend to be evacuated much earlier, noted with the widespread use of ultrasound, and may lack the pronounced histologic features of complete moles seen at a later gestational age. Features of earlier complete moles include redundant bulbous terminal villi, hypercellular villous stroma, a labyrinthine network of villous stromal canaliculi, focal cyto- and syncytiotrophoblastic hyperplasia of villi and undersurface of the chorionic plate, and enlarged hyperchromatic implantation-site trophoblast[589]. Genest and colleagues have shown that antibody to P57, which is a paternally imprinted, maternally expressed protein, will stain in all types of gestations (including partial moles) except complete moles[590]. They have shown further that villous dysmorphism and cisterns can be associated with triploidy; and villous hydrops, absent cord, absent fetal tissue, and absent anucleate erythrocytes can be associated with trisomy; however, these findings had low positive-predictive values. In a study by Redline and colleagues[591], autoimmune markers, chronic intervillositis, and increased perivillous fibrin were seen in abortions associated with normal karyotype, and dysmorphic villi with abnormal karyotype. The patients with recurrent spontaneous abortion and normal karyotype were more likely to have one or more of the histological features described than either patients with normal karyotype and no prior abortions, or patients with recurrent abortion and abnormal karyotype. In normal karyotype, lesions suggestive of an immune-mediated process, such as chronic vasculitis of maternal vessels, chronic intervillositis, and villous infarcts, may be seen[592]. Doss and associates[348] reported a patient with ten recurrent spontaneous abortions with massive chronic intervillositis.

PREMATURE LABOR AND DELIVERY

Introduction This complication (Table 12) can be associated with a number of obstetrical conditions including abruptio placentae, pre-eclampsia, maternal hypertension or other disease, and premature rupture of the membranes secondary to or following acute chorioamnionitis.

Pathology Findings in the placenta may correspond to the accompanying condition, or the placenta may be unremarkable and appropriate for the gestational age. Hansen and colleagues[142] found an association between acute inflammation and villous edema with preterm labor. In many cases, no etiology of the premature labor is evident. Women with incompetent cervix usually have painless cervical dilatation and deliver in their second trimester. The most common cause of premature delivery is acute chorioamnionitis. Recent literature has supported an increased risk of fetal neurological damage if there is an accompanying fetal inflammatory response in the fetal umbilical or chorionic plate vessels[538]. In pregnancies of less than 32 weeks, antenatal corticosteroids were found to be associated with increased severity of villous fibrosis and stromal mineralization with decreased villous infarcts[593]. It has been recommended that premature placentas be examined, with criteria variously set as ≤32 or 34 weeks, although obstetrically, a pregnancy is not considered a term gestation until after 36 completed weeks.

POSTMATURITY

Introduction Postmaturity (Table 12) is defined as gestational age over 42 weeks. It should be noted that the clinical assessment of gestational age may be inaccurate.

Gross findings Grossly, there may be no findings, or the placenta may be of increased weight. Meconium is more frequently present in postmature gestations, and the risk for meconium aspiration in these infants is increased. Infarcts and calcifications are frequently seen, but are no more severe than in a term gestation.

Microscopic findings Histologically, stromal fibrosis of villi, prominent syncytial knots, slight cytotrophoblast proliferation, and trophoblast basement membrane thickening may be seen. Fetal stem vessels may show obliterative endarteritis, and there may be hypovascular villi. It is unclear whether the changes are ischemic, or due to physiologic senescence. Fox[3] does not subscribe to there being aging in the placenta.

POLYHYDRAMNIOS AND OLIGOHYDRAMNIOS

Amniotic fluid allows for fetal movement and it cushions the fetus against trauma. Amniotic epithelial secretions and fetal urine are the main components of amniotic fluid. Cellular and non-cellular debris from the fetal skin and respiratory and urinary tracts are also present. The amount of fluid in mid-pregnancy is about 400 ml, and at term about 1000 ml; however, due to the relative size of the fetus, the second-trimester fetus has a great deal more mobility.

Amniotic fluid over 2000 ml is considered to be polyhydramnios (Table 12). It may be associated with fetal anomalies that impair normal physiologic swallowing, such as esophageal atresia, or may reflect twin–twin transfusion syndrome, anencephaly with increased fluid transudation from exposed meninges, maternal diabetes, or placental chorangioma. The weight of the placenta may be increased. There are no characteristic histologic findings.

Marked reduction of the amniotic fluid may be due to chronic leakage, often associated with chorioamnionitis, or may be due to decreased production of fluid due to fetal urinary tract obstruction or anomalies. The characteristic gross and microscopic finding in severe cases is amnion nodosum (Table 12) (see section on 'Amnion nodosum' in Chapter 12).

PREMATURE PRETERM AND PROLONGED RUPTURE OF THE MEMBRANES

Premature rupture of the membranes (Table 12) is multifactorial, with maternal enzymes, mechanical forces, membrane phospholipid content, collagen disruption, amniotic cytokines, bacterial phospholipases and collagenases, and prostaglandins all playing a role[594]. The acronym PPROM is often applied to this condition, and stands for preterm premature rupture of the membranes. PPROM may be due to chorioamnionitis, or chorioamnionitis may develop after PPROM, and it is often difficult to determine which came first. Premature rupture indicates rupture before the onset of labor, preterm indicates rupture before 38 weeks' gestation, and prolonged indicates duration greater than 24 h. Abruptio placentae is associated with PPROM. In one study, Arias and colleagues[595] found two distinct subgroups of patients with preterm labor and preterm ruptured membranes, a group associated with infection, and one with maternal placental vasculopathy.

MATERNAL FEVER

One study of intrapartum fever in term gestations showed histologic chorioamnionitis in fewer than half the cases, suggesting that ascending infection is often not the cause[596]. There may be no placental findings with maternal fever, or, depending on a causative organism, chorioamnionitis, funisitis, and/or villitis may be seen (Table 12). Malarial organisms can be identified in maternal erythrocytes in the intervillous space in cases of maternal malaria (Figure 69).

MATERNAL SUBSTANCE ABUSE

Substances potentially abused in pregnancy include cigarettes, alcohol, and a variety of drugs. Placentas from pregnancies associated with maternal substance abuse often show no specific histopathologic alterations associated with the abuse (Table 12), and the deleterious effects are likely pathophysiologic. Cocaine has been associated with placental abruption[597] and premature rupture of the membranes[598], but no diagnostic gross or histopathologic features have been identified in placentas from gestations complicated by maternal cocaine abuse[599]. Higher incidences of acute chorioamnionitis, low weight, villitis, abruption, and meconium staining have been described in some cases of ethanol abuse[600]. Alcohol can readily cross the placenta and lead to IUGR and fetal alcohol syndrome. Reduced placental weight, hypovascularity relating to ischemia, and increased incidence of single umbilical artery have been described in placentas from women who smoke cigarettes[4], but again, these placentas may be normal. Ultrastructural and histomorphometric studies of the villi have demonstrated reduced trophoblastic elements[601,602]. Acute chorioamnionitis, meconium staining, and IUGR were the principal findings in a study of heroin-abusing mothers[603]. It should be noted that the increased ACA in the placentas of substance-abusing mothers may relate to life-style factors rather than the substance abuse itself.

ABRUPTIO PLACENTAE

This clinical syndrome (Table 12) has been discussed in the section on 'Retroplacental hematoma', Chapter 8.

LUPUS, LUPUS ANTICOAGULANT, AND ANTICARDIOLIPIN

The parenchymal lesions associated with maternal autoantibodies of systemic lupus erythematosus (SLE) (Table 12), and the antiphospholipid syndrome (lupus anticoagulant and anticardiolipin), are often ischemic changes induced by maternal vasculopathy seen in the decidua. Lesions can include decreased weight, acute atherosis, ischemic changes, infarcts, villous fibrosis, increased syncytial knots, X cell proliferation, chronic villitis, decreased vasculosyncytial membranes, and abruption[103,573,604,605].

Deposition of complement (C3) and IgM in the wall of affected blood vessels has been described[606]. SLE is often associated with pre-eclampsia, and the atherosis may relate to the pre-eclampsia. Other associated lesions include coagulation-related lesions, including thrombi of fetal vessels of the chorionic plate, stem and villous vessels, and maternal decidual vessels, and avascular terminal villi[573]. Massive perivillous fibrin and maternal floor infarct have also been reported[607]. There is increased fetal loss.

Antiphospholipid antibodies are present in about 30–40% of SLE patients. The presence of both anticardiolipin antibody and lupus anticoagulant in patients with SLE was shown to be a risk factor for fetal death, with extensive infarction secondary to decidual vasculopathy and thrombosis[604].

Other immune-mediated maternal disorders have been evaluated. Scleroderma is rarely associated with successful pregnancies. In one series, Doss and colleagues[480] reported a high prevalence of maternal decidual vasculopathy and poor outcomes.

THROMBOPHILIAS

Thrombi in fetal vessels may be a reflection of a heritable thrombophilic condition[220,608,609] that includes a potential protein S deficiency, protein C deficiency, MTHFR mutation, hyperhomocysteinemia, and factor V Leiden mutation. In cases of extensive thrombi with no other explanation, thrombophilia screening should be considered for the mothers and possibly the infants in these situations. In addition, cranial ultrasound of the infant may pick up infarcts caused by thrombi that have crossed the foramen ovale by paradoxical embolization.

15

Findings and lesions of the placenta reflecting fetal conditions

MULTIPLE GESTATION PREGNANCIES

Twin placentas

Twinning may result in:

(1) A single placental disk with two umbilical cords with separate insertion sites;

(2) Partial to complete fusion of the chorioamniotic sacs and/or disks;

(3) Entirely separate disks.

The pattern of placentation will depend upon zygosity of the twins and site of blastocyst implantation. The development of the placenta was addressed at the beginning of this manual, and the reader is referred to this chapter, because recollection of the timing of formation of the chorion, amnion, and cord is key to understanding twin (multiple) placentation patterns.

The diagram of twinning (Figure 100) is a representation of the most widely accepted view of the twinning process and of the overwhelming majority of twin placental configurations. However, it does not account for rarely reported instances in which chorionic anastomoses have been identified between dichorionic twins' sacs[610], or the exceedingly rare recognition and implications of non-identical twins sharing a single placenta[611], or portray the rarest types of monozygotic twinning. Nevertheless, the diagram provides a valuable and plausible explanation of what has been observed about twinning and chorionicity, and what has been buttressed by genetic and X-inactivation studies[3,8,610,612].

The diagram shows that a single zygote may undergo 'fission' or 'splitting' prior to formation of the blastocyst stage (≤ 4 days), and thereby form two separate gestational sacs; these sacs may remain separate, or fuse, following implantation and growth within the uterus. Since each monozygotically derived morula gives rise to its own gestational sac, each twin develops its own chorion, amniotic sac, yolk sac, and cord, and the resulting placentation is diamniotic dichorionic (DiDi). The abbreviation 'DiDi', refers to cases in which the sacs are entirely separate, or in which they are fused at the membranes and/or chorionic plate. The diagram further shows that these same DiDi configurations result from *dizygotic* events. However, as is evident from the *right* side of the diagram, monozygotic twins will share components of chorionic vasculature (i.e. be monochorionic) if 'division' occurs after formation of the blastocyst. If 'fission' also occurs before about day 7, each monochorionic twin will have its own amniotic sac, and placentation will be diamniotic monochorionic (DiMo). 'Splitting' after day 7 or 8 will result in a single, shared amniotic sac and a single shared chorion, or a monoamniotic monochorionic (MoMo) placenta. Aberrations of monozygotic

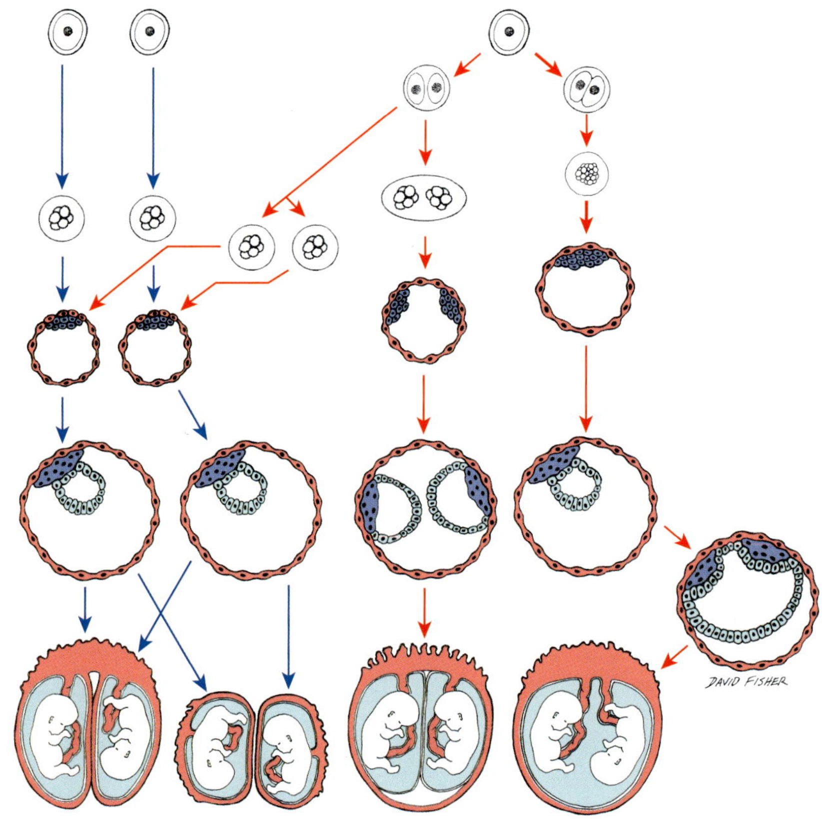

Figure 100 Diagram of twinning. The left side of this diagrammatic representation of twinning shows the placentation patterns of dizygotic twinning (blue arrows). Each morula gives rise to a blastocyst, which implants separately, and each conceptus generates its own chorion and amnion. If the implantation sites are proximate to one another, the chorions may abut, interdigitate, or grossly fuse, but true vascular anastomoses are extremely rare. The right side of the diagram shows the possible pathways of monozygotic twinning. If the morula splits prior to the formation of the blastocyst, then two solid balls of cells are formed that are capable of forming two separate blastocysts, and therefore following an implantation sequence that is identical to that of a dizygotic twin set. Hence, the far left schema denoted in red shows notched arrows and overlap with the blue arrows of the diamniotic dichorionic (DiDi)placentation patterns. In cases in which there is morular division after accumulation of blastocyst fluid and/or division of the inner cell mass after formation of the blastocyst, but before day 7 and formation of the amnion, the placentation is diamniotic monochorionic (DiMo) as depicted in the central, red arrow schema. If the inner cell mass does not divide until after day 7 or 8, and, therefore, after the generation of the amnion, the two embryos share a single amniotic cavity and the placentation is monoamniotic monochorionic (MoMo); this schema is seen in red, on the far right

twinning, after day 12, will result in yolk sac unity and/or conjoined twins (see below).

Twinning and the pathologic examination of twin placentas

The rate of spontaneous twinning is about 1/90 births in the USA[612], and twins constitute about 2.5% of the population in this country[613]. However, due to the rise in use of assisted reproductive technologies (ART) in the USA, about 50% of twin gestations currently result from infertility treatment programs, and about 1/43 pregnancies resulting from ART are twin gestations. Hence, the overall incidence of twins is predicted to continue to increase to the point where twin gestations have been speculated to outnumber singleton ones significantly, by 2015, in some developed countries[613]. Whether this will occur, of course, remains to be seen, but the need for placental examinations in twin gestations will likely not decline, especially since twins are at significantly increased risks over singletons for perinatal morbidity and mortality. Twins have higher rates of prematurity and IUGR (12–47% versus 5–7% for singletons) and structural and chromosomal anomalies, and are at a 3–7 times higher risk for perinatal mortality, such that they account for 12.6% of perinatal deaths[613]. Cerebral palsy is also more frequent among twin survivors[612]. Moreover, as will be noted in the subsequent discussions of chorionicity, the relative severities and frequencies of these risks are related to placentation[610,612–614]. Thus, there are three main objectives of pathologic examination of twin placentas:

(1) To determine the type of placentation (mono- or dichorionic) (and, thereby, zygosity, if possible);

(2) To identify anastomoses that exist between the twins' chorionic plate vessels (superficial) or chorionic plate vascular patterns that indicate shared portions of deep chorionic villous tree ('deep anastomoses'), since the latter are the major determinants of unbalanced shunting of blood in twin–twin transfusion syndrome (TTTS) (TTTS is a significant concern for DiMo twins, but MoMo twins may also rarely develop TTTS[613]);

(3) To document carefully the presence of other gross or histologic abnormalities associated with increased risks of perinatal morbidity and mortality.

For example, Redline and colleagues[615] found that peripheral umbilical cord insertion (insertion within or beyond the outer 10% of the placental plate to include marginal, paramarginal, and velamentous insertions) and villous avascularity were linked to increased risks of small for gestational age (SGA) and discordant fetal growth. Peripheral cord insertion was seen in 33% of cases of SGA, 29% of cases of discordant growth (versus 18% of cases with neither), and in 52% of cases with both SGA and growth discordance. Villous avascularity was more common in the smaller placentas of discordant twins (9%) versus those from cases without discordancy or SGA associations (4%). Chorangiosis and relatively increased chorionic villous vascularity for period of gestation are not uncommon in twin placentas, but Redline and colleagues[615] did not find its prevalence (5–6% in all types) to be increased over that observed for singletons.

With very rare exceptions[611], monochorionic placentas should be regarded as representing a monozygotic gestation. Dichorionic placentas may represent mono- or dizygotic twinning; of note is that some 25% of monozygotic twins have dichorionic placentas[612]. When two separate placental disk specimens are received, the type of placentation is obviously dichorionic, but the pathologic examination of these separate placentas is not helpful in determining the zygosity, if the twins are of like sex. Zygosity in these instances, and in instances of same-sex twins and a fused dichorionic placenta, is determined by laboratory studies. These include comparison of blood group antigens between the twins, and in some cases, the use of molecular techniques to detect the identity of genetic sequences[612,613].

Examination technique The placental specimen(s) should be weighed and its (their) overall dimensions measured, and recorded per clinical identification of the umbilical cords. If the cords are not labeled or specifically marked, the obstetrician should be contacted and requested to do so. The placental combined weight should be compared with the ranges of combined placental weights for twin placentas (as matched for gestational week), provided in Table 14[224].The size of each placental compartment should be measured; the areas of the chorionic plate territories may be unequal, and this should be noted as relative percentages of the total placental surface. Sites of dichorionic fusion may involve only the membranes, or partially or completely involve apposing

Table 14 Mean weights and centiles for twin placentas. Adapted from reference 224

Gestational week	*10th–90th centile*	*Cases (n)*
19	161–263	2
20	166–270	3
21	176–286	2
22	191–310	5
23	210–343	2
24	232–382	3
25	257–426	5
26	284–475	4
27	314–528	8
28	345–584	7
29	377–641	12
30	409–700	17
31	441–758	13
32	472–815	29
33	503–870	27
34	531–923	53
35	558–971	52
36	582–014	66
37	602–1051	58
38	619–1082	54
39	631–1105	38
40	639–1118	47
41	642–1123	12

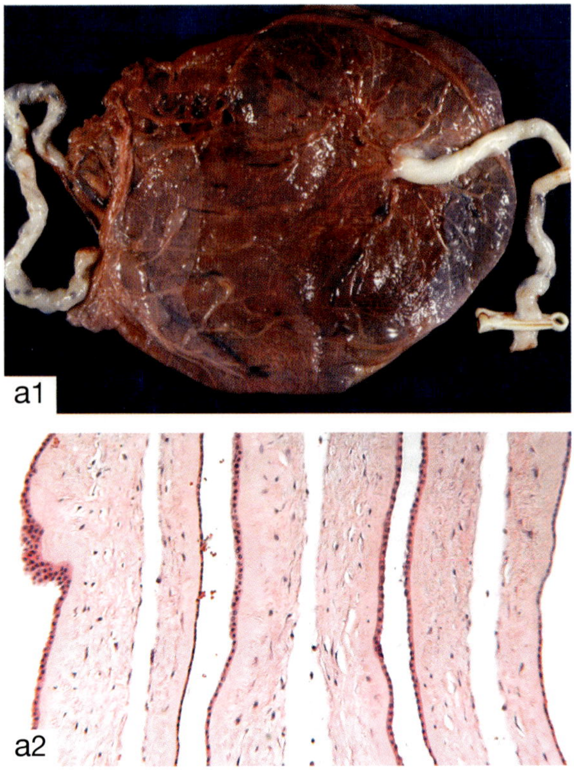

Figure 101 Twin placentations. (a-1) Diamniotic monochorionic (DiMo) placenta. The dividing membrane is spread over the left aspect of the disk, but its transparent character is obvious. Note the marginal to near velamentous insertion of the cord on the left. (a-2) Microscopic appearance of three sections of the DiMo dividing membrane showing amnion and basement membrane apposed to basement membrane and amnion. (a-3 and a-4) These photographs show that even in cases in which the DiMo dividing membrane is partially to fully avulsed, if the membrane can be located, its identity can be grossly confirmed. The membranous components can be peeled apart to reveal two delicate transparent amnions. (b-1) Diamniotic dichorionic (DiDi) placenta. An opaque dividing membrane is present. (b-2) The dividing membrane shows amnion, interposed fused layers of chorion, and a second layer of amnion

aspects of the placental disks, such that a 'single' diskoid configuration is seen.

Single disk specimens may show one or two amniotic sacs. When there are two amniotic sacs, the fetal surface of the placenta shows a septum. Additional details of the morphology of the septum will be addressed further, below, under features of DiDi and DiMo placentas, but, if the septum is transparent or translucent (Figure 101a-1), the placentation is most likely DiMo, with the septum composed of two apposed, delicate amnions (Figure 101a-2). If the septum is opaque, the placentation is likely DiDi (Figure 101b-1), with the septum composed of a lamination of amnion–chorion–chorion–amnion (Figure 101b-2). When there is a single placental disk with two amniotic sacs, histologic confirmation of grossly determined chorionicity is required and accomplished by microscopic examination of the sections of the dividing septum at its site of attachment to the chorionic plate surface. This so-called 'T zone' is best sampled by carefully incising the septum at about 3 cm above its attachment line and then

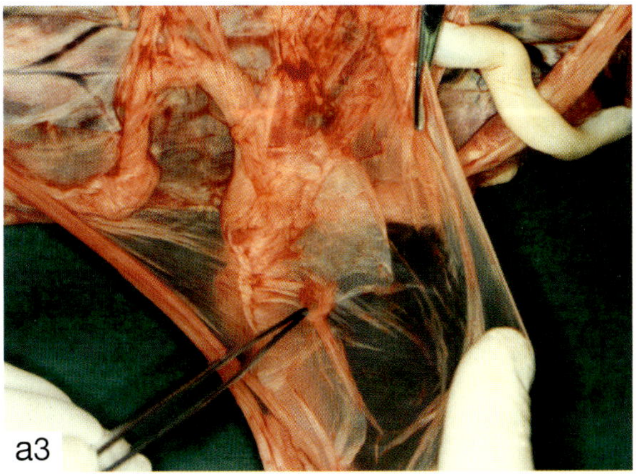

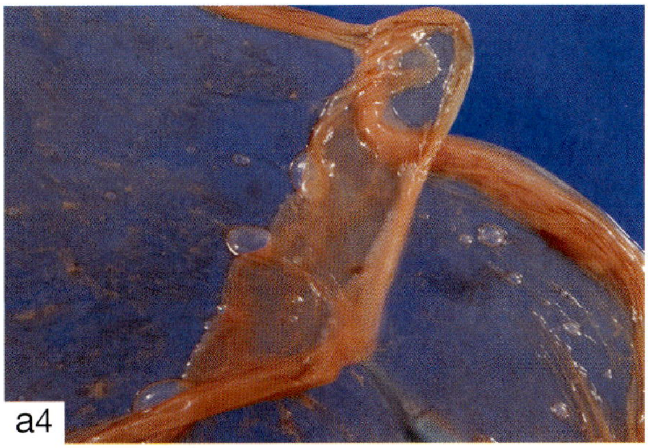

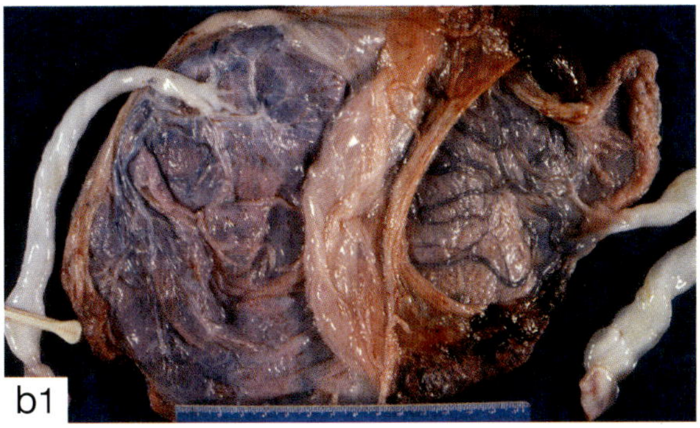

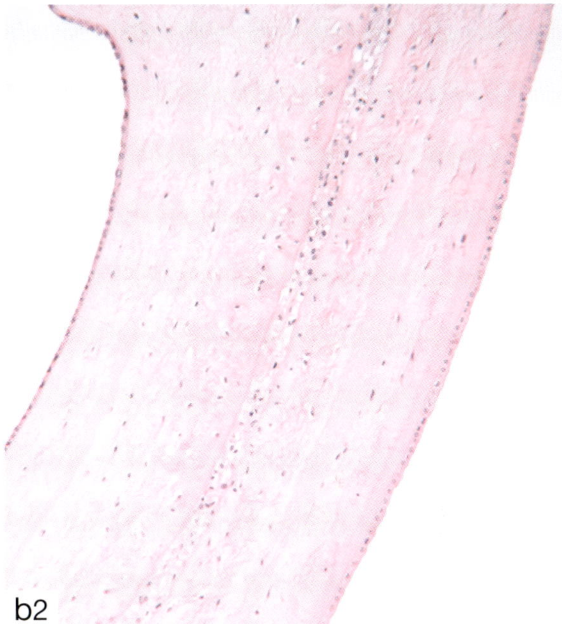

Figure 101 *Continued*

cutting sections, at right angles to this 'newly shortened' septum, that include the chorionic plate tissue below, on both sides of the septum. Inclusion of the chorionic plate tissue, in the inverted 'T section', serves to stabilize it during sampling and to preserve its orientation during histologic processing. Submission of two such sections is recommended to insure that a valid sample of the septum is available for microscopic interpretation.

In addition, assessment of the vascular equator of the twins should be determined. This 'equator' is that irregular interface of the limits of the branches of each twin's chorionic plate ramifications, and lies between the two cord insertion sites. Despite its name, it may not be a midline division (Figure 102a-2), and it often does not directly underlie the position of the septum in DiMo placentations (Figure 101a-1). The caliber and patency of the vessels at the equator should be assessed, and the appearance of the interface described (e.g. presence of dense subchorionic fibrinoid deposition in a DiMo placenta or abnormal fixation and plication of a DiDi septum to suggest circumvallation). A DiDi equator will have a rim of fibrinoid on either side of the septum, due to the apposition of the two placental margins.

The umbilical cord insertion sites should be recorded and the distance from the insertion of each cord to the nearest respective placental margin, *and* the dividing membrane, should be documented. Cord dimensions, morphology, color, and character, and vessel number, patency, and integrity, should also be documented. The incidences of single umbilical

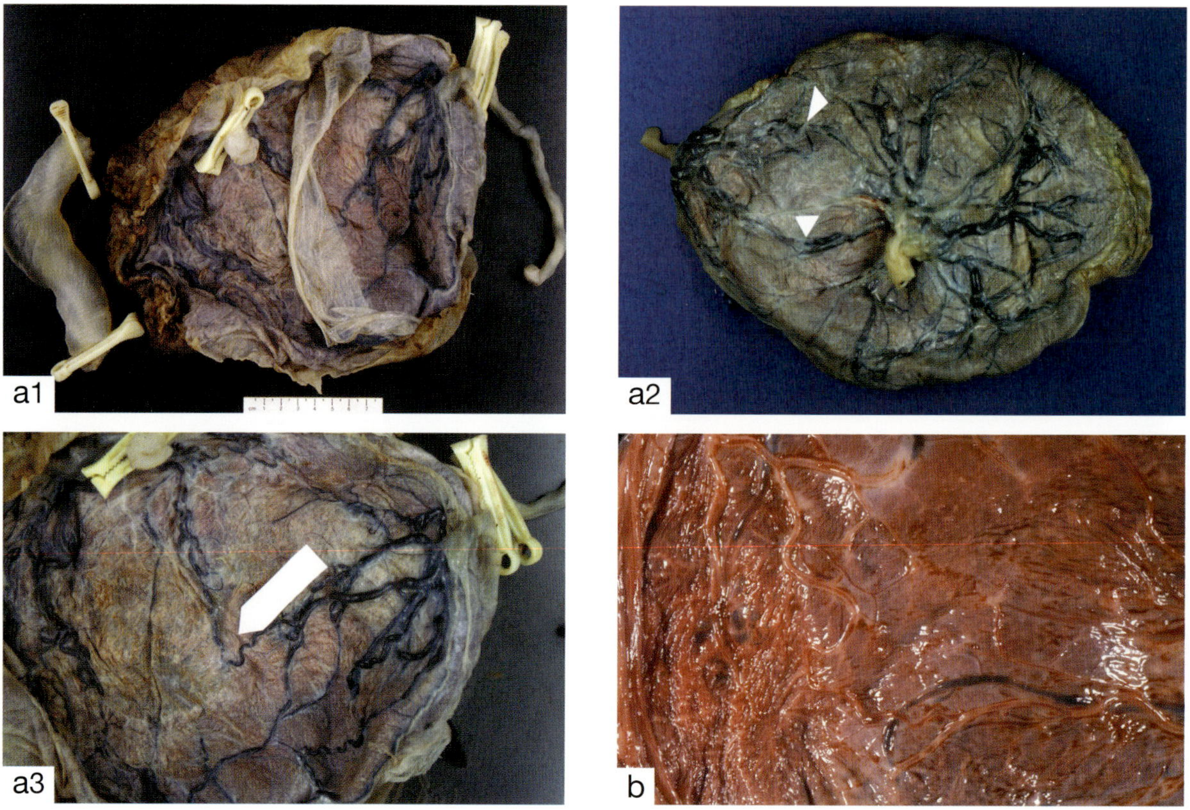

Figure 102 Diamniotic monochorionic (DiMo) placentation, vascular communications, and twin–twin transfusion syndrome (TTTS). (a-1) DiMo placenta from a clinically diagnosed case of 'stuck twin syndrome' with donor twin side on right with thin cord and recipient on left with thick, edematous cord segment. (a-2) The dividing membrane and amnion have been removed and two of several potential sites of vascular communication along the equator are shown (arrows). (a-3) The donor twin side on the left shows a venous vessel that courses to a shared lobule that is supplied by an artery from the recipient (arrow), and this was confirmed with dissection. This vascular pattern is unexpected, since the vein 'should' be connected to the cord of the recipient and the artery to the cord of the donor. This arrangement underscores the importance of the overall balance of shunting that occurs among the number of communications that exist between twin domains in DiMo placentas, and the necessity of a thorough pathologic examination in such cases. (b) This is a demonstration of a chorionic artery to artery (A–A) anastomosis on the placenta seen in Figure 101a-1

artery and cord insertional abnormalities are higher in twins than in singletons, regardless of zygosity, and associated with smaller placentas[616]. In addition, the incidence of abnormalities of cord insertion increases as the proximity of the placentas decreases. Peripheral cord insertions are seen in up to 36–45% of monochorionic placentas (Figures 101a-1, 102a-1 and a-2), and fused DiDi placentas more commonly show peripheral cord insertions than do separate DiDi placentas (up to 16–22% and between 3 and 15%, respectively)[615,616]. Color and translucency of the fetal surface of each twin's domain should be recorded, particularly if there has been fetal demise of one or both twins, or clinical suspicion of chorioamnionitis. Serial cross-sections of the placenta should be examined for all the features of a singleton placenta, with special documentation of discrepant findings between the respective twins' domains.

An important gross feature seen in virtually all DiMo placentas is the presence of vascular anastomoses between the two territories on either side of the septum (Figure 103, and Figure 102a-1, a-2, a-3 and b). Such vascular anastomoses are extremely rare in dichorionic, fused placentas. There are two basic

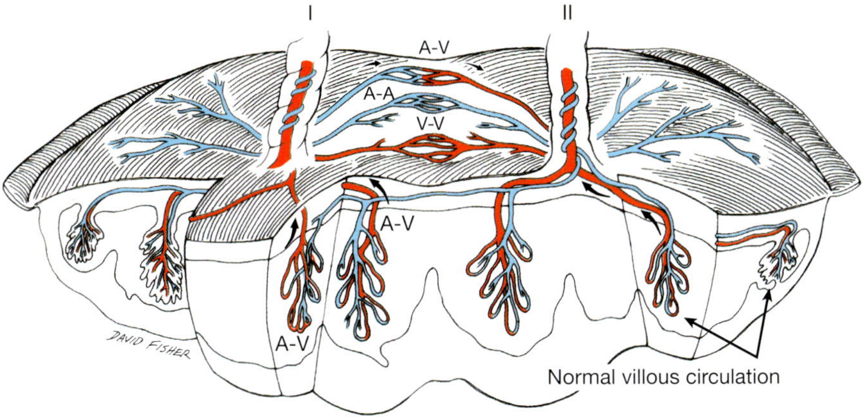

Figure 103 Patterns of vascular communications in monochorionic twin placentas. The diagrammatic representation shows chorionic plate anastomotic connections between the venous branches of twin I and twin II (V–V, arterial branches of twin I and twin II (A–A), and arterial branches of twin I and venous branches of twin II (A–V). The arrows indicate the flow of blood from twin I to twin II in the arteriovenous connection. However, in addition, deep communications at the lobular level are shown. An artery (blue) from twin II supplies at least one segment of chorionic villous tree that is ultimately drained by a vein (red) from twin I, the direction of blood flow denoted by arrows. The deep communications are generally of greater clinical significance and can contribute to the development of twin–twin transfusion syndrome (see text)

types of anastomoses: superficial and 'deep'. The superficial anastomoses are direct connections between chorionic plate vascular branches and are usually of small caliber and easily visualized, but their presence is highlighted by injection studies. They can exist between two arteries (A–A, most common) (Figure 102b), two veins (V–V, less common), or between an artery of one twin and a vein of the other (A–V, uncommon). 'Deep anastomoses' are not really anastomoses *per se*, since they consist of the artery from one twin's territory that supplies a lobule of chorionic villous capillaries that are drained, following oxygenation, by the vein of the contralateral twin (Figure 102a-3). Imbalances in the blood volumes shunted through these anastomoses between the twins' circulations, particularly of the deep type, can lead to chronic TTTS (Table 15). Demonstration of these anastomoses is addressed below. However, in general, transmural sections should be taken from the vascular equator of single disk placentas. In addition, sections from the two placental territories should be submitted and appropriately identified as to side, as well as to relative position within the respective territory. Clinical provision of fetal/neonatal weights and presence of growth discrepancy is important correlative information. Classically, hemoglobin (> 5 g/dl) and hematocrit discrepancies are present between the two twins, and the twin weights differ by > 20%, with the recipient twin exhibiting plethora and large size. However, hemoglobin and hematocrit are less reliable indictors of TTTS, since delivery of one twin can result in a rapid change in hematocrit of the second twin[612].

Demonstration of vascular anastomoses

Superficial anastomoses consist of arterial (A–A, most common), venous (V–V, least common), or arteriovenous (A–V, uncommon) types. The 'deep anastomoses' are of the A–V type, and, in these types, the afferent and efferent anastomotic branches of chorionic vessels enter vertically into the placental parenchyma within millimeters of each other (Figure 102a-3), and are the only vessels supplying and draining that portion of the villous tree; therefore, the arterial branch from and venous branch to each

Table 15 Twin–twin transfusion syndrome (TTTS) (see text for details and for exceptions)

Incidence

15–30% of diamniotic monochorionic (DiMo) placentas

Pathogenesis

Superficial and deep arteriovenous (A–V) anastomoses are present between both placental territories of virtually all DiMo twin placentas. However, clinically significant transfusion occurs only when there is an imbalance in the blood volumes exchanged between the twins, through a significantly higher proportion of deep A–V shunts from one twin's vascular domain to the other's. The donor twin chronically transfuses the recipient twin during gestation. TTTS is a dynamic process dependent upon fluctuations in arterial pressure in the donor twin and those in the venous pressure in the recipient twin

Diagnostic criteria

(1) Prenatal period: discrepant sac size in DiMo gestation, with 'stuck twin' or 'TOPS' sign on ultrasonographic examination (smaller sac size of one twin due to oligohydramnios and therefore associated with reduced movement of this twin, and larger polyhydramniotic sac often containing larger twin);

(2) At birth: classically, difference in hemoglobin of > 5 g/dl and/or in birth weight of > 20% between the twins with plethoric twin also being the larger twin;

(3) Placenta: superficial and especially deep A–V anastomoses between the placental territories of the twins. Pallor of placental territory of donor twin and congestion of recipient twin is often present

Sequelae

High perinatal morbidity and mortality of both twins, in general. *In utero* death more common in the donor twin, but if donor twin survives, it does better postnatally, after transfusions. *In utero*, recipient twin at risk for congestive heart failure, but may also die from transfused thromboplastins released with demise of donor twin. Postnatally, recipient twin at risk for hemolysis, hyperbilirubinemia, and respiratory distress

Treatment

Supportive management at birth (prenatal laser occlusion of A–V anastomoses can be done in selected medical centers)

TOPS, twin oligohydramnios–polyhydramnios syndrome

twin are *unpaired*[616–618]. Careful examination and documentation of the number, size, and type of each of these connections is key. In order to visualize best the vascular patterns, the amnion should be peeled back, except in the line of dividing septum, to expose the chorion. Vessels should be milked toward the umbilical cord, to remove intravascular blood, and all vessels inspected (arteries are superficial to veins) and traced. Use of injection studies is very helpful and strongly recommended. A variety of fluids have been used for injection, including radiopaque dyes, and latex tubing has been used to cannulate umbilical vessels; prewarming of the specimen in a 37°C saline bath has also been found to be helpful[619]. However, we prefer to use milk, since it is non-toxic, easily available, and food coloring can be added to it, if desired, to distinguish the vascular arterial distribution of one twin from the other. In addition, 'backwash' can be easily wiped from the chorionic surface in the event that overzealous pressure is applied with the injection study. The arteries should be gently and slowly injected, using a small-caliber needle (19–20 gauge) attached to a 10-ml syringe. We have found that by injecting vessels more distal from the cord insertion site, and applying gentle 'anterograde' pressure (in the direction toward the vascular equator) on the injected vessel, we are able to demonstrate both superficial and deep anastomoses, with deep A–V connections revealed by filling of the efferent vein. Careful description and mapping of these connections on a diagram or photograph are key; photographs should be taken to document various phases of the injection study, to insure against loss of clarity of vascular patterns as more injections are performed.

Histologic features

The sections made from the roll of the dividing septum and of the 'T zone', i.e. the site of the chorionic plate to which the septum is attached perpendicularly, show the absence of chorion in monochorionic placentas or the presence of two fused chorions between the two amnions in dichorionic placentas, respectively. The histologic features of the various tissues from the two placental territories show no difference in most cases, except as noted by Redline and colleagues[615] for growth-restricted twins. There are four exceptions:

(1) In a DiDi placenta, only one twin's membranes may show ACA; in a DiMo placenta, ACA affects both sacs;

(2) In a DiMo placenta with TTTS, the villous capillaries of the recipient twin are congested. Those of the donor twin are collapsed but, TTTS being a dynamic process, they may be congested if, at the time of delivery, there is no blood flow to the recipient (Figure 104);

(3) Capillaries of the villi of the shared lobules show evidence of or presence of the injected solutions, when deeper A–V anastomoses are present;

(4) In the event of death of one of the twins, the placental villi of the territory of the dead twin show various abnormalities secondary to the fetal death (see below, 'Features of intrauterine retention'), and, in the parenchyma of the recipient twin in a gestation affected by TTTS, thromboemboli, compatible with a disseminated coagulopathy, may be seen.

TYPES OF PLACENTAS IN TWIN PREGNANCY

Diamniotic monochorionic (DiMo) placenta

Zygosity Twins of a DiMo placenta are monozygotic, except in very rare instances[611].

Incidence DiMo placentas are found in about 20–30% of twin gestations[616].

Gross features The DiMo placenta consists, by definition, of a single placental disk and two amniotic sacs. The two sacs may be of similar or discordant size, and the position of the dividing septum may or may not mark the midline of the placenta or the vascular equator between the chorionic ramifications of each twin's umbilical vasculature. The dividing septum, which consists only of the reflections of two apposed amnions and no intervening chorionic tissue, is characteristically transparent to translucent (Figures 101a-1 and 102a-1), unless inflammation or meconium staining are present. Because of its structure, the two amniotic membranes of the septum can be easily peeled apart (Figure 101a-3 and a-4), and

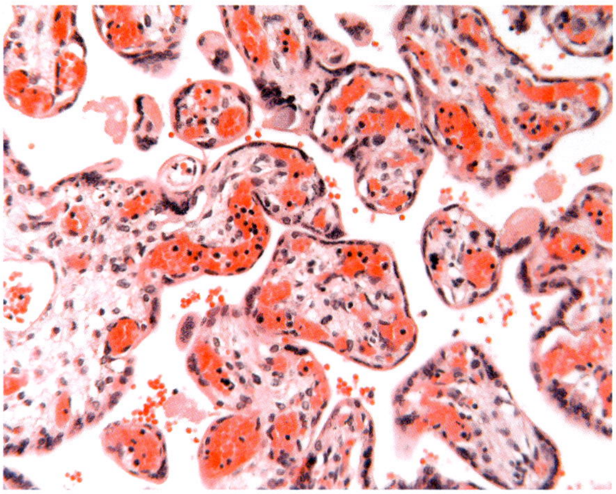

Figure 104 Chorionic villi of donor twin domain in this case of twin–twin transfusion syndrome (TTTS) show capillary congestion, numerous circulating nucleated red blood cells, and some villous edema. Thus, histopathology of the chorionic villi of the donor and recipient domains in a given placental case will reflect the balance in blood flow among the shunts at the time of delivery

the dissection can be carried across the fetal surface[4]. Moreover, since the dividing membrane is so tenuously attached to the chorionic surface, it can be easily dislodged with manipulation during delivery of the placenta or placental examination (Figure 101a-3). This can lead to an erroneous diagnosis of a MoMo placenta (see below) by the obstetrician or the pathologist. Cord abnormalities are more frequent in DiMo twins than in DiDi or singleton placentas from singleton deliveries; about 45% of cases of SUA, 56% of marginal insertions, and 42% of velamentous insertions occur in DiMo twins, compared with all DiDi placentations: SUA 45% (29% in fused); marginal insertion 42% (23.4% in fused) (Figure 101a-1); velamentous insertion 41% (Figure 105) (38.5% in fused) and singleton placentas from singleton pregnancies (SUA ~ 1%; marginal insertion ~ 7%)[610]. The rates of these abnormalities are even more striking when the relative frequency of DiDi placentations is taken into account, i.e. DiDi twin placentas are 3–4 times more common than DiMo placentas. When examining the DiMo placenta, the distance between the cord insertions and their relative distances from the dividing membrane should be documented. In addition, the integrity and length of velamentous vessels should be described, particularly since all cord anomalies in DiMo placentas are associated with a significantly higher perinatal mortality rate[610].

As stated above, essentially all DiMo placentas have vascular anastomoses (chorangiopagous vessels). The clinical detection of moderately to markedly discrepant sac sizes by prenatal ultrasonography of a DiMo twin placenta is referred to as 'twin oligohydramnios–polyhydramnios syndrome (TOPS)' or 'stuck twin syndrome' (Figure 102a-1), and denotes oligohydramnios in the sac of the donor twin and/or the appearance of the twin of being 'stuck' to the amniotic surface of its placenta, and polyhydramnios and enlargement of the sac of the clinically identified recipient twin. The identification of discrepant compartment size and amnion nodosum of the surface of the smaller sac on pathologic examination of a DiMo placenta may represent the sequelae of TTTS. Even in the absence of a clinical history of TTTS, careful search for

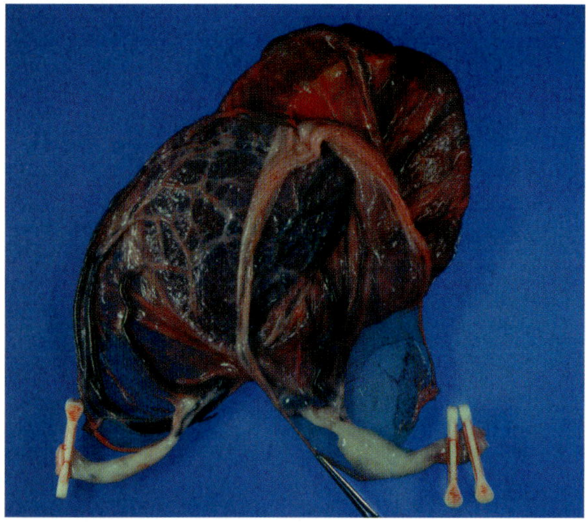

Figure 105 Diamniotic monochorionic (DiMo) twin placenta with velamentous insertion of both umbilical cords and that of twin 2, into the dividing membrane

chorangiopagous vessels should always be performed. It is also important to remember that:

(1) It is a paucity of anastomoses that are associated with TTTS (since there is greater chance for chronic unbalanced blood volume exchange delivered to one twin);

(2) It is the small-caliber vessels that are most often involved;

(3) Deep anastomoses are especially pathologic.

Injection studies should also be carried out, as described above, in cases of TTTS or discrepant sac size. Examination of the maternal surface, in cases of TTTS, may reveal an irregular line of demarcation between pale and dark red-brown congested tissue, denoting the donor's and recipient's sides, respectively (Figure 106a-1). Transmural sections may also reveal relatively reduced mural thickness, and pale friable parenchyma in the donor's territory and plethoric relatively thick parenchyma of the recipient's (Figure 106a-2 and a-3). However, as will be addressed below, the presence of this 'classic' discrepant appearance of chronic TTTS between the two domains of the DiMo placenta in TTTS may not always be evident, since it depends on a fairly

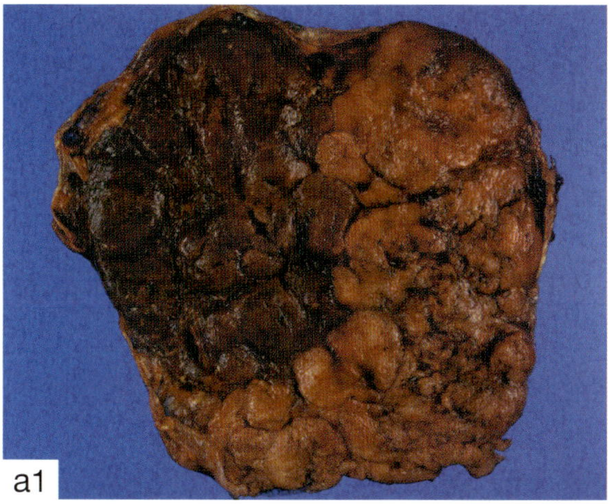

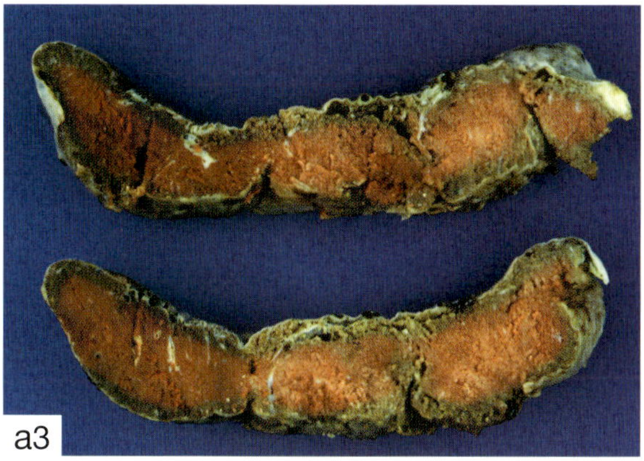

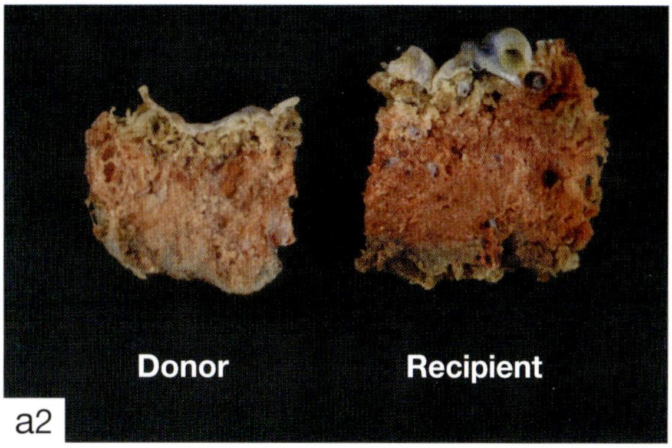

Figure 106 Additional gross features of diamniotic monochorionic (DiMo) placenta in twin–twin transfusion syndrome (TTTS). (a-1) In classic TTTS, the maternal surface will show a pale, firm, and somewhat friable tissue on the donor side in contrast to a dark, congested, firm, and relatively bulging surface of the domain of the recipient. (a-2) Sections show a relatively distinct difference in the dark congested parenchyma of the recipient's domain versus the paler villous tissue of the donor's. The demarcation is not a straight line, since the lobules interdigitate. (a-3) In some areas, the difference in mural appearance includes a marked difference in mural thickness, as well

consistent 'unidirectional' net excess of blood flow to the recipient.

While the most important concern regarding a DiMo placentation is TTTS, a small sac size (i.e. oligohydramnios) may also be due to a primary fetal renal anomaly or bladder outlet obstruction or vascular accident. Polyhydramnios may be due to a fetal gastrointestinal obstruction. Monosomy X and hydrops and a variety of syndromes may affect only one twin of the DiMo gestation[610].

Histologic features The dividing septum is composed of two apposing amnions, in a mirror-image-like arrangement, in which their basement membranes are separated by a narrow, acellular clear space (Figure 101a-2). In general, in cases of TTTS, capillaries of the villi of the donor territory are collapsed, and those of the recipient twin are congested. However, depending upon the status of the recipient and fluctuations in the shunting of blood between the various anastomoses, as discussed below, the chorionic villi of the donor may also show some edema, in addition to excessive normoblastemia or erythroblastosis due to anemia (Figure 104).

Clinical significance of vascular anastomoses in DiMo placentas and the pathogenesis of TTTS

As noted in the sections above, virtually all DiMo placentas have chorangiopagous vessels. However, TTTS develops in a only a small percentage of DiMo twins (10–30%)[618–620], since it requires the development of a net imbalance in blood volume exchange between the two twins. The pathogenesis of TTTS appears to involve variations in vascular size and number of anastomoses, and the development of placental asymmetry. Superficial A–A and V–V anastomoses are generally of little consequence in the development of TTTS because both types permit bidirectional shunting. However, 'deep anastomoses' (with unpaired afferent arterial and efferent venous branches) and a *paucity* of intertwin connections increase the risk of imbalances occurring in blood volumes transfused between the twins, and the development of TTTS[616–618].

In the example shown in Figure 103, an arterial vessel from twin II is supplying two adjacent segments of the chorionic villous tree, each drained by a venous branch (red for oxygenated blood following exchange at the villous surface) of twin I. The net effect is twin–twin transfusion from twin II to twin I. However, if several different shared lobules are present, they may effect shunting of blood in the same direction (i.e. twin II to twin I) or in the opposite direction (twin I to twin II), and thereby offset imbalances. In addition, the superficial anastomoses, if numerous enough, could effect a balance. All of the vascular anastomoses are formed during the early angiogenic phase of development of the placenta. However, it should also be noted that fetal thrombosis can cause acute TTTS in a previously balanced circulation[621].

It is tempting to view TTTS as a chronic, unidirectional, and continuous condition of blood volume siphon from donor to recipient twin. However, while the early and continued net result is preferential blood delivery to 'the recipient', TTTS is not a static condition. Moreover, while imbalanced blood flow is the principal cause, other factors appear to contribute to the pathogenesis and pathologic effects of TTTS. Fluctuations in arterial and venous blood pressures in the twins, due to volume exchange, affect the volume of blood flow across the anastomoses. As a 'donor fetus' (i.e. in this case, twin II of Figure 103) becomes hypovolemic, its perfusion pressure to the arterial deep anastomoses falls, and the effective transfusion to twin I declines. Then, as it recovers its intravascular blood volume, twin II's cardiac function may return, its systemic blood pressure 'recover', and perfusion of the deep anastomosis return. Conversely, the 'recipient twin' (twin I) becomes hypervolemic and may go into congestive failure, and be less able to 'accommodate' the volume of blood transfused from twin II. Therefore, in TTTS, dynamics of blood pressure fluctuations in each twin's arteries; fluctuations in their respective central venous pressures; the number of these connections; and the respective ratios of arteriovenous twin II→twin I : twin I→twin II connections all contribute to the net effect of blood volumes passed between the DiMo twins.

As noted above, superficial A–A anastomoses may be protective, in that they may allow, via arterial blood pressure differences, for blood to be 'sent back' to the other twin's territory, and effect a form of compensation. In addition to the volumetric considerations in TTTS, there is also evidence that activation of physiologic mechanisms may play a role in the pathology of TTTS. Mahieu-Caputo and colleagues[620] observed hypovolemia-related up-regulation of the rennin–angiotensin system (RAS) in the donor twin, and down-regulation of RAS in the recipient, in TTTS gestations. They found that RAS activation exacerbates oligohydramnios, and postulated that it may increase systemic arterial resistance in the donor, and thereby contribute to placental dysfunction (by poor perfusion of the fetal vasculature), and IUGR of the donor. They also postulated that transfusion of RAS effectors, through A–V anastomoses, may be involved in pathogenesis of cardiomyopathy (cardiac failure) in the recipient (a paradoxical effect). The polyhydramnios of the sac of the recipient twin may in part reflect the polyuria of the fetus, but the higher colloid osmotic pressure of the recipient also leads to passive absorption of water from the maternal blood[618].

The dynamics of chronic TTTS are incompletely understood, but, left untreated, it is associated with an approximate 90% perinatal mortality rate for both twins[622]. For uncompensated and worsening TTTS, laser fetoscopic occlusion of chorionic anastomoses and arterial unpaired vessels has been effective[617,623]. The placental pathology of this procedure is addressed below (Chapter 19, 'Placental features following intrauterine vascular laser ablation procedures'). Other effective methods have included serial amnioreduction[618].

Dichorionic diamniotic (DiDi) placenta

Zygosity The twins of DiDi placentas can be mono- or dizygotic.

Incidence DiDi placentas are found in about 70–80% of twin gestations[610].

Gross features The two placental disks may be entirely separate or intimately fused, resembling the DiMo placenta. The pathology of separate DiDi placentas is the same as that of singleton placentas, except for the higher rates of cord anomalies and perinatal mortality outlined above for the DiMo placenta. The fusion may be partial, so that only the membranes are fused along part of their fetal aspects, while the disks are prominently separated. Alternatively, the disks may be closely aligned and connected by intervening membranes. The dividing membranous septum between the intimately fused DiDi placentas is thick and opaque (Figure 101b-1). In contrast to the DiMo placenta, peeling the dividing membrane apart disrupts its connection to the chorionic plate surface. Vascular anastomoses are extremely rare.

Histologic features The dividing membranous septum of the intimately fused DiDi placenta shows chorion (Figure 101b-2), which may include ghost-like remnants of chorionic villi interposed between the two mirror-image amnions. The chorionic tissue overwhelmingly represents fused chorion from both placentas.

Clinical significance TTTS is *extremely* rare in fused DiDi placentas.

Monochorionic monoamniotic (MoMo) placenta

Zygosity The twins are monozygotic.

Incidence MoMo placentation is found in 1–2% of all twins or about 1/10 000–1/16 000 pregnancies[4].

Gross features This is the least common type of twin placenta. There is only one amniotic sac. Consequently, there is no dividing septum on the fetal surface (Figure 107a-1 and a-2). There is a single placental disk with two closely inserting umbilical cords. It is *highly* unusual for the cords to insert more than a few centimeters apart, and adjacent or near common insertions may be seen (Figure 107a-3). However, in occasional cases, a small amniotic fold or plica may be present on the fetal surface that intersects the cord insertion site(s). It may represent an early, interrupted attempt to form amniotic sacs. Vascular anastomoses are extensive and easily visualized between the large peri-insertional branches of each cord and between more distal branches; all types (A–A, V–V, and A–V) can be seen (Figure 107a-4 and a-5). The cord insertions may be wrapped in a drape of amnion; the proximity of the cord insertions and the large peri-insertional anastomoses are very useful features in differentiating MoMo from DiMo placentations in which the membranes have become avulsed; DiMo placentas and DiDi placentas have significantly greater interinsertional distances; and DiMo placentas rarely show peri-insertional anastomoses.

Histologic features The fold that may be present on the fetal surface is composed of amnion. If one of the twins dies *in utero*, the corresponding placental tissue may become atrophic, or its circulation may persist via the extensive anastomoses with the blood vessels of the surviving twin. However, intrauterine fetal demise of one twin is rarely associated with survival of the other twin, and thromboemboli due to initiation of disseminated coagulopathy may be seen in the cord and chorionic plate vessels.

Clinical significance Because of fetal movements in a common sac, the two umbilical cords can become entangled; this is the most common cause of fetal death and is most often found early on, presumably because of the relatively smaller size of the fetuses and the relatively greater possibility for movement in the fluid-filled sac. Cord entanglement produces venous obstruction and leads to intrauterine fetal demise in early gestation (Figure 108), but is infrequently the cause of death in late third trimester. Other causes of intrauterine fetal demise are coagulopathy and exsanguination through placental anastomoses. The fetal mortality rate of MoMo gestations is 68% and dual survival is only about 16%. Discordant malformations are common, and likely reflect the effects on intrafetal blood flow variations due to the

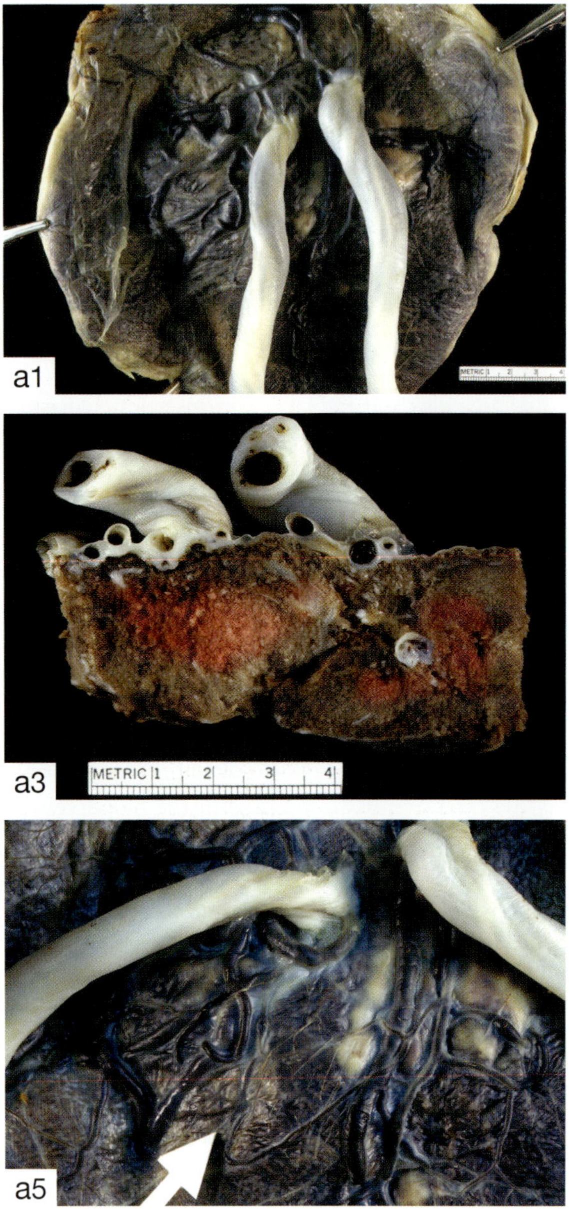

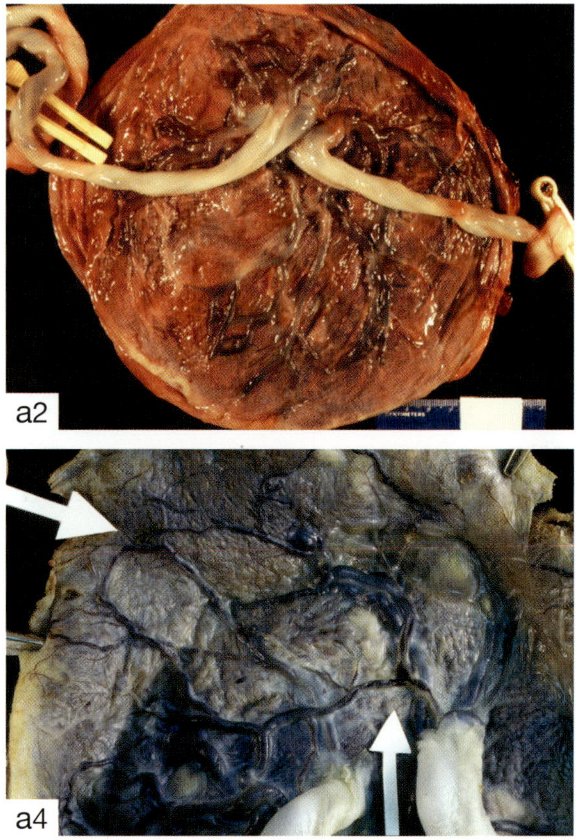

Figure 107 Monoamniotic monochorionic (MoMo) twin placentation. (a-1) and (a-2) show typical juxtaposition of cord insertions of MoMo placentas. The late division of the cell mass after generation of the amnion results in close approximation of the cord insertion sites. (a-3) Cross-section of cord insertion site of 500-g placenta in (a-1), delivered at 32 weeks of gestation. Close-up of artery to artery (A–A) anastomosis (lower arrow) and a shared lobule (upper arrow) of the two cord vascular domains (a-4), and artery of right cord supplies lobule drained by vein from left cord (a-5) in these images from placenta of (a-1)

anastomoses, as well as other mechanisms. TTTS is uncommon in MoMo gestations, because of the extensive placental anastomoses[4,610]. However, reversal of blood flow within the anastomoses, after intrauterine fetal demise of one twin, may result in exsanguination of the survivor's blood into the relaxed vasculature of the dead, smaller twin. Such situations may result in a smaller, but *lethoric-appearing* twin (original donor) and a larger *pale* twin (original recipient) (F. Kraus, MD, personal communication). In most cases of MoMo gestations, neonatal death is related to prematurity[4,610].

Vanishing twins

This term is used to indicate the birth of a single child to a mother for whom sonographic diagnosis of multiple pregnancy was made during the first 15 weeks of gestation. The phenomenon occurs much more

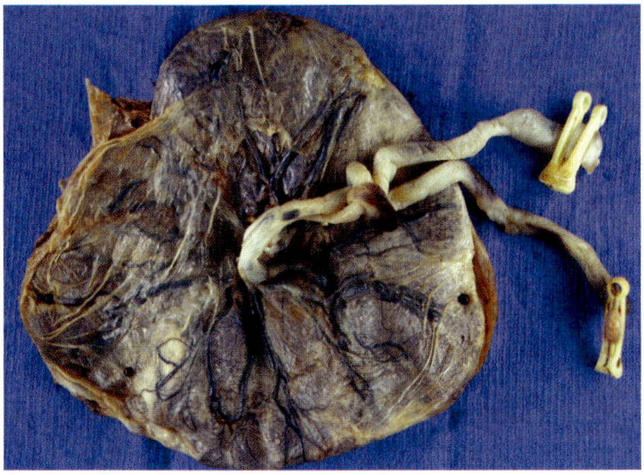

Figure 108 Monoamniotic monochorionic (MoMo) placenta with cord entanglement. The twins were live-born, but were preterm, at 32 weeks' gestational age

frequently in spontaneous pregnancies than was appreciated prior to the use of first-trimester ultrasonography; the rate of spontaneous twinning is about 12%. However, only about 14% of twins both survive to term, with most demises occurring prior to the second trimester (21–63%)[33]. In addition, as noted above, monochorionic twins have a significantly higher risk of abortion than do dichorionic twins. In medically assisted pregnancies, each twin/fetus has about a 17–19% risk of demise[624,625], with first-trimester loss predominating. There are few reports of pathologic examination of the placenta. Plaques of perivillous fibrinoid deposition, with or without embryonic remnants on the membranes, have been described by Jauniaux and colleagues[626]. Evidence of a second sac, with or without a small embryo, may be found. The embryo/fetus may appear as a flattened tan-yellow plaque, with or without retinal pigment. In some instances, the placental disk itself is detectable, and a dividing membrane remnant may be identifiable, particularly if sections are taken through plaque-like elevations at the perimeter of the placenta[610]. Vaginal bleeding occurs frequently in early pregnancy in patients with vanishing twin, and the vanishing twin may be aborted during one of these events, especially in the case of first-trimester dichorionic gestations. Pathologic examination of the placenta will fail to reveal the twin in such cases. However, the placenta and the membranes should be carefully examined for the presence of a second sac and/or the remnants of a dead embryo in cases of vanishing twin. Determination of chorionicity may help to explain the presence of structural abnormalities in the surviving twin, since a DiMo placentation may implicate TTTS. The cause of demise of the embryo/fetus is seldom clear, but in spontaneous and assisted reproductions an abnormal karyotype of the embryo/fetus may be responsible.

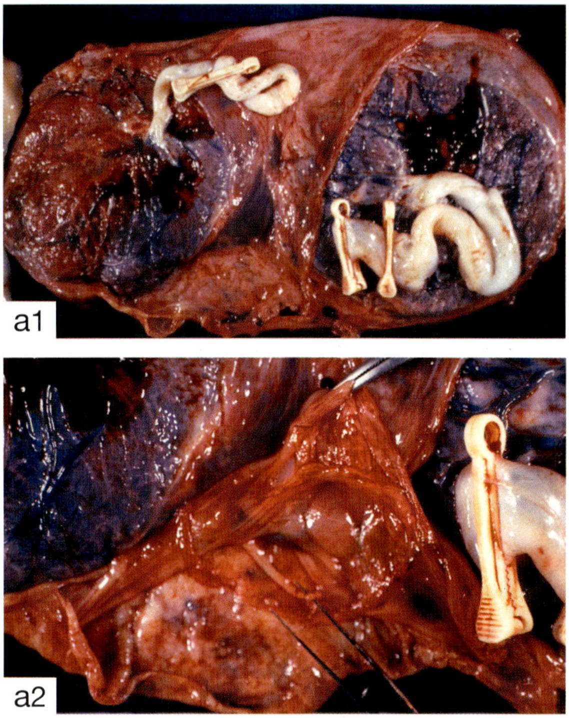

Figure 109 Fetus compressus/fetus papyraceus. (a-1) This fused diamniotic dichorionic (DiDi) placenta showed a marginal area of yellow-tan gritty infarction on the maternal surface, which on the fetal surface showed this pale, firm, infarcted area that resembled an accessory lobe. (a-2) Upon dissection, a remnant of umbilical cord was found, but no other fetal parts were grossly confirmed. Radiography of the placenta revealed collapsed skull, vertebral, and long bone remnants in the plaque. Thus, this was originally a triplet gestation

Fetus papyraceus/fetus compressus

Vanishing twin and fetus papyraceus/fetus compressus (FP/FC) form a continuum. In FP/FC, one of the twins dies and is identifiable as a plaque composed of the compressed, dehydrated remnant of the dead fetus, or of some identifiable fetal parts. This plaque may be missed if a careful gross examination is not done, especially of the placental margin (Figure 109). X-radiography of the plaque will demonstrate the skeleton of the fetus. The placenta may be mono- or dichorionic. The cause of death or the presence of congenital anomalies of the FP/FC may be demonstrable (e.g. umbilical cord torsion, mid-facial clefting), but most often, a prolonged period of retention precludes such determinations. Prolonged retention may also lead to calcification of the FP/FC and formation of a lithopedion. The use of selective reduction procedures in multiple gestation pregnancies, of course, also results in FP/FC and the need for pathologic documentation by placental examination[627].

Acardiac twin

This is a rare abnormality (occurring in ~ 1/34 600 deliveries or about 1/100 monozygotic twin gestations)[4] that is almost exclusively confined to monochorionic monoamniotic twinnings, and one in which the acardiac twin develops and is maintained as viable *in* utero because of an artery-to-artery and a vein-to-vein anastomosis with the normal donor twin. The specimen of acardiac twin may be submitted with the placenta. It characteristically consists of a large, spheroid, skin-covered soft tissue mass which may have a cephalocaudal polarity with poorly formed lower limbs and severely hypoplastic, malformed-to-absent upper limbs; a malformed head may or may not be present. The heart is absent or a very rudimentary structure (Figure 110). The acardius variations are termed *acardius acephalus* (failure or disruption of the development of a head), *acardius myelocephalus* (a head and rudimentary limbs present), and *acardius amorphous* (no structures identifiable). A wide number of visceral abnormalities have been identified, but the most common are hepatic absence or malformations (~ 90%)[628] and omphaloceles[629]. These malformations are particularly associated with sites of vascular connections and blood flow to and from the embryo, and their frequencies support the hypothesis that acardius represents the sequelae of a large, early artery-to-artery chorionic shunt between the twin embryos. Presumably the arterial pressure of one embryo exceeds that of the other such that the recipient twin receives arterial (suboptimally oxygenated blood) through iliac-level arteries (umbilical arteries are branches of the internal iliacs). The venous connections do not supply oxygenated blood, and the liver, which would normally be the first organ to encounter oxygenated blood, is characteristically very abnormal to absent in acardius. The preferential blood flow to the caudal aspects of the developing acardiac twin presumably permits some development of the lower limbs, the gastrointestinal tract, and portions of the vertebral column (that can be documented by X-ray of the specimen), but the upper portions of the embryo fail to develop or exhibit disrupted growth. Since the arterial blood flow to and within the acardiac twin is reversed, the term 'TRAP sequence' is often applied (twin reversed arterial perfusion) to these cases[4,610]. A rudimentary umbilical cord-like structure can be seen connecting the acardius to the placental vascular conduits with the donor twin. The donor twin is nearly always structurally and genetically normal, but, due to the parasitic relationship of the acardius, there is a high risk of mortality (50–75%) in the donor twin, without obstetrical intervention[33]. Cord entanglement may also occur due to the MoMo placentation. The placenta will show a large, often marginal, vascular pedicle containing an arterial and venous connection from the donor to the cord structure of the acardius recipient, and the placenta may be hydropic. Intrauterine fetal demise of the donor twin will be accompanied by secondary changes of intrauterine retention (see below, 'Features of intrauterine retention').

Conjoined twins

These are also rare occurrences (1 in 33 000 to 1 in 165 000 deliveries in North America) of monozygotic twinning and a MoMo placentation, but are symmetric duplications (acardius represents asymmetric duplication). Twins of roughly equal size share

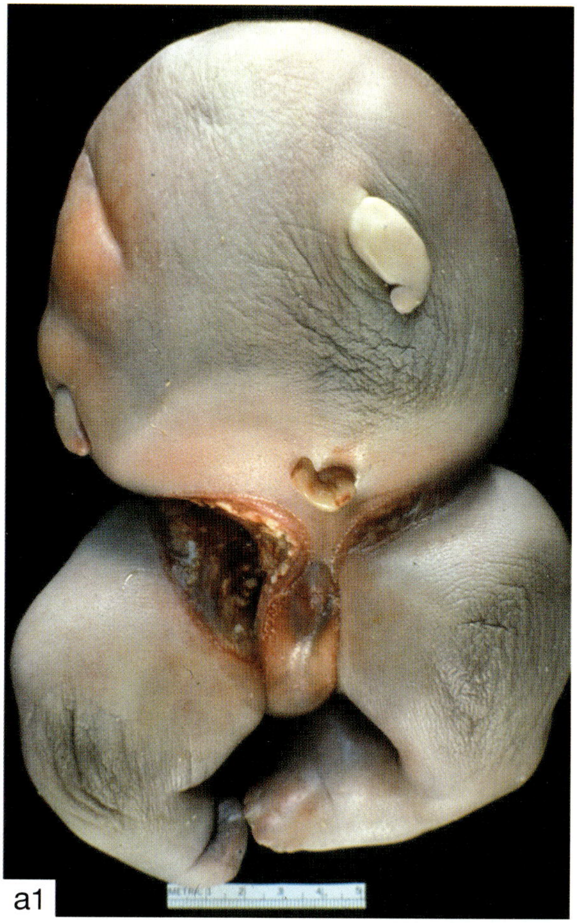

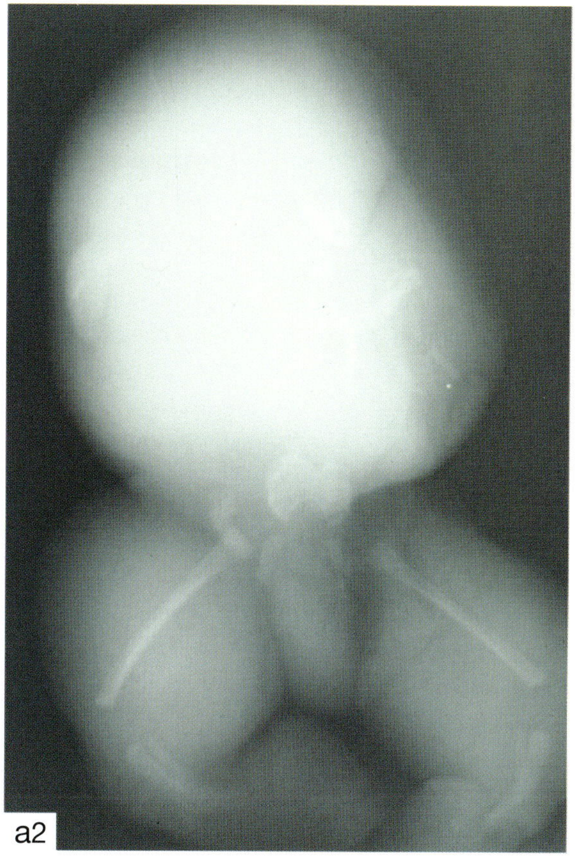

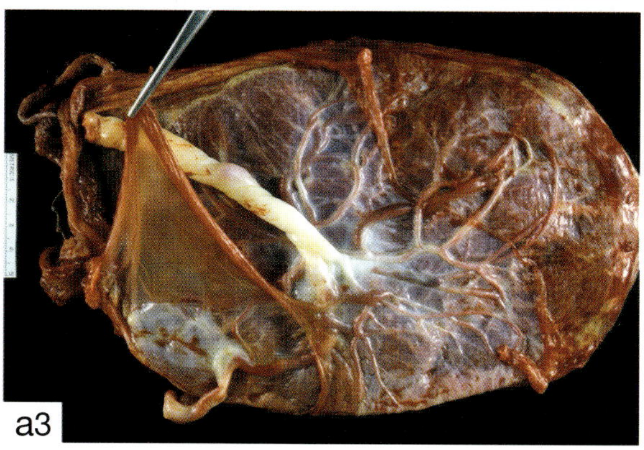

Figure 110 Acardiac twin. (a-1) Acardius acephalus with cephalocaudal polarity with malformed lower limbs, a spheroid upper mass with rudimentary upper limbs, and no head. The umbilical cord structure supplied a branching vascular tree, but no heart was present. Internal organs consisted of few dysplastic ribs, a tiny portion of liver, a small spleen, proximal gastrointestinal tract, a single, multicystic dysplastic kidney, two adrenals, and two ovaries. The soft tissue was edematous and fatty. (a-2) X-ray image of the acardius acephalus. (a-3) The placenta shows the presence of a communicating artery and vein at the margin (the amnion is retracted to expose the vessels) that supplied the acardius acephalus

portions of trunk and/or cranium, and these sites most likely represent regions of failed separation of the two embryonic disks. The cause(s) of this condition is not understood but the findings are compatible with disturbance of division of the cell masses after day 13 of development. The extent and site of the shared body region are variable, as are the number of limbs, and the terminology applied is complex. However, most have thoraco-omphalopagus (thoracoabdominal fixation; 28.4%) or thoracopagus (thoracic fixation; 18.5%) connections, and most are duplicated above and below the common region such that there are eight extremities and two facing heads, or anakatadidyma types (Greek for 'up' and 'down' 'twins'; 59.3%). Conjoined twins are found at a surprisingly high frequency in triplet pregnancies. In addition, the majority of conjoined twins are female and there is a high rate of stillbirth (or abortion). Visceral arrangement is most commonly mirror-image and the cardiovascular trees are highly complex but incompletely duplicated; secondary (those related to incomplete twinning) and primary malformations occur, with discordant major malformations seen in 20%. The umbilical cord is multivascular and singular, and most often fused at the insertional end, although separate adjacent insertions with fusion within a short distance from the amniotic surface may be seen. Depending upon the region of shared anatomy, it may remain fused, but usually it is furcated at the abdomen(s) with separate mirror-image branching of its venous vessels to the respective domains of the liver mass(es), and of its arteries with the iliac arteries of each twin in the anakatadidyma thoracopagus/thoraco-omphalopagus pair. In cases of katadidyma twins, with a single lower body, the umbilical vein will be 'normal' but the umbilical artery may be single or 'normal' and bilateral. Thus, from the standpoint of the placental examination, the number of umbilical vessels in the cord will differ, but since most conjoined twins are anakatadidyma type and since SUA is common, most cords from conjoined twins will show five vessels, consisting of three arteries and two veins[610]. For reasons related to timing of its formation (roughly days 11–12), the MoMo placenta of conjoined twins will show only a single yolk sac[4]. The reader interested in a discussion of the mechanisms believed to be responsible for producing the various conjoined twin types is referred to the fascinating treatise by Machin[630].

Figure 111 shows two examples of the external and some of the internal anomalies of thoraco-omphalopagus conjoined twins.

Triplet and multiple deliveries

Triplet pregnancy may be monzygotic (a single zygote replicating into two zygotes, with subsequent replication of one of these two zygotes), dizygotic (due to subsequent monozygotic twinning of one of the zygotes), or trizygotic. Prior to the use of assisted reproductive technologies, dizygotic sets were 2–3 times more common than monozygotic or trizygotic sets. Examination of the triplet placental case, while somewhat time-consuming, is only an extension of the principles applied to the twin placenta. Chorionicity needs to be established and umbilical cord vascularity, insertion, and integrity need to be determined for each triplet component. In addition, while a monochorionic triamniotic, a monochorionic diamniotic, or a monochorionic monoamniotic placenta represents a monozygotic replication, *none* of the other patterns can be used to determine zygosity. If the cords are not clinically designated, the obstetrician should be contacted to identify the compartments. Most triplet placentas exhibit a triamniotic trichorionic pattern (Figure 112a), and most of these show fusion of two of the three disks, but the placentas may all be separate. The next most common pattern is triamniotic dichorionic placentation with two disks. Figure 112b shows a triamniotic dichorionic placentation with a single disk. A dichorionic diamniotic configuration, in which one of the sacs contains *two* triplets, is the least common type[610]. The pathologist should sample all dividing membranes, carefully documenting which relationship he/she is examining (i.e. triplet 1 to 2, triplet 2 to 3, and triplet 1 to 3) and examine and sample the fetal, maternal, and cut surfaces of each triplet's domain. In addition, care should be taken to ensure that a FP/FC is not present, particularly in cases of medically assisted pregnancies. Placentas from higher multiple gestations should be approached in a similar manner, with documentation of chorionicity and cord morphology.

INTRAUTERINE GROWTH RESTRICTION

It should be noted that most investigations of IUGR have been focused on singleton gestations, and the focus of this section is the singleton infant. However, studies of twin (multiple) gestations have indicated that intrauterine growth of twins parallels that of singletons to 32 weeks of gestation[610,631] and that, after 32 weeks, differences between twins and singletons probably reflect placentation (dichorionic dizygotic twins are larger than monochorionic twins), site of placentation, and/or TTTS[610]. The issue of whether twins are constitutionally smaller than singletons remains unclear. Some studies have shown that fetal growth after 32 weeks is markedly slowed, whereas others have shown that unless there is growth discordance, twins are of comparable weights to singletons, and that in cases of growth discordance, the weight of the larger twin is comparable to that of a gestationally age-matched singleton. What is not disputed is that IUGR and prematurity remain the most significant parameters of increased risks of neonatal morbidity and mortality for singletons and multiples[631].

Low birth weight is defined as a weight < 2500 g. Very low birth weight is < 1500 g, and extremely low birth weight is < 1000 g. Low birth weight may be due to prematurity, but it may also be due to IUGR. IUGR is defined as fetal/infant weight < 10th centile expected for gestational age (Table 10). There has been ongoing research into the myriad mechanisms involved in the development of fetal IUGR, including differences in mechanisms and outcome with gestational period of onset and the implications of IUGR for development of adult onset of coronary arterial and cardiovascular disease and glucose intolerance. A discussion of this research is beyond the scope of this manual; however, the reader is referred to the superb review by Cetin and colleagues[632].

Briefly, IUGR may be related to the following:

(1) Maternal factors: pre-eclampsia and/or hypertension, or other conditions that result in underperfusion of the placental bed, severe malnutrition, and maternal substance abuse. Of late, the potential roles of maternal thrombophilia and autoimmune diseases have been aggressively explored[632]. Maternal thrombophilia, with thrombosis in vessels of the placental bed together with increased coagulation in the maternal space, have been implicated in the development of IUGR[59,633].

(2) Fetal factors: chromosomal disorders, intrauterine infection (e.g. CMV, toxoplasmosis), and severe structural anomalies or anomalous syndromes or associations, such as VACTERL (association of vertebral anomalies, anal atresia, cardiac malformation, tracheoesophageal fistula, and renal and limb anomalies), and genetic factors, such as genomic imprinting, are implicated.

(3) Placental factors: lesions such as extrachorial placenta, marginal and velamentous insertion of the umbilical cord, multiple infarcts (usually involving more than 30% of the term placenta), extensive perivillous fibrinoid deposition and MFI, VUE, large chorangioma, and confined placental mosaicism, etc.

The placenta of the growth-restricted fetus/infant is often of small size. The small size of the placenta may be a reflection of a generalized growth disturbance of the fetus, since the placenta is a fetal organ. In most cases, however, the small placental size is a manifestation of the sequelae of an underlying maternal disorder or pathologic process that damages the placenta and reduces its functional volume. Placental lesions seen in cases of IUGR will reflect the underlying conditions, such as poor perfusion of the placental bed; however, the placenta may appear completely normal. In some cases, the cause of the IUGR cannot be determined.

PLACENTA IN FETAL HYDROPS AND ERYTHROBLASTOSIS FETALIS

The differential diagnoses in hydrops fetalis is extensive, but is basically divided into immune-mediated and non-immune-mediated etiologies. Immune-mediated hydrops fetalis (IMHF) may be due to ABO, Rh (D), C and E, and Kell blood group isoimmunization, but the overwhelming majority of cases of hydrops fetalis are due to non-immune-mediated causes (i.e. non-immune fetal hydrops or NIFH). Rates of NIHF-complicating gestations have ranged from 0.04%[308,634,635] to 0.5%[636]. As the causes of

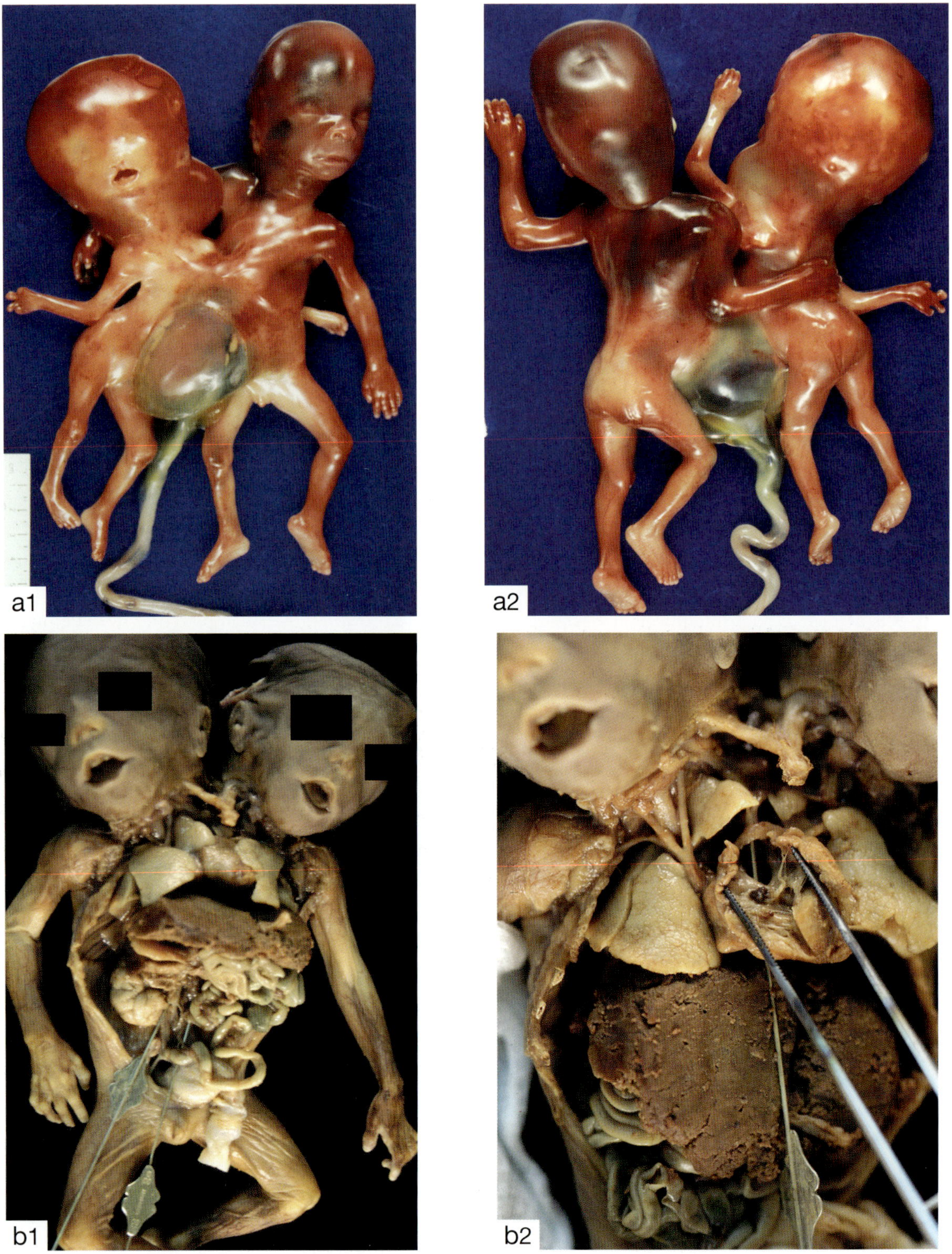

Figure 111 *See opposite for legend*

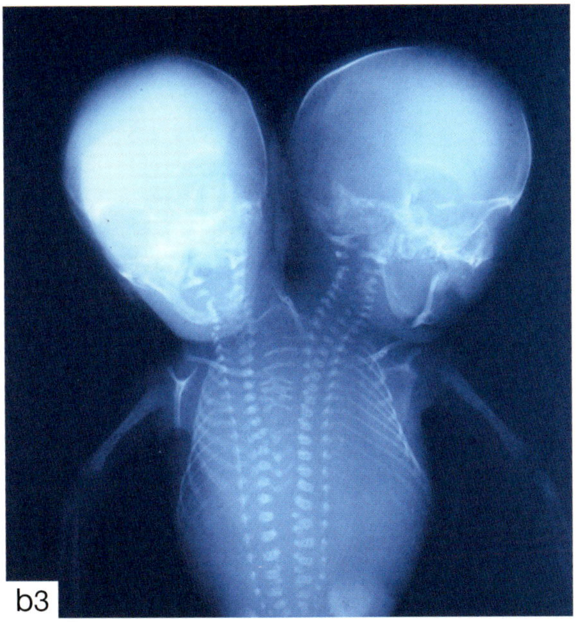

Figure 111 Conjoined twins. These are examples of thoraco-omphalopagus type conjoined twins with fusion of the thorax and portions of the abdomen. (a-1 and a-2) Conjoined twins at 18 weeks of gestational age with a single, somewhat short umbilical cord that had five vessels. Both twins had kyphoscoliosis, with thoracolumbar vertebral anomalies, and the left twin was more severely affected, with cervical anomalies and a nuchal hygroma, hydrocephalus, alobar holoprosencephaly, arrhinencephaly, cleft palate, anophthalmia, and low-set, dysplastic ears. There was mirror-image duplication of the thoracic structures and most of the gastrointestinal tract; the liver was shared, but there were two gallbladders and the anus of the left twin was imperforate. (b-1–b-3) These conjoined twins at 24 weeks of gestational age demonstrate the spectrum of shared and mirror-image arrangement of organs of the thoracoabdominal cavity in thoraco-omphalopagus type of anomalous twinning. There was left and right lung morphology with a central fused lung mass behind an extremely complex, malformed, fused heart that included a common midline atrium (note probe within chamber in b-2) with a three-chamber ventricle that gave rise to mirror-image aortae and arches. The proximal gastro-intestinal tract was duplicated, to the level of the cecum (probes at cecum and behind colon in b-1). There were two kidneys and a normal pelvis and genitourinary tract. (b-3) The X-ray image shows the extent of duplication of the vertebral columns

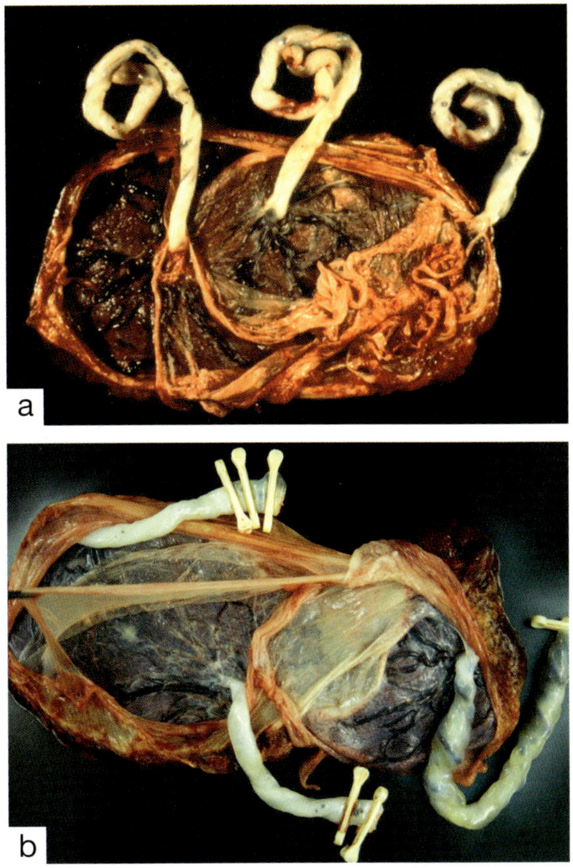

Figure 112 Triplet placentations. (a) The most common is triamniotic trichorionic placentation, with fusion of at least two of the disks. This case shows fusion of all three disks. (b) This triplet placenta shows diamniotic dichorionic (DiDi) placentatation between triplets 1 and 2, DiDi between 1 and 3, and diamniotic monochorionic (DiMo) between triplets 2 and 3; note the translucent dividing membrane between the domains of 2 and 3

IMHF have declined due to institution of Rh immune globulin therapy, non-immune etiologies have correspondingly risen, and currently account for about 87% of clinically identified cases[636,637]. NIFH may be due to a large number of conditions including, but not limited to, a variety of genetic, metabolic, cardiac, pulmonary, and hematologic disorders, infections (particularly CMV and PVB19), fetomaternal hemorrhage, and fetal tumors. The etiology of the hydrops may not be determined in 5.2–16% of clinically detected cases. However, in the study of stillbirth by Rodriguez and colleagues[638], in which 6% of cases were due to NIFH, placental examination provided the explanation for perinatal loss in nearly one-fifth of cases and helped to confirm the causal diagnosis in an additional 63%; the combination of a thorough autopsy examination and placental examination resulted in a very low rate of cases for which a cause could not be determined (3.92%).

The placenta in cases of hydrops fetalis and erythroblastosis fetalis (EBF) will show varying degrees of hydropic change depending on the severity of the fetal hydrops, with edema of the cord, increased placental weight, and pale bulky parenchyma (see Figure 43a). Microscopic examination in NIFH will show edematous chorionic villi, but other features will be dependent upon the etiology (e.g. CMV or PVB19 inclusions and/or villitis). Generally, abundant nucleated orthochromic normoblasts and, in some cases, earlier stages of the erythroid series are seen in fetal vessels (Figure 43b and c). When circulating, more immature forms of erythrocytes are seen, the pathologic term *erythroblastosis fetalis* is most appropriately applied. EBF is more frequently seen in IMHF. EBF due to IMHF generally shows synchronous villous immaturity, prominence of Hofbauer cells, and intervillous thrombi (up to 30% of cases), and hemosiderin may be present in macrophages.

CHROMOSOMAL DISORDERS

In trisomies 13, 18 and 21, both the fetus and placenta tend to be small. Single umbilical artery is a common finding in trisomies. The villi may show delayed maturation, with decreased vascularity, and the presence of large atypical cells of unclear origin in the stroma. In monosomy 45X, the villi may show variable cellularity and stromal fibrosis, with trophoblastic hypoplasia with deficient syncytial budding. Over 98% of monosomy-X conceptuses are spontaneously aborted, and massive fetal and placental hydrops are characteristic in the second trimester[522]. The placentas of triploidy have been previously described, and tetraploid gestations are similar. In a study of fetuses between 18 and 23 weeks, placentas from gestations with abnormal karyotype showed a significant decrease in small muscular artery counts in villi[639]. However, abnormalities of placental histology have been shown to be poor predictors of chromosomal abnormalities[640].

METABOLIC DISORDERS

Placental changes have been described in gangliosidoses[641], mucopolysaccharidoses, mucolipidoses, Gaucher's disease, Niemann–Pick disease, Wolman's disease, Zellweger's syndrome, glycogen storage disease type II, ceroid liopfuscinosis, etc. On gross examination, the placenta as well as the fetus may be hydropic. The accumulated metabolites of these disorders are soluble in water or xylene; hence, in routine histologic sections of the placenta, empty vacuoles may be seen in the syncytiotrophoblast, intermediate trophoblast, Hofbauer cells, endothelium, and fetal white blood cells in villous capillaries. Specific categorization of a metabolic disorder is not possible by placental examination. Electron microscopy may provide additional information in these cases. Jones and colleagues have described ultrastructural features of placentas and chorionic villus biopsy samples from a variety of metabolic disorders[642], such as myelin bodies in Niemann–Pick disease, and intralysosomal glycogen accumulation in glycogen storage disease type II. Prompt fixation for electron microscopy aids in avoiding artifacts. Biochemical investigation of fresh tissue is critical to demonstrate the enzyme defect and establish the appropriate diagnosis; hence, fresh placental tissue should be snap-frozen when there is any indication of a metabolic disease.

INTRAPARTUM FETAL DEATH

In contrast to antepartum fetal death, there is no maceration in the fetus and there is insufficient time for any of the placental changes associated with retention after fetal death to occur. The placenta may be normal or may show lesions that may relate to the demise, such as retroplacental hematoma, velamentous insertion of the umbilical cord, with or without rupture of vasa previa (the membranous vessels coursing over the internal os), nuchal cord, and true knot of the cord (see Figure 80). In cases of nuchal cord or true knot of the cord, the pathologist should seek evidence of true obstruction to flow (stricture, thrombosis) before concluding that these findings caused the demise. Placenta previa and placenta accreta may also be associated with intrapartum stillbirth.

FEATURES OF INTRAUTERINE RETENTION FOLLOWING INTRAUTERINE FETAL DEMISE

Pathologic examination of the placenta is an integral part of the autopsy examination of the stillborn fetus. There are three types of placental findings:

(1) Placental lesions that cause intrauterine fetal death;

(2) Lesions related to maternal and fetal diseases that are the cause of fetal demise;

(3) Placental lesions that are secondary to fetal death.

In the first category are lesions such as massive infarction, retroplacental hematoma, large chorangioma, true knot, torsion and stricture of the umbilical cord, nuchal cord, and intrauterine infection. These are not common but, when present, provide the explanation for fetal death. In rare cases, the stillbirth (or IUGR) may be associated with confined placental mosaicism (CPM)[225]. CPM is characterized by a discrepancy between the fetal and placental karyotypes; most often, the placenta has a trisomic cell line in the cytotrophoblast, stroma, or both, that is not present in the fetus. Such a discrepancy is observed in 1–2% of pregnancies and involves trisomy 2, 3, 8, 9, or 16. The significance of CPM in fetal development is unclear, but IUGR may be severe and intrauterine fetal demise has also been noted[643–645]. The aneuploid cell line(s) presumably interferes with placental function and affects fetal growth and survival. Karyotyping for CPM should be done on cultured cells obtained from chorionic villous sampling (i.e. not from amniotic fluid; see the Appendix) from multiple sites, since CPM is not uniformly distributed[646]. The placenta in CPM may not show any specific morphologic abnormalities on routine examination, but is often small. In the second category are lesions related to maternal diseases such as pre-eclampsia and maternal hypertension (retroplacental hematoma and acute atherosis and/or arteriosclerosis of decidual uteroplacental maternal arteries), and fetal diseases such as EBF and congenital anomalies with IUGR.

After fetal death, the placenta remains viable, since the villi receive their oxygen and nutrients from the maternal circulation in the intervillous space. However, there is cessation of fetal circulation, which results in the following lesions:

(1) Progressive sclerosis of blood vessels in the stem villi followed by obliteration;

(2) Hypovascularity followed by stromal fibrosis of terminal villi;

(3) An increased number of syncytial knots;

(4) Villous edema.

In addition, cytotrophoblastic hyperplasia and trophoblastic basement membrane thickening secondary to uteroplacental ischemia are seen, since there is a reduction in maternal blood flow after fetal death. It is possible that villous 'pulse' may be a factor influencing circulation of blood in the intervillous space, and when lost with fetal demise, this contributes to stagnation of maternal blood and a rise in pressure in the intervillous space. However, with fetal demise, there is a reduction in maternal blood flow to the placenta. Focal calcification of villi, particularly of the trophoblastic basement membrane, is frequently seen. The main importance of knowledge of these placental changes is that these should not be considered as the cause of intrauterine fetal demise.

Changes seen in the placenta may help in determining the time interval between demise and delivery. However, as some may show overlap with features seen in FTV and HEV (see Chapter 9), the pathologist should exercise caution in interpreting the presence of chorionic plate and stem villous vascular occlusions as representing only postmortem change in the placenta of a stillborn. The most widely used schema of assessment of the period of intrauterine retention was developed by Genest[109], in his

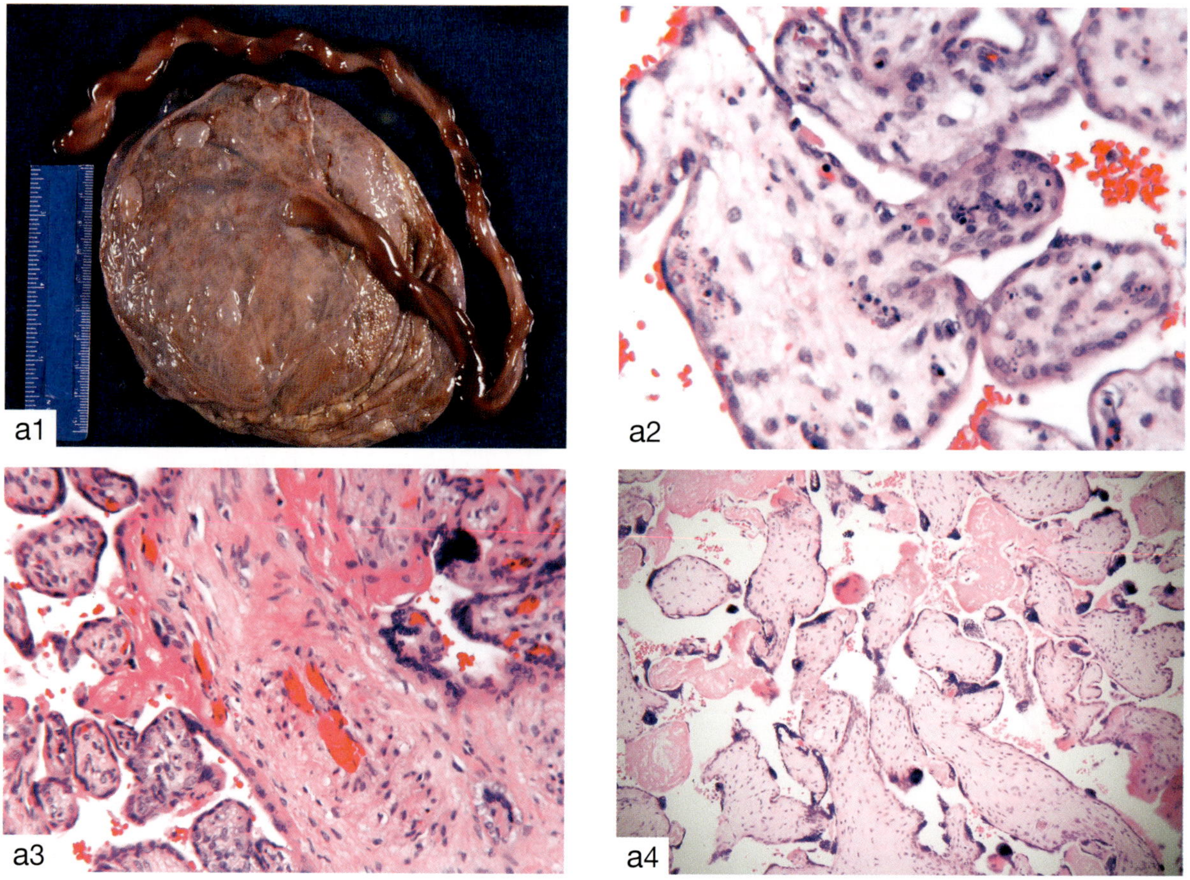

Figure 113 Features of retention. (a-1) The umbilical cord of this placenta is red-brown discolored. The fetal surface is still pale pink-tan, although opacified, due to the presence of chorioamnionitis, which was the cause of the intrauterine fetal demise in this case. (a-2) Karyorrhexis of the stromal endothelial cell and/or blood cell nuclei is the earliest histologic feature of retention. (a-3) The stem villus shows 'septation', or ingrowth of fibroblasts. (see also Figure 42 for additional features of retention). (a-4) This field of chorionic villi shows diffuse involutional change with diffuse villous sclerosis and syncytial knot formation

study of 71 stillborns and placentas from cases in which the time of fetal demise had been clinically ascertained. He identified the following as reliably predictive features of duration of retention;

(1) Gross brown-red cord discoloration (> 8–12 h) (Figure 113a-1);

(2) Histologic villous intravascular karyorrhexis (6 or more hours after demise) (Figure 113a-2);

(3) The appearance of stem villous vascular luminal abnormalities of 'septation' and total obliteration (Figure 113a-3).

Luminal septation, due to ingrowth of fibroblasts, was multifocal at ≥ 48 h and extensive by 2 weeks; extensive stromal sclerosis of terminal villi was also seen after 2 weeks (Figure 113a-4). Altemani[647] evaluated placentas from stillborns and normal liveborns for the presence of thrombi in stem villous vessels. Placentas from stillborns delivered within a day of demise and from normal newborns showed rare organizing thrombi and, when occlusive, associated avascular villi. Their presence in placentas from the live-born infants suggested that they represented an antemortem process. Retention *in utero* for 2–7 days following fetal demise was associated with organizing stem villous 'thrombi' in 78.5% of cases, but rarely with avascular villi. After 7 days, however, the luminal occlusions appeared to be totally organized. Altemani interpreted these findings as indicating that most organizing thrombi in placental vessels, associated with macerated stillbirth, are due to postmortem change.

Jaques and colleagues[648] evaluated second-trimester placentas in cases for which the time of death was known. They divided their cases into time intervals < 12 h, 12–24 h, 24–36 h, and > 36 h. Degeneration of the smooth muscle of the umbilical cord was seen in a third of cases with a < 12-h death to delivery interval, but was detected in 100% of cases in all groups with retention of ≥ 12 h, and in increasing degrees with increasing time intervals. Intravascular karyorrhexis was seen in about two-thirds of cases retained for < 36 h (75% at < 12 h, 73% at 12–24 h, and 64% at 24–36 h, respectively), and increased to 100% when the time interval exceeded 36 h. Villous blood vessel luminal changes were present in 25%, 7%, 21%, and 67%, respectively. They concluded that these three features (umbilical mural degeneration, villous intravascular karyorrhexis, and villous vascular luminal changes) are the earliest changes in placentas from cases of second-trimester intrauterine fetal death, but that these findings could not be used to predict timing accurately to the degree of the short time intervals evaluated. Genest and colleagues[566] had previously evaluated second-trimester stillbirth placentas, and cautioned against the over-interpretation of umbilical vessel smooth muscle degeneration seen with retention, which they termed 'pseudo-vasculitis', as representing umbilical vasculitis.

16

Iatrogenic lesions of the placenta, umbilical cord, and membranes

A number of diagnostic and therapeutic procedures may be performed during pregnancy that may affect the placenta, including chorionic villus sampling, amniocentesis, umbilical cord blood sampling (cordocentesis), and intraperitoneal and intravascular fetal transfusion. Intrauterine fetal transfusion for hemolytic anemias (e.g. immune-mediated hemolysis) via a sonographically directed transfusion through an umbilical cord vessel is efficacious and safe. Cordocentesis is considered when fetal blood sampling may provide a diagnosis not obtainable by other methods, or in lieu of other methods (such as amniocentesis); tests may include fetal karyotyping, hemoglobin concentration determination and electrophoresis, liver transaminase evaluation, and serologic tests for IgM specific antibodies to infectious agents[33]. Examination of the umbilical cord from a case for which intrauterine transfusion or fetal blood sampling was performed may show recent or more chronic evidence of localized extravasation in Wharton's jelly, corresponding to sites of the procedure(s), and potentially, even vascular sites of repair as well (Figure 114). Sikovanyecz and colleagues[649] evaluated the amount of fetomaternal bleeding resulting from cordocentesis, and found that the amount correlated with procedural time, fetal post-procedural bleeding time, puncture site, and transplacental penetration. There was increased bleeding if the puncture site was at the cord insertion rather than a cord loop, and more bleeding occurred with transplacental penetration. The amount was nearly always < 1 ml in their series. There may be hematoma formation in the cord after puncture as well as bleeding into the amniotic sac. Trauma to the placenta from a procedure may result in intra-amniotic bleeding or fetomaternal hemorrhage. This injury to the placenta may lead to premature delivery and fetal loss. It is incumbent on the obstetrician to provide the pertinent clinical information, and a diligent search for these lesions should be made by the pathologist in such cases.

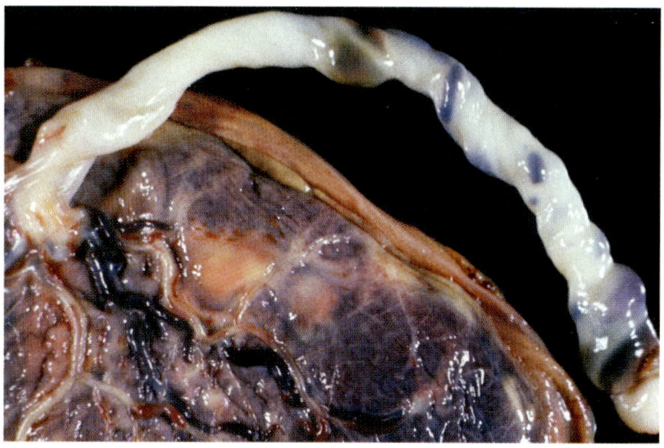

Figure 114 Iatrogenic lesion. Two sites of prior intrauterine transfusion, performed 2–3 weeks prior to delivery for fetal rhesus immune-mediated anemia, are seen as greenish brown patches of old extravasation, on this umbilical cord

17

Traumatic lesions of the placenta

Abdominal trauma, most commonly by motor vehicle accident, can result in placental abruption and fetal–maternal hemorrhage. If contusion and tears of the placenta occur, there may be extensive intravillous hemorrhage, and bleeding into the amniotic sac. Concurrent fetal injuries including skull fractures, with or without cranial hemorrhages, have also been described. Fetal death can occur associated with placental abruption, infarction, and laceration of the placenta[650]. Fetomaternal hemorrhage can cause acute Rh isoimmunization[651].

18

Placentas after assisted reproductive technologies

Assisted reproduction (ART) currently includes a variety of technologies; the two most frequently used are *in vitro* fertilization and embryo transfer (IVF/ET), and intracytoplasmic sperm injection and embryo transfer (ICSI/ET)[652]. There are few studies of the placentas from these assisted gestations and the majority of studies have evaluated IVF/ET. The incidences of abnormal placental shapes, such as bilobate and accessory lobated placentas, have been found to be significantly increased in IVF/ET singleton pregnancies, in some non-blinded and/or non-controlled studies[68,653], but the incidences of these gross findings were not identified to be significantly different in the blinded and controlled study of ART placentas by Daniel and colleagues[652]. Histology was also not identified to be significantly different between study and control placentas in their study, nor was it appreciated to be different in the IVF/ET placentas evaluated by others[68,653]. However, all investigators have noted an increased incidence of marginal (< 2 cm from the placental margin) and/or velamentous insertion of the cord[68,652,653]. These changes may relate to orientation of the blastocyst at implantation or to abnormalities of the reproductive tract (e.g. leiomyomas, endometriosis, sequelae of pelvic inflammatory disease) that were responsible for the infertility problem that led to the need for ART in the first place. Superficial implantation has also been proposed to be a factor, but, since Daniel and colleagues[652] found no differences in the rates of abnormal placental shape, this remains a debated cause. Increased placental : fetal weight ratio and placental thickness have been identified in one study[652], and postulated to be due to ART-related endometrial hyperstimulation from hormonal administration and multiple embryo transfer procedures that may alter the endometrium both histologically and biochemically. Of note is that infertility *per se* increases the risk of low birth weight and preterm birth, so it seems plausible that the effects of hormonal stimulation and/or multiple embryo transfer may confer 'advantage' in assisted gestations, including, perhaps, continuation to term. Gavrill and colleagues[653] found no differences between spontaneous twin gestations and those of IVF/ET in terms of pregnancy complications. Multiple pregnancies are more common in pregnancies achieved with IVF/ET and ICSI/ET, and vanishing twins or other multiples may occur spontaneously, or artificial reduction may have been performed. In these cases, particularly after artificial reduction, remnant nodules may be seen on the fetal surface. Radiography of these placentas may show fetal skeletal remnants on the surface.

19

Placental features following intrauterine vascular laser ablation procedures

Fetoscopic or ultrasonographically guided laser ablation procedures are performed for pathologically significant shunting of fetal blood flow in cases of large (or multiple) chorangioma, acardius, and TTTS. Laser surgery of pathologic vascular supply to chorangiomas[428,440,441] and acardiac twins[4] can result in the resolution of shunting and of fetal cardiac failure. In TTTS, which has an extremely high mortality rate of one or both twins of at least 80%, fetoscopic ablation of chorangiopagous vessels has gained acceptance as an effective treatment. Since in TTTS the system of placental vascular anastomoses is not in equilibrium, this intervention aims at rapid photocoagulation of all fetoscopically identifiable anastomoses on the vascular equator as soon after diagnosis of TTTS as possible[618]. (An average of eight anastomoses are seen in TTTS[610,617]). Infant outcomes are related to the gestational period of onset and severity. However, even in cases of severe and early TTTS, laser treatment in mid-gestation has been associated with a 68% overall survival rate, an 81% survival of at least one twin, 42–57% dual twin survival, and continuation of pregnancy for an additional 10–13-week period[617]. Severe neurologic morbidity/cerebral palsy rates have been reported to be from 3.4–4.3%[623] to 9–13%[622,654]. Therefore, while perinatal mortality and morbidity with laser surgery are not insignificant, it has proved to be a very valuable mode of treatment.

Laser surgeries are performed at select, medical centers, but, as pointed out by DePaepe and colleagues[619], the treated women may return to their primary obstetricians for continued clinical care and delivery at a more local hospital. Thus, the practicing pathologist may encounter such post-ablation placentas despite the fact that the procedure was not performed in his/her institution, and he/she may be asked to verify occlusion of the sites photocoagulated, by injection studies, determine the patency and type of remaining anastomoses, and interpret the placental findings with reference to infant outcomes*. In so doing, the pathologist should remember that the locations of anastomoses often do not correspond to the position of the dividing membranous attachment, that injection studies are required, and that he/she should strive to document carefully the type and caliber of non-coagulated chorangiopagous vessels.

Gross and light microscopic features of ten DiMo placentas delivered within 1 month and more than 1 month of laser ablation procedures were recently documented by DePaepe and colleagues[619]. In placentas delivered within 1 month of the procedure, the sites of photocoagulation (which lay on the recipient's side of the dividing septum) appeared focally hemorrhagic, with a beaded pattern of alternating dark-red (blood-filled) to white (bloodless) segments downstream of the coagulation site. Luminal occlusion was evidenced by abrupt interruption of dye passage, upon injection study. Microscopically, these recent sites of photocoagulation showed a spectrum

*If adequate facilities for performing injection studies and/or their interpretation are not available in the pathology department, gross photographs of the fetal surface of the unfixed placenta should be taken and, together with the fresh placenta (packed in a box containing adequate dry ice), sent by overnight mail to the medical center where the intervention was performed.

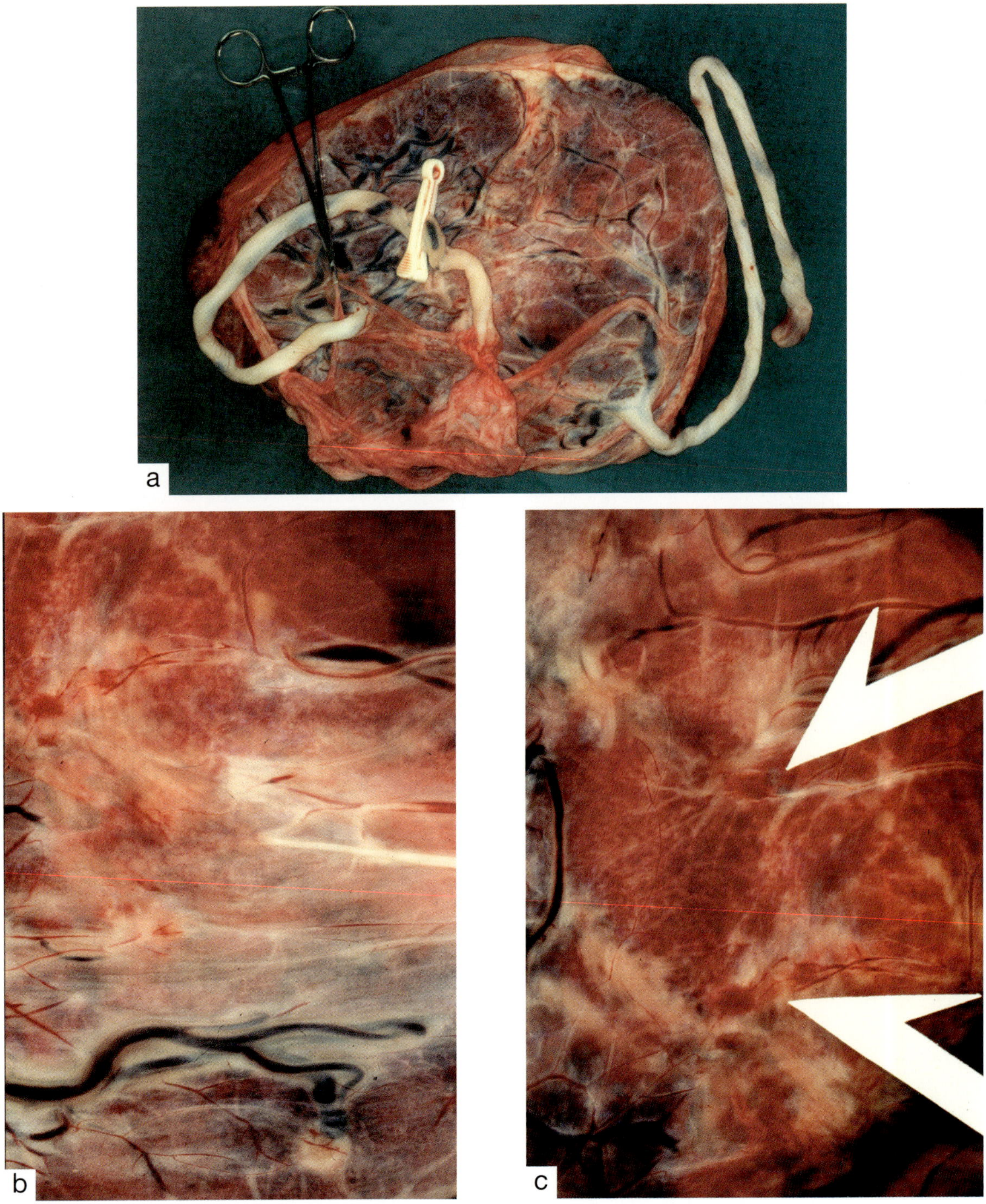

Figure 115 Features of intraurerine laser ablation procedure. (a) The sites of laser ablation of this diamniotic monochorionic placenta with twin–twin transfusion syndrome are visible near the vascular equator as small yellow-white plaques with erythematous borders near the center of the placenta. The donor twin cord is the cord without the clamp; the vessels of the recipient fetus' placental domain are darker and more congested. (b) Several laser sites are shown in closer detail and the upper, 8 mm in total dimension, lesion in this field is further magnified with another, more superior adjacent site in (c) (arrows). Histology of such sites may show dense fibrinoid deposition, coagulative necrosis, and thrombosis

of subchorionic hemorrhage: to transmural coagulative necrosis, and underlying villous avascularity and perivillous fibrin(oid) deposition; to thrombosis with hemosiderosis. Placentas from gestations in which the laser procedure had been performed more remotely showed grossly a paucity of vessels, patchy subchorionic fibrin(oid) deposition, and an absence of demonstrable anastomoses in the intervening area between the two domains. Histologic examination revealed this central area to contain necrotic remnants of vessels with early dystrophic mineralization, surrounded by organizing subchorionic thrombohematoma. Dye injection studies revealed small, residual anastomoses at the periphery of the 'bare area' between the vascular domains. Of note is that six of eight of their fully evaluated cases showed between one and six residual A–V anastomoses, and microscopically there was villous edema. Three of these cases culminated in the intrauterine fetal demise of five twins and one perinatal death. Hence, such residual anastomoses may be responsible for suboptimal resolution of TTTS, following laser surgery. Moreover, even residual A–A anastomoses may secondarily become important as shunts[618] (and personal communication).

The DiMo twin placenta shown in Figure 115a-1 is an example of the gross findings of photocoagulation performed 8 weeks prior to delivery. The placenta was examined in the presence of the maternal–fetal medicine specialist, Dr Julian DeLia, who performed the procedure. The asymmetry of the placental regions is evident. The laser sites are evident as small, yellow plaques of subchorionic fibrinoid with congested-appearing borders and delicate adjacent vessels (Figure 115b and c). No residual patency of the prior anastomotic site was identified by injection studies. One twin, the donor (birth weight 760 g; hematocrit 58%), died on day 8 of life, during surgery for necrotizing enterocolitis. The other twin, the recipient (birth weight 1090 g; hematocrit 42%), was hospitalized in intensive care for nearly 10 weeks, but thereafter did well, and is now a healthy, teenage male[617].

20

Final comment

As indicated in the 'Introduction', the placenta is not a favorite subject of surgical pathologists. Unlike in other areas of the field, placental examination seldom yields precise pathologic diagnoses that have direct and immediate clinical impact. The clinician may feel that placental examination is a way of confirming conditions previously clinically diagnosed with the assistance of laboratory and imaging techniques. There are, however, instances in which the placenta has immediate or remote clinical implications. An infection with a specific organism may first be picked up by placental examination, as may an indication of a thrombophilia. Appropriate therapy can be instituted, or a stillbirth explained. Recurrent conditions such as thrombophilias and maternal floor infarctions may be picked up by placental examination, and categorize the mother as high risk, allowing for appropriate interventions in her future pregnancies. The role of examination of the placenta in explaining suboptimal perinatal outcome, as well as in medicolegal investigations, has been emphasized in the literature.

However, placentas submitted to the laboratory may show no changes in the face of maternal or fetal conditions, or may show non-specific, inconclusive, or non-contributory changes. Conversely, placental lesions may be detected in placentas from normal pregnancies. The following suggestions may be of help to the surgical pathologist:

(1) Develop a list of indications for examination at your institution. Input, from the obstetricians and neonatologists, is extremely important.

(2) Placentas meeting the above indications should be submitted. If a pathologist with perinatal expertise/interest is on staff, some institutions may consider submission of all placentas.

(3) Familiarization with the normal gross and microscopic findings in placentas will enhance appreciation of the abnormal.

(4) Findings expected in normal placentas, such as $< 5\%$ infarcts in a term placenta, may be recorded in the gross or microscopic description, but do not need to be reported in the final diagnosis.

(5) Estimation of the percentage of the placenta involved with a lesion such as infarcts or massive perivillous fibrin is important in predicting clinical significance. While subjective, and estimated from evaluating the placental slices, practice will yield consistency.

(6) Standardize the number, and locations of placental sections taken for histology, as well as the gross and histologic descriptions. A template such as the one provided in the Appendix is helpful for dictation.

(7) Be familiar with the common gross and microscopic lesions that are encountered.

(8) The provided tables are meant to assist in gross and microscopic evaluation.

(9) Assigning a single pathologist on staff to sign out the placentas will yield more consistency.

(10) When evaluating placental specimens, as is the case with other surgical pathology specimens, communication with clinical colleagues is key. Appropriate clinical history regarding the gestation, maternal presentation at the time of hospital admission, the period of labor and delivery, and status and characteristics of the infant are critical to ensuring a meaningful assessment of the placenta. If such information is not provided, the pathologist should seek out the obstetrician or neonatologist and obtain it. The pathologist is part of the diagnostic team for the mother and infant, and the responsibility of the accuracy and completeness of the report is, in a very real sense, shared by the obstetrician and pediatrician. Moreover, there may have been developments that occurred after the submission of the placenta to pathology, in the baby or the mother, which may be explained by findings in the placenta. Therefore, the pathologist may have an important role in determining the appropriate management of the mother or infant, parental education regarding their child, or counseling regarding future pregnancies.

For those who specialize in placental pathology, after examining many thousands of specimens and making the correlations, it can be said that placental pathology does grow on one and provides a very real sense of satisfaction and contribution.

Appendix

PLACENTAL GROSS TEMPLATE

Singleton

Clinical history

The patient is a _ year-old, para _ female with an intrauterine pregnancy at a clinically estimated period of gestation of _ weeks. _ Gestational complications are/are not given. These include pre-eclampsia/diabetes mellitus/hypertension/fetal anomaly (describe)/etc. _ Intrapartum complications included _ (describe). A(n) _ induced/spontaneous/vaginal/cesarean section delivery was accomplished. The placenta was _ spontaneously delivered/manually extracted. A _ g/lb, stillborn fetus/live-born infant was delivered. Apgar scores were _ and _, at 1 and 5 min, respectively.

The major clinical problem(s) of concern is/are _ (e.g. IUGR, intrauterine fetal demise, neonatal encephalopathy, etc.)/ _ not otherwise specified.

Gross description

The specimen is received fresh, labeled with the patient's name and medical record number, '_'. It consists of a(n) _ intact/disrupted/fragmented, singleton, _ g (trimmed weight/aggregate), _ × _ cm placenta with a _ three-/two-vessel umbilical cord.

(_ An accessory lobe, _ × _ × _ cm is present _ cm from the main placental disk; its vascular supply appears _ intact/describe.)

The umbilical cord is _ glistening _ white/yellowish-white/greenish/red-brown discolored and shows _ central/eccentric/paramarginal/marginal/velamentous insertion, _ cm away from the nearest placental margin. It now measures _ cm in length, _ cm in diameter, and is free of lesions/shows small white-yellow punctate lesions, etc. (describe).

(Velamentous vascular segments are _ to _ cm long, and appear _ intact/disrupted/thrombosed and the surrounding membranes _ show no/show evidence of acute intramembranous/chronic hemorrhage/hematoma.)

Also accompanying the specimen is a separate, _ cm long, _ cm in diameter segment of similar-appearing umbilical cord. Cross-sections of both segments show _ patent vessels/ _ acute/chronic/ thrombosis of the umbilical _ vein/artery(s)/features of necrotizing funisitis (describe). True cord knots _ are not/are identified.

(_ The knot is _ loose/tight, _ × _ × _ cm, and _ (describe appearance of cord jelly and any dilatation or compression of vein and arteries on both sides of the knot, and within the tightest part of the knot, itself, respectively designating which is the placental and the fetal side).)

The fetal membranes display _ marginal insertion/circum-marginate/circumvallate insertion and are _ translucent/pink-tan/opacified/greenish. The point of rupture is _ identified _ cm away from the nearest placental margin.

(_ Circumvallation affects _ % of circumference, with a _ cm wide extrachorial rim of _ tissue.)

The fetal surface shows a _ scant/moderate amount/plaque-like distribution of subchorionic fibrinoid deposition. *The chorionic plate vessels* radiate _ evenly/describe and _ are patent/exhibit apparent acute/chronic thrombosis of the _ arterial/ venous branches.

(_ A _ × _ × _ cm, _ bulging, _ acute/ laminated/chronic-appearing, subchorionic thrombohematoma/intra-amnionic hematoma is identified.)

The maternal surface displays _ intact/disrupted cotyledons, and a _ scant amount of adherent decidua (if disrupted describe). _ Scattered/punctate/patchy/plaque-like/gritty maternal surface infarctions are noted and affect _ % of the maternal surface. _ No marginal/retroplacental hematoma _ is/are identified.

(_ An acute/incidental-appearing/recent/chronic marginal hematoma is present that is _ × _ × _ cm, involves _ % of the marginal circumference; it does _ not appear to dissect into the adjacent chorionic villous tissue.)

(There is _ a(n) acute/recent/chronic retroplacental hematoma that affects _ % of the maternal surface; it is _ × _ ×_ cm in maximal dimensions, _loosely adherent/firm/red-brown/friable/describe. A _ × _ ×_ cm underlying depression in the maternal surface _ with adjacent compressed/congested/ infarcted parenchyma _ is/is not observed.)

Serial sections of the placenta reveal _ spongy/red-brown/congested/pale/edematous tissue with an average mural thickness of _ cm. _ No parenchymal infarctions are appreciated.

(Acute red-brown/firm pale/white to tan infarctions/infarctions of varying age are noted in the _ subchorionic, middle, and basal _ parenchyma and affect _ % of the total parenchymal volume.)

(Areas of mural attenuation _ are not seen/are seen and mural thickness ranges from _ to _ cm, and _ (describe parenchymal appearance and texture).)

(_ Intervillous thrombus is _ not appreciated/_ × _ × _ cm, _ acute/chronic-appearing, and located _.)

Block summary

A1: membrane roll, umbilical cord from insertion site.

A2: membrane roll, umbilical cord from fetal end.

A3/A4: representative transmural sections.

A5: sections from separate segment of umbilical cord.

A6/etc.: additional sections from _ .

Microscopic description

The following features are noted in the:

(1) Free membranes including decidua capsularis;

(2) Umbilical cord;

(3) Chorionic plate membranes, vessels;

(4) Stem and chorionic villi including vessels, stroma, vascularity, maturation;

(5) Intervillous space, cell islands;

(6) Placental septa and decidua, including decidual (maternal) arteries, inflammatory cell numbers and types, tissue viability and presence of myometrial smooth muscle.

Diagnosis

METHOD OF OBTAINING PLACENTAL TISSUE FOR CYTOGENETIC STUDY

Indications: recurrent abortions and/or stillbirths, syndromic or non-syndromic fetal structural anomaly(ies), fetal syndrome not otherwise specified, non-immune fetal hydrops, osteochondrodysplasia, large-for-gestational-age infant in the absence of history of diabetes, unexplained fetal growth restriction.

Specimen: appropriate viable tissue (cells) obtained by sterile technique is the basic requirement. (Sterile instruments, gloves, Petri dishes, etc. are needed, and sample selection under a laminar flow hood is optimal.) The specimen should be placed in tissue culture medium (RPMI) (Roswell Park Memorial Institute) medium supplemented with bovine serum and antibiotics. Hank's balanced salt solution or sterile saline may be used as substitutes in exceptional circumstances.

Specimen selection:

(1) *Products of conception*: select pale pink to translucent, delicate fronds of soft tissue representing chorionic villi (confirmed by examination under stereomicroscope or with hand-held magnifying lens) from among the fragments of smooth decidua and blood clot. Floating the selected tissue in sterile saline helps to separate the delicate branches of a true chorionic villous tree fragment and enables the pathologist to distinguish chorionic villous tissue from shredded decidual tissue. Remove any bloody strands of tissue, from the sample to be submitted, since they commonly represent adherent decidua and will result in 'contamination' of the karyotypic results. Rinse the selected villous tissue sample several times in sterile saline. Submit small mirror-image section of the tissue selected for cytogenetics, in a cassette, for correlative histologic verification of villous tissue. This will ensure that the subsequent karyotypic results can be interpreted as representing those of the conceptus (especially if a normal female karyotype is returned).

(2) *Placental fetal surface:*

   (a) Stroke wipe an area midway between cord insertion site and placental margin by five unidirectional strokes using a fresh alcohol wipe each time (do not use an iodine-containing solution to clean the surface);

   (b) Incise amnion after 'tenting' it up with a forceps and peel it back;

   (c) Excise a section of the chorionic plate, rinse at least three times in sterile saline, and place in tissue culture medium.

References

1. American College of Obstetricians and Gynecologists. Clinical Management Guidelines for Obstetrician–Gynecologists. Antepartum Fetal Surveillance, ACOG Practice Bulletin 9, Washington, DC: ACOG, 1999
2. Langston C, Kaplan C, McPherson T, et al. Practice guidelines for examination of the placenta. Arch Pathol Lab Med 1997; 121: 449–76
3. Fox H. Pathology of the Placenta, 2nd edn, Vol 7, Major Problems in Pathology. Philadelphia: WB Saunders, 1997
4. Benirschke K, Kaufmann P. Pathology of the Human Placenta, 4th edn. New York: Springer, 2000: 242–8
5. Frank HG, Malekzadeh F, Kertschanska S, et al. Immunohistochemistry of two different types of placental fibrinoid. Acta Anat (Basel) 1994; 150: 55–68
6. Mayhew TM, Bowles C, Orme G. A stereological method for testing whether or not there is random deposition of perivillous fibrin-type fibrinoid at the villous surface: description and pilot applications to term placentae. Placenta 2000; 21: 684–92
7. Khong TY. What's in fibrin? Pediatr Dev Pathol 2002; 5: 106–7
8. Perrin EDVK. Pathology of the Placenta. Contemporary Issues in Surgical Pathology 5. New York; Churchill Livingstone, 1984
9. Kaplan C, Blanc WA, Elias J. Identification of erythrocytes in intervillous thrombi: a study using immunoperoxidase identification of hemoglobins. Hum Pathol 1982; 13: 554–7
10. Altshuler G. A conceptual approach to placental pathology and pregnancy outcome. Semin Diagn Pathol 1993; 10: 204–21
11. Manning FA, Platt LD, Sipos L. Antepartum fetal evaluation: development of a fetal biophysical profile. Am J Obstet Gynecol 1980; 136: 787–95
12. Harris RD, Alexander RD. Ultrasound of the placenta and cord. In Callen PW, ed, Ultrasound in Obstetrics and Gynecology, 4th edn. Philadelphia: WB Saunders 2000: 597–625
13. Apgar V. A proposal for a new method of evaluation of newborn infant. Curr Res Anesth 1953; 32: 260–7
14. Fox GE, Wesep RV, Resau JH, Sun CC. The effect of immersion formaldehyde fixation on human placental weight. Arch Pathol Lab Med 1991; 115: 726–8
15. Khong TY, Bendon RW, Qureshi F, et al. Chronic deciduitis in the placental basal plates: definition and interobserver reliability. Hum Pathol 2000; 31: 292–5
16. Khong TY, Werger AC. Myometrial fibers in the placental basal plate can confirm but do not necessarily indicate clinical placenta accreta. Am J Clin Pathol 2001; 116: 703–8
17. Kraus FT. Perinatal pathology, the placenta, and litigation. Hum Pathol 2003; 34: 517–21; discussion 522–7
18. Zini J-M, Murray SC, Graham CH, et al. Characterization of urokinase receptor expression by human placental trophoblasts. Blood 1992; 79: 2917–29
19. Multhaupt HA, Mazar A, Cines DB, et al. Expression of urokinase receptors by human trophoblast. A histochemical and ultrastructural analysis. Lab Invest 1994; 71: 392–400
20. Monzon-Bordonaba F, Wang CL, Feinberg RF. Fibronectinase activity in cultured human

trophoblasts is mediated by urokinase-type plasminogen activator. Am J Obstet Gynecol 1997; 176: 58–65
21. Liu YX, Hu ZY, Liu K, et al Localization and distribution of tissue type and urokinase type plasminogen activators and their inhibitors type 1 and 2 in human and rhesus monkey fetal membranes. Placenta 1998; 19: 171–80
22. Floridan C, Nielsen O, Sunde L, et al. Localization and significance of urokinase plasminogen activator and its receptor in placental tissue from intrauterine, ectopic and molar pregnancies. Placenta 1999; 20: 711–21
23. Feng Q, Liu Y, Liu K, et al. Expression of urokinase, plasminogen activator inhibitors and urokinase receptor in pregnant rhesus monkey uterus during early placentation. Placenta 2000; 21: 184–93
24. Bendon RW, Hommel AB. Maternal floor infarction in autoimmune disease: two cases. Pediatr Pathol Lab Med 1996; 16: 293–7
25. Vogt E, Ng A-K, Rote NS. Antiphosphatidylserine antibody removes annexin-V and facilitates the binding of prothrombin at the surface of a choriocarcinoma model of trophoblast differentiation. Am J Obstet Gynecol 1997; 177: 964–72
26. Baergen RN, Chacko SA, Edersheim T, et al. The placenta in thrombophilias: a clinicopathologic study. Mod Pathol 2001; 14: 213A
27. Becker V, Röckelein G. Pathologie der weiblichen Genitalorgane I. Pathologie der Plazenta und des Abortes. Heidelberg: Springer-Verlag, 1989
28. Redline RW, O'Riordan MA. Placental lesions associated with cerebral palsy and neurologic impairment following term birth. Arch Pathol Lab Med 2000; 124: 1785–91
29. Redline RW. Placental inflammation. Semin Neonatol 2004; 9: 265–74
30. Shanklin DR, Scott JS. Massive subchorial thrombohematoma (Breus' mole). Br J Obstet Gynaecol 1975; 82: 476–87
31. Heller DS, Rush D, Baergen RN. Subchorionic hematoma associated with thrombophilia: report of three cases. Pediatr Dev Pathol 2003; 6: 261–4
32. Mooney EE, Shunnar AA, O'Reagan MO, Gillan JE. Chorionic villous hemorrhage is associated with retroplacental hemorrhage. Br J Obstet Gynaecol 1994; 101: 965–9
33. Cunningham FG, Gant NF, Leveno KJ, et al. Williams Obstetrics, 21st edn. New York: McGraw-Hill, 2001
34. Sheiner E, Shoham-Vardi I, Hadar A, et al. Incidence, obstetric risk factors and pregnancy outcome of preterm placental abruption: a retrospective analysis. J Matern Fetal Neonatal Med 2002; 11: 34–9
35. Sheiner E, Shoham-Vardi I, Hallak M, et al. Placental abruption in term pregnancies: clinical significance and obstetric risk factors. J Matern Fetal Neonatal Med 2003; 13: 45–9
36. Lowe TW, Cunningham FG. Placental abruption. Clin Obstet Gynecol 1990; 33: 406–13
37. Sibai BM, Lindheimer M, Hauth J, et al. Risk factors for pre-eclampsia, abruptio placentae, and adverse neonatal outcomes among women with chronic hypertension. National Institute of Child Health and Human Development Network of Maternal–Fetal Medicine Units. N Engl J Med 1998; 339: 667–761
38. Goddjin-Wessel TA, Wouters MG, van de Molen EF, et al. Hyperhomocysteinemia: a risk factor for placental abruption or infarction. Eur J Obstet Gynecol Reprod Biol 1996; 66: 23–9
39. Agorastos T, Karavida A, Lambropoulos A, et al. Factor V Leiden and prothrombin G20210A mutations in pregnancies with adverse outcome. J Matern Fetal Neonatal Med 2002; 12: 267–73
40. Prochazka M, Happach C, Marsal K, et al. Factor V Leiden in pregnancies complicated by placental abruption. Br J Obstet Gynaecol 2003; 110: 462–6
41. Brenner B, Kupferminc MJ. Inherited thrombophilia and poor pregnancy outcome. Best Pract Res Clin Obstet Gynaecol 2003; 17: 427–39
42. Walker MC, Ferguson SE, Allen VM. Heparin for pregnant women with acquired or inherited thrombophilias. Cochrane Database Syst Rev 2003; CD003580
43. Holmes VA. Changes in haemostasis during normal pregnancy: does homocysteine play a role in maintaining homeostasis? Proc Nutr Soc 2003; 62: 479–93
44. Many A, Kupferminc MJ. Thrombophilias and adverse pregnancy outcome. Haematologica 2003; 88: 729–31
45. Facchinetti F, Marozio L, Grandone E, et al. Thrombophilic mutations are a main risk factor for placental abruption. Haematologica 2003; 88: 785–8
46. Liu DF, Dickerman LH, Redline RW. Pathologic findings in pregnancies with unexplained increases in midtrimester maternal serum human chorionic gonadotropin levels. Am J Clin Pathol 1999; 111: 209–15
47. Hladky K, Yankowitz J, Hansen WF. Placental abruption. Obstet Gynecol Surv 2002; 57: 299–305

48. Rushton DI. Placenta as a reflection of maternal disease. In Perrin EDVK, ed. Pathology of the Placenta, Contemporary Issues in Surgical Pathology 5. New York: Churchill Livingstone, 1984: 70
49. Kayani SI, Walkinshaw SA, Preston C. Pregnancy outcome in severe placental abruption. Br J Obstet Gynaecol 2003; 110: 679–83
50. Nagy S, Bush M, Stone J, et al. Clinical significance of subchorionic and retroplacental hematomas detected in the first trimester of pregnancy. Obstet Gynecol 2003; 102: 94–100
51. Howorka E, Kapczynski W. Marginal circular haematoma disrupting the chorionic plate of the placenta. J Obstet Gynaecol Br Commonw 1971; 78: 280–2
52. Harris BA Jr, Gore H, Flowers CE Jr. Peripheral placental separation: a possible relationship to premature labor. Obstet Gynecol 1985; 66: 774–8
53. Takeda S, Baba K, Kojima T, et al. Ultrasonographic monitoring of the placenta in patients with bleeding during the first and second trimesters. Asia Oceania J Obstet Gynaecol 1990; 16: 211–18
54. Stabile I, Campbell S, Grudzinskas JG. Threatened miscarriage and intrauterine hematomas. Sonographic and biochemical studies. J Ultrasound Med 1989; 8: 289–92
55. Abu-Yousef MM, Bleicher JJ, Williamson RA, Weiner CP. Subchorionic hemorrhage: sonographic diagnosis and clinical significance. Am J Roentgenol 1987; 149: 737–40
56. Bendon RW, Bornstein S, Faye-Petersen OM. Two fetal deaths associated with maternal sepsis and with thrombosis of the intervillous space of the placenta. Placenta 1998; 19: 385–9
57. Becroft DM, Thompson JM, Mitchell EA. Placental infarcts, intervillous fibrin plaques, and intervillous thrombi: incidences, cooccurrences, and epidemiological associations. Pediatr Dev Pathol 2004; 7: 26–34
58. Kline BS. Microscopic observations of the placental barrier in transplacental erythrocytotoxic anemia (erythroblastosis fetalis) and in normal pregnancy. Am J Obstet Gynecol 1948; 56: 226–37
59. Sugimura M, Ohashi R, Kobayashi T, Kanayama N. Intraplacental coagulation in intrauterine growth restriction: cause or result? Semin Thromb Hemost 2001; 27: 107–13
60. Rolschau J. Infarctions and intervillous thrombosis in placenta, and their association with intrauterine growth retardation. Acta Obstet Gynecol Scand Suppl 1978; 72: 22–7
61. Moldenhauer JS, Stanek J, Warshak C, et al. The frequency and severity of placental findings in women with preeclampsia are gestational age dependent. Am J Obstet Gynecol 2003; 189: 1173–7
62. Batcup G, Tovey LA, Longster G. Fetomaternal blood group incompatibility studies in placental intervillous thrombosis. Placenta 1983; 4: 449–53
63. Soma H, Watanabe Y, Osawa H, Hata T. A clinicopathological aspect of chorionic villous hemorrhage leading to formation of intervillous thrombosis. Semin Thromb Hemost 1998; 24: 497–501
64. Hoogland HJ, de Haan J, Vooys GP. Ultrasonographic diagnosis of intervillous thrombosis related to Rh isoimmunization. Gynecol Obstet Invest 1979; 10: 237–45
65. Spirt BA, Gordon LP, Kagan EH. Intervillous thrombosis: sonographic and pathologic correlation. Radiology 1983; 147: 197–200
66. Biankin SA, Arbuckle SM, Graf NS. Autopsy findings in a series of five cases of fetomaternal haemorrhages. Pathology 2003; 35: 319–24
67. Salafia CM, Silberman L, Herrera NE, Mahoney MJ. Placental pathology at term associated with elevated midtrimester maternal serum alpha-fetoprotein concentration. Am J Obstet Gynecol 1988; 158: 1064–6
68. Jauniaux E, Englert Y, Vanesse M, et al. Pathologic features of placentas from singleton pregnancies obtained by in vitro fertilization and embryo transfer. Obstet Gynecol 1990; 76: 61–4
69. Fischer RL, Kuhlman K, Grover J, et al. Chronic massive fetomaternal hemorrhage treated with repeated fetal intravascular transfusions. Am J Obstet Gynecol 1990; 162: 203–4
70. Hartung J, Chaoui R, Bollmann R. Nonimmune hydrops from fetomaternal hemorrhage treated with serial fetal intravascular transfusion. Obstet Gynecol 2000; 96: 844
71. Bakas P, Liapis A, Giner M, et al. Massive fetomaternal hemorrhage and oxytocin contraction test: case report and review. Arch Gynecol Obstet 2004; 269: 149–51
72. Naulaers G, Barten S, Vanhole C, et al. Management of severe neotatal anemia due to fetomaternal transfusion. Am J Perinatol 1999; 16: 193–6
73. Gori A, Tamim M, Moore J. Index of suspicion. Case 1. Diagnosis: a fetomaternal hemorrhage (FMH). Pediatr Rev 2001; 22: 135–40
74. Sueters M, Arabin B, Oepkes D. Doppler sonography for predicting fetal anemia caused by massive fetomaternal hemorrhage. Ultrasound Obstet Gynecol 2003; 22: 186–9

75. Mentzer WC, Glader BE. Erythrocyte disorders in infancy. In: Taeusch HW, Ballard RA, Gleason CA, Eds. Avery's Diseases of the Newborn, 8th edn. Philadelphia; Elsevier Saunders, 2005: 1185–6
76. Samadi R, Greenspoon JS, Gviazda I, et al. Massive fetomaternal hemorrhage and fetal death: are they predictable? J Perinatol 1999; 19: 227–9
77. Murphy KW, Venkatraman N, Stevens J. Limitations of ultrasound in the diagnosis of fetomaternal haemorrhage. Br J Obstet Gynaecol 2000; 107: 1317–19
78. Balderston KD, Towers CV, Rumney PJ, Montgomery D. Is the incidence of fetal-to-maternal hemorrhage increased in patients with third-trimester bleeding? Am J Obstet Gynecol 2003; 188: 1615–18
79. Lau MS, Tan JV, Tan TY, et al. Idiopathic chronic fetomaternal haemorrhage resulting in hydrops – a case report. Ann Acad Med Singapore 2003; 32: 642–4
80. Dayal AK, Manning FA, Berck DJ, et al. Fetal death after normal biophysical profile score: an eighteen-year experience. Am J Obstet Gynecol 1999; 181: 1231–6
81. Hoag RW. Fetomaternal hemorrhage associated with umbilical vein thrombosis. Case report. Am J Obstet Gynecol 1986; 154: 1271–4
82. Redline RW. Placental pathology: a neglected link between basic disease mechanisms and untoward pregnancy outcome. Curr Opin Obstet Gynecol 1995; 7: 10–15
83. Manoura A, Hatzidaki E, Christodoulaki M, et al. Anemia due to massive chronic foetomaternal hemorrhage. Haematologia (Budap) 1999; 29: 319–21
84. Kecskes Z. Large fetomaternal hemorrhage: clinical presentation and outcome. J Matern Fetal Neonatal Med 2003; 13: 128–32
85. de Almeida V, Bowman JM. Massive fetomaternal hemorrhage: Manitoba experience. Obstet Gynecol 1994; 83: 323–8
86. Fung KAFK, Giulivi A, Chisholm J, et al. Clinical usefulness of flow cytometry in detection and quantification of fetomaternal hemorrhage. J Matern Fetal Invest 1998; 8: 121–5
87. Lafferty JD, Raby A, Crawford L, et al. Fetal–maternal hemorrhage detection in Ontario. Am J Clin Pathol 2003; 119: 72–7
88. Kennedy GA, Shaw R, Just S, et al. Quantification of feto-maternal haemorrhage (FMH) by flow cytometry: anti-fetal haemoglobin labeling potentially underestimates massive FMH in comparison to labeling with anti-D. Transfus Med 2003; 13: 25–33
89. Pelikan DM, Mesker WE, Scherjon SA, et al. Improvement of the Kleihauer–Betke test by automated detection of fetal erythrocytes in maternal blood. Cytometry 2003; 54B: 1–9
90. Deans A, Jauniaux E. Prenatal diagnosis and outcome of subamniotic hematomas. Ultrasound Obstet Gynecol 1998; 11: 319–23
91. Sepulveda W, Aviles G, Carstens E, et al. Prenatal diagnosis of solid placental masses: the value of color flow imaging. Ultrasound Obstet Gynecol 2000; 16: 554–8
92. Benirschke K. What pediatricians should know about the placenta. Curr Prob Pediatr 1971; 2: 3–32
93. DeSa DJ. Rupture of fetal vessels on placental surface. Arch Dis Child 1971; 46: 495–501
94. Castelluci M, Kaufmann P. Basic structure of the villous tree. In Benirschke K, Kaufmann P, eds. Pathology of the Human Placenta, 4th edn. New York: Springer, 2000: 50–115
95. Huppertz B, Kaufmann P, Kingdom J. Trophoblastic turnover in health and disease. Fetal Matern Med Rev 2002; 13: 103–18
96. Demir R, Kaufmann P, Castelluci M, et al. Fetal vasculogenesis and angogenesis in human placental villi. Acta Anat (Basel) 1989; 136: 190–203
97. Chan CCW, Lao TT, Cheung ANY. Apoptotic and proliferative activities in first trimester placentae. Placenta 1999; 20: 223–7
98. Levy R, Nelson DM. To be or not be, that is the question: apoptosis in human trophoblast. Placenta 2000; 21: 1–13
99. Danihel L, Gomolcak P, Korbel M, et al. Expression of proliferation and apoptotic markers in human placenta during pregnancy. Acta Histochem 2002; 104: 335–8
100. Smith SC, Baker PN, Symonds EM. Placental apoptosis in normal human pregnancy. Am J Obstet Gynecol 1997; 177: 57–65
101. Austgulen R, Chedwick L, Vogt Isaksen C, et al. Trophoblast apoptosis in human placenta at term as detected by expression of a cytokeratin 18 degradation product of caspase. Arch Pathol Lab Med 2002; 126: 1480–6
102. Huppertz B, Kingdom J, Caniggia I, et al. Hypoxia favours necrotic versus apoptotic shedding of placental syncytiotrophoblast into maternal circulation. Placenta 2003; 24: 181–90
103. Magid MS, Kaplan C, Sammaritano LR, et al. Placental pathology in systemic lupus erythematosis: a

prospective study. Am J Obstet Gynecol 1998; 179: 226–34
104. Roberts D, Schwartz RS. Clotting and hemorrhage in the placenta – a delicate balance. N Engl J Med 2002; 347: 57–9
105. Ismail MR, Ordi J, Menendez C, et al. Placental pathology in malaria: a histological, immunohistochemical, and quantitative study. Hum Pathol 2000; 31: 85–93
106. Qureshi F, Jacques SM, Reyes MP. Placental histopathology in syphilis. Hum Pathol 1993; 24: 779–84
107. Sheffield JS, Sanchez PJ, Wendel GD Jr, et al. Placental histopathology of congenital syphilis. Obstet Gynecol 2002; 100: 126–33
108. Axt R, Meyberg R, Mink D, et al. Immunohistochemical detection of apoptosis in the human term and post-term placenta. Clin Exp Obstet Gynecol 1999; 26: 56–9
109. Genest D. Estimating the time of death in stillborn fetuses. II. Histologic evaluation of the placenta; a study of 71 stillborns. Obstet Gynecol 1992; 80: 585–92
110. Chua S, Wilkins T, Sargent I, Redman C. Trophoblastic deportation in pre-eclamptic pregnancy. Br J Obstet Gynecol 1991; 98: 973–9
111. DiFrederico E, Genbacev O, Fisher SJ. Preeclampsia is associated with widespread apoptosis of placental cytotrophoblasts within the uterine wall. Am J Pathol 1999; 155: 293–301
112. Allaire AD, Ballenger KA, Wells SR, et al. Placental apoptosis in pre-eclampsia. Obstet Gynecol 2000; 96: 271–6
113. Cockell AP, Learmont JG, Smarason AK, et al. Human placental syncytiotrophoblastic microvillous membranes impair maternal vascular endothelial function. Br J Obstet Gynaecol 1997; 104: 235–40
114. Knight M, Redman CW, Linton EA, Sargent IL. Shedding of syncytiotrophoblastic microvilli into maternal circulation in pre-eclamptic pregnancies. Br J Obstet Gynaecol 1998; 105: 632–40
115. Huppertz B, Frank HG, Reister F, et al. Apoptosis progresses during turnover of human trophoblast: an analysis of villous cytotrophoblast and syncytial fragments in vitro. Lab Invest 1999; 79: 1687–702
116. Redman C, Sargent I. Placental debris, oxidative stress and preeclampsia. Placenta 2000; 21: 597–602
117. Maynard SE, Min J-Y, Merchan J, et al. Excess placental soluble fms-like tyrosine kinase 1(sFlt1) may contribute to endothelial dysfunction, hypertension, and proteinuria of pre-eclampsia. J Clin Invest 2003; 111: 649–58
118. Levine RJ, Maynard SE, Qian C, et al. Circulating angiogenic factors and the risk of preeclampsia. N Engl J Med 2004; 350: 672–83
119. Solomon CG, Seely EW. Preeclampsia – searching for the cause. N Engl J Med 2004; 350: 641–2
120. Marcuse PM. Pulmonary syncytial giant cell embolism. Report of maternal death. Obstet Gynecol 1954; 3: 210–13
121. Roffman BY, Simons M. Syncytiotrophoblastic embolism associated with placenta increta and pre-eclampsia. Am J Obstet Gynecol 1969; 104: 1218–20
122. Baker AM, Morey MK, Berg KK, Crosson J. Trophoblastic microemboli as a marker for pre-eclampsia–eclampsia in sudden unexpected maternal death: a case report and review of the literature. Am J Forensic Med Pathol 2000; 21: 354–8
123. Delmis J, Pfeifer D, Ivanisevic M, et al. Sudden death from trophoblastic embolism in pregnancy. Eur J Obstet Gynecol Reprod Biol 2000; 92: 225–7
124. Caniggia I, Winter JL. Hypoxia inducible factor-1: oxygen regulation of the trophoblast differentiation in normal and pre-eclamptic pregnancies – a review. Placenta 2002; 23 (Suppl A,Trophoblastic Research 16): S47–57
125. Sen DK, Kaufmann P, Schweikhart G. Classification of human placental villi. II Morphometry. Cell Tissue Res 1979; 200: 425–34
126. Altshuler G. Placental infection and inflammation. In Perrin EVDK, ed. Pathology of the Placenta. New York: Churchill Livingstone, 1984: 141–63
127. Galbraith GM, Galbraith RM, Paulsen EP. Placental immunopathology in gestational diabetes. Placenta Suppl 1981; 3: 183–91
128. Burstein R, Frankel S, Soule SD, Blumenthal HT. Aging of the placenta: autoimmune theory of senescence. Am J Obstet Gynecol 1973; 116: 271–6
129. Bulmer JN, Rasheed FN, Morrison L, et al. Placental malaria. II. A semi-quantitative investigation of the pathological features. Histopathology 1993; 22: 219–25
130. Thliveris JA, Baskett TF. Fine structure of the human placenta in prolonged pregnancy. Preliminary report. Gynecol Obstet Invest 1978; 9: 40–8
131. Ernst LM, Parkash V. Placental pathology in fetal Bartter syndrome. Pediatr Dev Pathol 2002; 5: 76–9
132. Kasznica JM, Petcu EB. Placental calcium pump: clinical-based evidence. Pediatr Pathol Mol Med 2003; 22: 223–7

133. McDermott M, Gillan JE. Trophoblastic basement membrane haemosiderin in the placental lesions of fetal artery thrombosis: a marker for disturbance of maternofetal transfer. Placenta 1995; 16: 171–8
134. Varma VA, Kim KM. Placental calcification: ultrastructural and X-ray microanalytic studies. Scan Electron Microsc 1985; 4: 1567–72
135. Salafia CM, Minior VK, Pezzullo JC, et al. Intrauterine growth restriction in infants of less than thirty-two weeks' gestation: associated placental pathologic features. Am J Obstet Gynecol 1995; 173: 1049–57
136. Overstreet K, Benirschke K, Scioscia A, Masliah E. Congenital nephrosis of Finnish type. Pediatr Dev Pathol 2002; 5: 179–83
137. Naeye RL, Maisel M, Loren J, Botti JJ. The clinical significance of placental villous edema. Pediatrics 1983; 71: 588–94
138. Kovalovszki L, Villanyi E, Benko G. Placental villous edema: a possible cause of antenatal hypoxia. Acta Pediatr Hung 1990; 30: 209–15
139. Ilagen NB, Elias EG, Liang KC. Perinatal and neonatal significance of bacteria-related placental villous edema. Acta Obstet Gynecol Scand 1990; 69: 287–90
140. Naeye RL. Disorders of the Placenta, Fetus, and Neonate. St Louis: Mosby Year Book, 1992
141. Salafia CM, Minior VK, Lopez-Zena JA, et al. Relationship of histologic features and umbilical cord gases in preterm gestation. Am J Obstet Gynecol 1995; 173: 1058–64
142. Hansen AR, Collins MH, Genest D, et al. Very low birthweight infant's placenta and its relation to pregnancy and fetal characteristics. Pediatr Dev Pathol 2000; 3: 419–30
143. Redline RW, Wilson-Costello D, Borawski E, et al. The relationship between placental and other perinatal risk factors for neurologic impairment in very low birth weight children. Pediatr Res 2000; 47: 721–6
144. Ogino S, Redline RW. Villous capillary lesions of the placenta: distinctions between chorangioma, chorangiomatosis, and chorangiosis. Hum Pathol 2000; 31: 945–54
145. Franciosi RA. Placental pathology casebook. Chorangiosis of the placenta increases the probability of perinatal mortality. J Perinatol 1999; 19: 393–4
146. Baergen RN, Malicki D, Behling CA, Benirschke K. Morbidity, mortality, and placental pathology in excessively long umbilical cords. Pediatr Devel Pathol 2001; 4: 144–53
147. Redline RW, Boyd T, Campbell V, et al. Maternal vascular underperfusion: nosology and reproducibility of placental reaction patterns. Pediatr Dev Pathol 2004; 7: 237–49
148. DeSa DJ. Infection and amniotic aspiration of middle ear in stillbirths and neonatal deaths. Arch Dis Child 1973; 48: 872–80
149. Redline RW, Pappin A. Fetal thrombotic vasculopathy: the clinical significance of extensive avascular villi. Hum Pathol 1995; 26: 80–5
150. Kraus FT. Placenta: thrombosis of fetal stem vessels with fetal thrombotic vasculopathy and chronic villitis. Pediatr Pathol Lab Med 1996; 16: 143–8
151. Kraus FT, Acheen VI. Fetal thrombotic vasculopathy in the placenta: cerebral thrombi and infarcts, coagulopathies, and cerebral palsy. Hum Pathol 1999; 30: 759–69
152. Kraus FT. Cerebral palsy and thrombi in placental vessels of the fetus: insights from litigation. Hum Pathol 1997; 28: 246–8
153. Hebisch G, Bernasconi MT, Gmuer J, et al. Pregnancy-associated recurrent hemolytic uremic syndrome with fetal thrombotic vasculopathy in the placenta. Am J Obstet Gynecol 2001; 185: 1265–6
154. Khong TY, Hague WM. Biparental contribution to fetal thrombophilia in discordant twin intrauterine growth restriction. Am J Obstet Gynecol 2001; 185: 244–5
155. Ariel I, Anteby E, Hamani Y, Redline RW. Placental pathology in fetal thrombophilia. Hum Pathol 2004; 35: 729–33
156. Oppenheimer EH, Esterly JR. Thrombosis in the newborn: comparison between infants of diabetic and nondiabetic mothers. J Pediatr 1965; 67: 549–56
157. Ornoy A, Crone K, Altshuler G. Pathological features of the placenta in fetal death. Arch Pathol Lab Med 1976; 100: 367–71
158. Saldeen P, Olofsson P, Laurini RN. Structural, functional and circulatory placental changes associated with impaired glucose metabolism. Eur J Obstet Gynecol Reprod Biol 2002; 105: 136–42
159. Khong TY. Placental vascular development and neonatal outcome. Semin Neonatol 2004; 9: 255–63
160. Dahms BB, Boyd T, Redline RW. Severe perinatal liver disease associated with fetal thrombotic vasculopathy. Pediatr Dev Pathol 2002; 5: 80–5
161. Shen-Schwarz S, Macpherson TA, Mueller-Heubach E. The clinical significance of hemorrhagic

endovasculitis of the placenta. Am J Obstet Gynecol 1988; 159: 48–51
162. Altemani AM, Sarian MZ. Hemorrhagic endovasculitis of the placenta. A clinical–pathological study in Brazil. J Perinat Med 1995; 23: 359–63
163. Stevens NG, Sander CH. Placental hemorrhagic endovasculitis: risk factors and impact on pregnancy outcome. Int J Gynaecol Obstet 1984; 22: 393–7
164. Sander CH, Stevens NG. Hemorrhagic endovasculitis of the placenta: an in depth morphologic appraisal with initial clinical and epidemiologic observations. Pathol Annu 1984; 19: 37–79
165. Sander CM, Gilliland D, Akers C, et al. Livebirths with placental hemorrhagic endovasculitis: interlesional relationships and perinatal outcomes. Arch Pathol Lab Med 2002; 126: 157–64
166. Rayburn W, Sander C, Compton A. Histologic examination of the placenta in the growth-retarded fetus. Am J Perinatol 1989; 6: 58–61
167. Salafia CM, Vintzileos AM, Silberman L, et al. Placental pathology of idiopathic intrauterine growth retardation at term. Am J Perinatol 1992; 9: 179–84
168. Sander CM, Gilliland D, Flynn MA, Swart-Hills LA. Risk factors for recurrence of hemorrhagic endovasculitis of the placenta. Obstet Gynecol 1997; 89: 569–76
169. Novak PM, Sander CM, Yang SS, von Oeyen PT. Report of fourteen cases of nonimmune hydrops fetalis in association with hemorrhagic endovasculitis of the placenta. Am J Obstet Gynecol 1991; 165: 945–50
170. Salafia CM, Pezzullo JC, Lopez-Zeno JA, et al. Placental pathologic features of preterm preeclampsia. Am J Obstet Gynecol 1995; 173: 1097–105
171. Silver MM, Yeger H, Lines LD. Hemorrhagic endovasculitis-like lesion induced in placental organ culture. Hum Pathol 1988; 19: 251–6
172. Sander CH, Harrison AK, Ayalya C. Mycoplasma-like particles within the placenta. A potential placentofetal pathogen. Ann NY Acad Sci 1988; 549: 81–102
173. Brosens I, Robertson WB, Dixon HG. The physiological response of the vessels of the placental bed to normal pregnancy. J Pathol Bacteriol 1967; 93: 569–79
174. DeWolf F, DeWolf-Peeters C, Brosens I. Ultrastructure of the spiral arteries in the human placental bed at the end of normal pregnancy. Am J Obstet Gynecol 1973; 117: 177–91
175. Pijnenborg R, Bland JM, Robertson WB, Brosens I. Uteroplacental arterial changes related to interstitial trophoblast migration in early human pregnancy. Placenta 1983; 4: 397–413
176. Kam EP, Gardner L, Loke YW, King A. The role of trophoblast in the physiological change in decidual spiral arteries. Hum Reprod 1999; 14: 2131–8
177. Zhou Y, Fisher SJ, Janatpour M, et al. Human cytotrophoblasts adapt a vascular phenotype as they differentiate. A strategy for successful endovascular invasion? J Clin Invest 1997; 99: 2139–51
178. Pijnenborg R. Implantation and immunology: maternal inflammatory and immune cellular responses to implantation and trophoblast invasion. Reprod Biomed Online 2002; 4 (Suppl 3): 14–17
179. Zhou Y, Bellingard V, Feng KT, et al. Human cytotrophoblasts promote endothelial survival and vascular remodeling through secretion of Ang2, PlGF, and VEGF-C. Dev Biol 2003; 263: 114–25
180. Dekken GA, Sibai BM. Etiology and pathogenesis of pre-eclampsia: current concepts. Am J Obstet Gynecol 1998; 179: 1359–75
181. Starzyk KA, Pijnenborg R, Salafia CM. Decidual and vascular pathophysiology in pregnancy compromise. Semin Reprod Endocrinol 1999; 17: 63–72
182. Drake PM, Red-Horse K, Fisher SJ. Chemokine expression and function at the human maternal–fetal interface. Rev Endocr Metab Disord 2002; 3: 159–65
183. Pang ZJ, Xing FQ. Expression profile of trophoblast invasion-associated genes in the pre-eclamptic placenta. Br J Biomed Sci 2003; 60: 97–101
184. Zhou Y, Genbacev O, Fisher SJ. The human placenta remodels the uterus by using a combination of molecules that govern vasculogenesis or leukocyte extravasation. Ann N Y Acad Sci 2003; 995: 73–83
185. Anteby EY, Greenfield C, Natanson-Yaron S, et al. Vascular endothelial growth factor, epidermal growth factor and fibroblast growth factor-4 and -10 stimulate trophoblast plasminogen activator system and metalloproteinase-9. Mol Hum Reprod 2004; 10: 229–35
186. O'Brien PM, Pipkin FB. The effect of essential fatty acid and specific vitamin supplements on vascular sensitivity in the mid-trimester of human pregnancy. Clin Exp Hypertens B 1983; 2: 247–54
187. Mallet A, Poston L. Vitamin C and E supplementation in women at risk of preeclampsia is associated with changes in indices of oxidative stress and placental function. Am J Obstet Gynecol 2002; 187: 777–84
188. Chappell LC, Seed PT, Kelly FJ, et al. Vitamin C and E supplementation in women at risk of

preeclampsia is associate with changes in indices of oxidative stress and placental function. Am J Obstet Gynecol 2002; 187: 778–84
189. Roberts JM, Balk JL, Bodnar LM, et al. Nutrient involvement in preeclampsia. J Nutr 2003; 133 (Suppl 2): 1684S–2S
190. Starzyk KA, Salafia CM, Pezzullo JC, et al. Quantitative differences in arterial morphometry define the placental bed in preeclampsia. Hum Pathol 1997; 28: 353–8
191. Zeek PM, Assalinsi NS. Vascular changes in the decidua associated with eclamptogenic toxemia of pregnancy. Am J Clin Pathol 1950; 20: 1099–109
192. Labarrere CA. Acute atherosis. A histopathological hallmark of immune aggression? Placenta 1988; 9: 95–108
193. Roberts JM, Cooper DW. Pathogenesis and genetics of pre-eclampsia. Lancet. 2001; 357: 53–6
194. Roberts JM, Lain KY. Recent insights into the pathogenesis of pre-eclampsia. Placenta 2002; 23: 359–72
195. Zhou Y, McMaster M, Woo K, et al. Vascular endothelial growth factor ligands and receptors that regulate human cytotrophoblast survival are dysregulated in severe preeclampsia and hemolysis, elevated liver enzymes, and low platelets syndrome. Am J Pathol 2002; 160: 1405–23
196. Lim KH, Zhou Y, Janatpour M, et al. Human cytotrophoblast differentiation/invasion is abnormal in pre-eclampsia. Am J Pathol 1997; 151: 1809–18
197. Said J, Dekker G. Pre-eclampsia and thrombophilia. Best Pract Res Clin Obstet Gynaecol 2003; 17: 441–58
198. Kupferminc MJ, Rimon E, Ascher-Landsberg J, et al. Perinatal outcome in women with severe pregnancy complications and multiple thrombophilias. J Perinat Med 2004; 32: 225–7
199. Branch DW, Khamashta MA. Antiphospholipid syndrome: obstetric diagnosis, management, and controversies. Obstet Gynecol 2003; 101: 1333–44
200. Brenner B. Thrombophilia and fetal loss. Semin Thromb Hemost 2003; 29: 165–70
201. Heilmann L, von Tempelhoff GF, Pollow K. Antiphospholipid syndrome in obstetrics. Clin Appl Thromb Hemost 2003; 9: 143–50
202. Chappell LC, Seed PT, Briley A, et al. A longitudinal study of biochemical variables in women at risk of preeclampsia. Am J Obstet Gynecol 2002; 187: 127–36
203. Heiskanen J, Romppanen EL, Hiltunen M, et al. Polymorphism in the tumor necrosis factor-alpha gene in women with preeclampsia. J Assist Reprod Genet 2002; 19: 220–3
204. Darmochwal-Kolarz D, Rolinski J, Leszczynska-Goarzelak B, Oleszczuk J. The expressions of intracellular cytokines in the lymphocytes of preeclamptic patients. Am J Reprod Immunol 2002; 48: 381–6
205. Pang ZJ, Xing FQ. Comparative study on the expression of cytokine-receptor genes in normal and preeclamptic human placentas using DNA microarrays. J Perinat Med 2003; 31: 153–62
206. Orange S, Horvath J, Hennessy A. Preeclampsia is associated with a reduced interleukin-10 production from peripheral blood mononuclear cells. Hypertens Pregnancy 2003; 22: 1–8
207. Many A, Hubel CA, Fisher SJ, et al. Invasive cytotrophoblasts manifest evidence of oxidative stress in preeclampsia. Am J Pathol 2000; 156: 321–31
208. Tempfer CB, Dorman K, Deter RL, et al. An endothelial nitric oxide synthase gene polymorphism is associated with preeclampsia. Hypertens Pregnancy 2001; 20: 107–18
209. Bilodeau JF, Hubel CA. Current concepts in the use of antioxidants for the treatment of preeclampsia. J Obstet Gynaecol Can 2003; 25: 742–50
210. Qiu C, Williams MA, Leisenring WM, et al. Family history of hypertension and type 2 diabetes in relation to preeclampsia risk. Hypertension 2003; 41: 408–13
211. Laivuori H, Lahermo P, Ollikainen V, et al. Susceptibility loci for preeclampsia on chromosomes 2p25 and 9p13 in Finnish families. Am J Hum Genet 2003; 72: 168–77
212. Francoual J, Audibert F, Trioche P, et al. Is a polymorphism of the apolipoprotein E gene associated with pre-eclampsia? Hypertens Pregnancy 2002; 21: 127–33
213. Winkler K, Wetzka B, Hoffmann MM, et al. Triglyceride-rich lipoproteins are associated with hypertension in preeclampsia. J Clin Endocrinol Metab 2003; 88: 1162–6
214. Broughton Pipkin F. What is the place of genetics in the pathogenesis of pre-eclampsia? Biol Neonate 1999; 76: 325–30
215. Lachmeijer AM, Dekker GA, Pals G, et al. Searching for preeclampsia genes: the current position. Eur J Obstet Gynecol Reprod Biol 2002; 105: 94–113
216. Luttun A, Carmeliet P. Soluble VEGF receptor Flt1: the elusive preeclampsia factor discovered? J Clin Invest 2003; 111: 600–2

217. Staff AC, Ranheim T, Halvorsen B. Augmented PLA2 activity in pre-eclamptic decidual tissue – a key player in the pathophysiology of 'acute atherosis' in pre-eclampsia? Placenta 2003; 24: 965–73
218. Sibai BM. Diagnosis and management of gestational hypertension and preeclampsia. Obstet Gynecol 2003; 102: 181–92
219. Ackerman J, Gonzalez EF, Gilbert-Barness E. Immunological studies of the placenta in maternal connective tissue disease. Pediatr Dev Pathol 1999; 2: 19–24
220. Many A, Schreiber L, Rosner S, et al. Pathologic features of the placenta in women with severe pregnancy complications and thrombophilia. Obstet Gynecol 2001; 98: 1041–4
221. Khong TY. Acute atherosis in pregnancies complicated by hypertension, growth retardation, and diabetes mellitus. Arch Pathol Lab Med 1991; 115: 722–5
222. Sebire NJ. Fetal postmortem weight loss in utero. Br J Obstet Gynaecol 2003; 110: 86–7
223. Gruenwald P, Minh HN. Evaluation of body and organ weights in perinatal pathology. II. Weight of body and placenta of surviving and of autopsied infants. Am J Obstet Gynecol 1961; 82: 312–19
224. Pinar H, Sung CJ, Oyer CE, Singer DB. Reference values for singleton and twin placental weights. Pediatr Pathol Lab Med 1996; 16: 901–7
225. Kalousek DK, Dill FJ. Chromosomal mosaicism confined to the placenta in human conceptions. Science 1983; 221: 665–7
226. Amiel A, Bouaron N, Kidron D, et al. CGH in the detection of confined placental mosaicism (CPM) in placentas of abnormal pregnancies. Prenat Diagn 2002; 22: 752–8
227. Masuzaki H, Miura K, Yoshiura KI, et al. Detection of cell free placental DNA in maternal plasma: direct evidence from three cases of confined placental mosaicism. J Med Genet 2004; 41: 289–92
228. Sistrom CL, Ferguson JE. Abnormal membranes in obstetrical ultrasound: incidence and significance of amniotic sheets and circumvallate placenta. Ultrasound Obstet Gynecol 1993; 3: 249–55
229. Ahmed A, Gilbert-Barness E. Placenta membranacea: a developmental anomaly with diverse clinical presentation. Pediatr Dev Pathol 2003; 6: 201–2
230. Armstrong CA, Harding S, Matthews T, Dickinson JE. Is placenta accreta catching up with us? Aust NZ J Obstet Gynaecol 2004; 44: 210–13
231. Dildy GA 3rd. Postpartum hemorrhage: new management options. Clin Obstet Gynecol 2002; 45: 330–44
232. American College of Obstetricians and Gynecologists, Committee on Obstetric Practice. Placenta accreta. ACOG Committee Opinion 266. Washington, DC: ACOG, January 2002
233. Khadra M, Obhrai M, Keriakos R, Johanson R. Placenta percreta revisited. J Obstet Gynaecol 2002; 22: 689
234. Imseis HM, Murtha AP, Alexander KA, Barnett BD. Spontaneous rupture of a primigravid uterus secondary to placenta percreta. A case report. J Reprod Med 1998; 43: 23323–6
235. Breen JL, Neubecker R, Gregori CA, Franklin JE Jr. Placenta accreta, increta, and percreta. A survey of 40 cases. Obstet Gynecol 1977; 49: 43–7
236. Esmans A, Gerris J, Corthout E, et al. Placenta percreta causing rupture of an unscarred uterus at the end of the first trimester of pregnancy: case report. Hum Reprod 2004; 18: 2401–3
237. Lin CC, Adamczyk CJ, Montag AG, et al. Placenta previa percreta involving the left broad ligament and cervix. A case report. J Reprod Med 1998; 43: 839–43
238. Cox SM, Carpenter RJ, Cotton DB. Placenta percreta: ultrasound diagnosis and conservative surgical management
239. Jacques SM, Qureshi F, Trent VS, Ramirez NC. Placenta accreta: mild cases diagnosed by placental examination. Int J Gynecol Pathol 1996; 15: 28–33
240. Sherer DM, Salafia CM, Minior VK, et al. Placental basal plate myometrial fibers: clinical correlations of abnormally deep trophoblast invasion. Obstet Gynecol 1996; 87: 444–9
241. Sarantopoulos GP, Natarajan S. Placenta accreta. Arch Pathol Lab Med 2002; 126: 1557–8
242. Katzman PJ, Genest DR. Maternal floor infarction and massive perivillous fibrin deposition: histological definitions, association with intrauterine fetal growth restriction, and risk of recurrence. Pediatr Dev Pathol 2002; 5: 159–64. Erratum in Pediatr Dev Pathol 2003; 6: 102
243. Bane AL, Gillan JE. Massive perivillous fibrinoid causing recurrent placental failure. Br J Obstet Gynaecol 2003; 110: 292–5
244. Andres RL, Kuyper W, Resnik R, et al. The association of maternal floor infarction of the placenta with adverse perinatal outcome. Am J Obstet Gynecol 1990; 163: 935–8
245. Naeye RL. Maternal floor infarction. Hum Pathol 1985; 16: 823–8
246. Redline RW, Jiang JG, Shah D. Discordancy for maternal floor infarction in dizygotic twin placentas. Hum Pathol 2003; 34: 822–4

247. Vernof KK, Benirschke K, Kephart GM, et al. Maternal floor infarction: relationship to X cells, major basic protein, and adverse perinatal outcome. Am J Obstet Gynecol 1992; 167: 1355–63
248. Mandsager NT, Bendon R, Mostello D, et al. Maternal floor infarction of the placenta: prenatal diagnosis and clinical significance. Obstet Gynecol 1994; 83: 750–4
249. Gersell DJ. Chronic villitis, chronic chorioamnionitis, and maternal floor infarction. Semin Diagn Pathol 1993; 10: 251–66
250. Redline RW. Clinically and biologically relevant patterns of placental inflammation. Pediatr Dev Pathol 2002; 5: 326–8
251. Tettey T, Wiredu EK. Autopsy studies on stillbirths in Korle Bu Teaching Hospital: pathological findings in stillbirths and their placentae. West Afr J Med 1997; 16: 12–19
252. Fuke Y, Aono T, Imai S, et al. Clinical significance and treatment of massive intervillous fibrin deposition associated with recurrent fetal growth retardation. Gynecol Obstet Invest 1994; 38: 5–9
253. Adams-Chapman I, Vaucher YE, Bajar RF, et al. Maternal floor infarction of the placenta: association with central nervous system injury and adverse neurodevelopmental outcome. J Perinatol 2002; 22: 236–41
254. Clewell WH, Manchester DK. Recurrent maternal floor infarction: a preventable cause of fetal death. Am J Obstet Gynecol 1983; 174: 346–7
255. Katz VL, Bowes WA, Sierkh AE. Maternal floor infarction of the placenta associated with elevated second trimester alpha fetoprotein. Am J Perinatol 1987; 4: 225–8
256. Robinson L, Grau P, Crandall BF. Pregnancy outcomes after increasing maternal serum alpha fetoprotein levels. Obstet Gynecol 1989; 74: 17–20
257. Gorbe E, Rigo J, Marton T, et al. Maternal floor infarct, simultaneous manifestation of intrauterine fetal retardation and high maternal AFP level [German]. Z Geburtsch Neonatol 1999; 203: 218–20
258. Sun CC, Revell VO, Belli AJ, Viscardi RM. Discrepancy in pathologic diagnosis of placental lesions. Arch Pathol Lab Med 2002; 126: 706–9
259. Lindoff G, Astedt B. Plasminogen activator of urokinase type and its inhibitor of placental type in hypertensive pregnancies and in intrauterine growth retardation: possible markers of placental function. Am J Obstet Gynecol 1994; 171: 60–4
260. Zhang JC, Sakthivel R, Kniss D, et al. The low density lipoprotein receptor-related protein/alpha2-macroglobulin receptor regulates cell surface plasminogen activator activity on human trophoblast cells. J Biol Chem 1998; 273: 32273–80
261. Floridon C, Nielsen O, Holund B, et al. Does plasminogen activator inhibitor-1 (PAI-1) control trophoblast invasion? A study of fetal and maternal tissue in intrauterine, tubal and molar pregnancies. Placenta 2000; 21: 754–62
262. Pierleoni C, Samuelsen GB, Graem N, et al. Immunohistochemical identification of the receptor for urokinase plasminogen activator associated with fibrin deposition in normal and ectopic human placenta. Placenta 1998; 19: 501–8
263. McCrae KR, DeMichele AM, Pandhi P, et al. Detection of antitrophoblast antibodies in the sera of patients with anticardiolipin antibodies and fetal loss. Blood 1993; 82: 2730–41
264. Katz VL, DiTomasso J, Farmer R, Carpenter M. Activated protein C resistance associated with maternal floor infarction treated with low-molecular-weight heparin. Am J Perinatol 2002; 19: 273–7
265. Sebire NJ. Early onset discordant growth in a successful monochorionic twin pregnancy. Br J Obstet Gynaecol 2002; 109: 1426
266. Matern D, Shehata BM, Sheljawa P, et al. Placental floor infarction complicating the pregnancy of a fetus with long-chain 3-hydroxyacyl-CoA dehydrogenase (LCHAD) deficiency [Brief communication]. Mol Genet Metabol 2001; 72: 265–8
267. Burton GJ, Watson AL. The structure of the human placenta: implications for initiating and defending against virus infections. Rev Med Virol 1997; 7: 219–28
268. Chan G, Hemmings DG, Yurochko AD, Guilbert LJ. Human cytomegalovirus-caused damage to placental trophoblasts mediated by immediate-early gene-induced tumor necrosis factor-alpha. Am J Pathol 2002; 161: 1371–81
269. Koi H, Zhang J, Parry S. The mechanisms of placental viral infection. Ann NY Acad Sci 2001; 943: 148–56
270. Koi H, Zhang J, Makrigiannakis A, et al. Syncytiotrophoblast is a barrier to maternal–fetal transmission of herpes simplex virus. Biol Reprod 2002; 5: 1572–9
271. Lecuit M, Nelson DM, Smith SD, et al. Targeting and crossing of the human maternofetal barrier by Listeria monocytogenes: role of internalin interaction with trophoblast E-cadherin. Proc Natl Acad Sci USA 2004; 101: 6152–7

272. Saji F, Samejima Y, Kamiura S, Koyama M. Dynamics of immunoglobulins at the feto-maternal interface. Rev Reprod 1999; 4: 81–9
273. Garcia-Lloret MI, Winkler-Lowen B, Guilbert LJ. Monocytes adhering by LFA-1 to placental syncytiotrophoblasts induce local apoptosis via release of TNF-alpha. A model for hematogenous initiation of placental inflammations. J Leukoc Biol 2000; 68: 903–8
274. Torres G, Garcia V, Sanchez E, et al. Expression of the HIV-1 co-receptors CCR5 and CXCR4 on placental macrophages and the effect of IL-10 on their expression. Placenta 2001; 22 (Suppl A): S29–33
275. Ben-Hur H, Gurevich P, Berman V, et al. The secretory immune system as part of the placental barrier in the second trimester of pregnancy in humans. In Vivo 2001; 15: 429–35
276. Zachar V, Fink T, Koppelhus U, Ebbesen P. Role of placental cytokines in transcriptional modulation of HIV type 1 in the isolated villous trophoblast. AIDS Res Hum Retroviruses 2002; 18: 839–47
277. Arias RA, Munoz LD, Munoz-Fernandez MA. Transmission of HIV-1 infection between trophoblast placental cells and T-cells takes place via an LFA-1-mediated cell to cell contact. Virology 2003; 307: 266–77
278. Dye JF, Jablenska R, Donnelly JL, et al. Phenotype of the endothelium in the human term placenta. Placenta 2001; 1: 32–43
279. Jordan JA, Butchko AR. Apoptotic activity in villous trophoblast cells during B19 infection correlates with clinical outcome: assessment by the caspase-related M30 Cytodeath antibody. Placenta 2002; 23: 547–53
280. Goldenberg RL, Thompson C. The infectious origins of stillbirth. Am J Obstet Gynecol 2003; 189: 861–73
281. Altshuler G, Russell P. The human placental villitides: a review of chronic intrauterine infection. Curr Top Pathol 1975; 60: 64–112
282. Parkash V, Morotti RA, Joshi V, et al. Immunohistochemical detection of Listeria antigens in the placenta in perinatal listeriosis. Int J Gynecol Pathol 1998; 17: 343–50
283. Centers for Disease Control. Multistate outbreak of listeriosis – United States, 2000. Morbid Mortal Weekly Rep 2000; 49: 1129–30
284. Bakardjiev AI, Stacy BA, Fisher SJ, Portnoy DA. Listeriosis in the pregnant guinea pig: a model of vertical transmission. Infect Immun 2004; 72: 489–97
285. Centers for Disease Control and Prevention. Sexually transmitted disease surveillance, 1999. Atlanta: Department of Health and Human Services, Centers for Disease Control and Prevention, September 2000
286. Riley BS, Oppenheimer-Marks N, Hansen EJ, et al. Virulent Treponema pallidum activates human vascular endothelial cells. J Infect Dis 1992; 165: 484–93
287. Radolf JD, Arndt LL, Akins DR, et al. Treponema pallidum and Borrelia burgdorferi lipoproteins and synthetic lipopeptides activate monocytes/ macrophages. J Immunol 1995; 154: 2866–77
288. Norgard MV, Riley BS, Richardson JA, Radolf JD. Dermal inflammation elicited by synthetic analogs of Treponema pallidum and Borrelia burgdorferi lipoproteins. Infect Immun 1995; 63: 1507–15
289. Young SA, Crocker DW. Occult congenital syphilis in macerated stillborn fetuses. Arch Pathol Lab Med 1994; 118: 44–7
290. Jacques SM, Qureshi F. Necrotizing funisitis: a study of 45 cases. Hum Pathol 1992; 23: 1278–83
291. Genest DR, Choi-Hong SR, Tate JE, et al. Diagnosis of congenital syphilis from placental examination: comparison of histopathology, Steiner stain, and polymerase chain reaction for Treponema pallidum DNA. Hum Pathol 1996; 27: 366–72
292. Machin GA, Honore LH, Fanning EA, Molesky M. Perinatally acquired neonatal tuberculosis: report of two cases. Pediatr Pathol 1992; 12: 707–16
293. Henderson CE. Management of tuberculosis in pregnancy. J Assoc Acad Minor Phys 1995; 6: 38–42
294. Duncan ME, Fox H, Harkness RA, Rees RJ. The placenta in leprosy. Placenta 1984; 5: 189–98
295. Horne HW, Hertig AT, Kundsin RB, Kosasa TS. Sub-clinical endometrial inflammation and T-mycoplasma: a possible cause of human reproductive failure. Int J Fertil 1973; 18: 226–31
296. Dische MR, Quinn PA, Czegledy-Nagy E, Sturgess JM. Genital mycoplasma infection. Intrauterine infection: pathologic study of the fetus and placenta. Am J Clin Pathol 1979; 72: 167–74
297. Schwartz DA, Khan R, Stoll B. Characterization of the fetal inflammatory response to cytomegalovirus placentitis. An immunohistochemical study. Arch Pathol Lab Med 1992; 116: 21–7
298. Kaplan C. The placenta and viral infections. Semin Diagn Pathol 1993; 10: 232–50
299. Sander CM. What is new in placental pathology? Pathol Annu 1995; 30: 59–93
300. Nakamura Y, Sakuma S, Ohta Y, et al. Detection of the human cytomegalovirus gene in placental

chronic villitis by polymerase chain reaction. Hum Pathol 1994; 25: 815–18

301. Centers for Disease Control. Risks associated with human parvovirus B19 infection. Morbid Mortal Weekly Rep 1989; 38: 81–97
302. Boley TJ, Rodis JF, Duff P, et al. Spring is parvovirus time: how to counsel your patients. Ask the perinatologist. Sarasota Memorial Hosp (Newslett) 1994; Spring: 1–5
303. Rogers BB, Mark Y, Oyer CE. Diagnosis and incidence of fetal parvovirus infection in an autopsy series: I. Histology. Pediatr Pathol 1993; 13: 371–9
304. Török TJ. Human parvovirus B19 infections in pregnancy. Pediatr Infect Dis J 1990; 9: 772–6
305. Kailasam C, Brennand J, Cameron AD. Congenital parvovirus B19 infection: experience of a recent epidemic. Fetal Diagn Ther 2001; 16: 18–22
306. Jordan JA, DeLoia JA. Globoside expression within the human placenta. Placenta 1999; 20: 103–8
307. Weigel-Kelley KA, Yoder MC, Srivastava A. Recombinant human parvovirus B19 vectors: erythrocyte P antigen is necessary but not sufficient for successful transduction of human hematopoietic cells. J Virol 2001; 75: 4110–16
308. Keeling JW. Hydrops fetalis and other forms of excess fluid collection in the fetus. In Wigglesworth JS, Singer DB, eds. Textbook of Fetal and Perinatal Pathology. Boston: Blackwell Scientific Publications, 1991: 429–54
309. Metzman R, Anand A, DeGuillo PA, Knisely AS. Hepatic disease associated with intrauterine parvovirus B19 infection in a newborn premature infant. J Pediatr Gastroenterol Nutr 1989; 9: 112–14
310. White FV, Jordan J, Dickman PS, Knisely AS. Fetal parvovirus B19 infection and liver disease of antenatal onset in an infant with Ebstein's anomaly. Pediatr Pathol Lab Med 1995; 15: 121–9
311. Krause JR, Penchansky L, Knisely AS. Morphologic diagnosis of parvovirus B19 infection. Arch Pathol Lab Med 1992; 116: 178–80
312. Rogers BB, Singer DB, Mak SK et al. Detection of human parvovirus B19 in early spontaneous abortuses using seroloy, histology, electron microscopy, in situ hybridization, and the polymerase chain reaction. Obstet Gynecol 1993; 81: 402–8
313. Mark Y, Rogers BB, Oyer CE. Diagnosis and incidence of fetal parvovirus infection in an autopsy series: II. DNA amplification. Pediatr Pathol 1993; 13: 381–6
314. Tolfvenstam T, Papadogiannakis N, Norbeck O, et al. Frequency of human parvovirus. B19 infection in intrauterine fetal death. Lancet 2001; 357: 1494–7
315. Morey AL, O'Neill HJ, Coyle PV, Fleming KV. Immunohistochemical detection of human parvovirus B19 formalin fixed paraffin embedded tissues. J Pathol 1992; 166: 105–8
316. Essary LR, Vnencak-Jone CL, Manning SS, et al. Frequency of parvovirus B19 infection in NIHF and utility of three diagnostic methods. Hum Pathol 1998; 29: 696–701
317. Altshuler G, Hyde SR. Clinicopathologic implications of placental pathology. Clin Obstet Gynecol 1996; 39: 549–70
318. Hyde SR, Giacoia GP. Congenital herpes infection: placental and umbilical cord findings. Obstet Gynecol 1993; 81: 852–5
319. Heifetz SA, Bauman M. Necrotizing funisitis and herpes simplex infection of placental and decidual tissues: study of four cases. Hum Pathol 1994; 25: 715–22
320. Bendon RW, Perez F, Ray MB. Herpes simplex virus: fetal and decidual infection. Pediatr Pathol 1987; 7: 63–70
321. Schwartz DA, Caldwell E. Herpes simplex virus infection of the placenta. The role of molecular pathology in the diagnosis of viral infection of placental-associated tissues. Arch Pathol Lab Med 1991; 115: 1141–4
322. Muhlemann K, Menegus MA. Placental examination in intrauterine coinfection with herpes simplex virus and cytomegalovirus. Pediatr Pathol Lab Med 1996; 16: 935–9
323. Zimmerman L, Reef SE. Incidence of congenital rubella syndrome at a hospital serving a predominantly Hispanic population, El Paso, Texas. Pediatrics 2001; 107: E40
324. Centers for Disease Control. Rubella among Hispanic adults – Kansas, 1998, and Nebraska, 1999. Morbid Mortal Weekly Rep 2000; 49: 225–8
325. Sheridan E, Aitken C, Jeffries D, et al. Congenital rubella syndrome: a risk in immigrant populations. Lancet 2002; 359: 674–5
326. Gall SA. Maternal immunization. Obstet Gynecol Clin North Am 2003; 30: 623–36
327. Crowcroft N, Pebody R. Prevention of congenital rubella infection: a challenge for every country in Europe. Euro Surveill 2004; 9
328. Tookey P. Rubella in England, Scotland and Wales. Euro Surveill 2004; 9
329. Lemos C, Ramirez R, Ordobas M, et al. New features of rubella in Spain: the evidence of an outbreak. Euro Surveill 2004; 9
330. Glismann S. Rubella in Denmark. Euro Surveill 2004; 9

331. Centers for Disease Control and Prevention. Rubella and congenital rubella syndrome – United States January 1, 1991–May 7th 1994. Morbid Mortal Weekly Rep 1994; 43: 391
332. Bar-Oz B, Levichek Z, Moretti ME, et al. Pregnancy outcome following rubella vaccination: a prospective controlled study. Am J Med Genet 2004; 130A: 52
333. Ornoy A, Segal S, Nishmi M, et al. Fetal and placental pathology in gestational rubella. Am J Obstet Gynecol 1973; 116: 949–56
334. Paryani SG, Arvin AM. Intrauterine infection with varicella-zoster virus after maternal varicella. N Engl J Med 1986; 314: 1542–6
335. Qureshi F, Jacques SM. Maternal varicella during pregnancy: correlation of maternal history and fetal outcome with placental histopathology. Hum Pathol 1996; 27: 191–5
336. Enders G, Miller E, Cradock-Watson J, et al. Consequences of varicella and herpes zoster in pregnancy: prospective study of 1739 cases. Lancet 1994; 343: 1548–51
337. Jones KL, Johnson KA, Chambers CD. Offspring of women infected with varicella during pregnancy: a prospective study. Teratology 1994; 49: 29–32
338. Chandra PC, Patel H, Schiavello HJ, Briggs SL. Successful pregnancy outcome after complicated varicella pneumonia. Obstet Gynecol 1998; 92: 680–2
339. Garcia AGP. Fetal infection in chickenpox and alastrim with histopathologic study of the placenta. Pediatrics 1963; 32: 895–901
340. Chow KC, Lee CC, Lin TY, et al. Congenital enterovirus 71 infection: a case study with virology and immunohistochemistry. Clin Infect Dis 2000; 31: 509–12
341. Basso NG, Fonseca ME, Garcia AG, et al. Enterovirus isolation from foetal and placental tissues. Acta Virol 1990; 34: 49–57
342. Batcup G, Holt P, Hambling MH, et al. Placental and fetal pathology in Coxsackie virus A9 infection: a case report. Histopathology 1985; 9: 1227–35
343. Garcia AG, Basso NG, Fonseca ME, et al. Enterovirus associated placental morphology: a light, virological, electron microscopic and immunohistologic study. Placenta 1991; 125: 533–47
344. Euscher E, Davis J, Holzman I, Nuovo GJ. Coxsackie virus infection of the placenta associated with neurodevelopmental delays in the newborn. Obstet Gynecol 2001; 98: 1019–26
345. Satosar A, Ramirez NC, Bartholomew D, et al. Histologic correlates of viral and bacterial infection of the placenta associated with severe morbidity and mortality in the newborn. Hum Pathol 2004; 35: 536–45
346. Altshuler G. Placental villitis of unknown etiology: harbinger of serious disease? A four month's experience of nine cases. J Reprod Med 1973; 11: 215–22
347. Labarrere CA, McIntyre JA, Faulk WP. Immunohistologic evidence that villitis in human normal term placentas is an immunologic lesion. Am J Obstet Gynecol 1990; 162: 515–22
348. Doss BJ, Greene MF, Hill J, et al. Massive chronic intervillositis associated with recurrent abortions. Hum Pathol 1995; 26: 1245–51
349. Redline RW, Patterson P. Villitis of unknown etiology is associated with major infiltration of fetal tissue by maternal inflammatory cells. Am J Pathol 1993; 143: 473–9
350. Altemani AM, Gonzatti AR. [Villitis of unknown etiology in placentas of pregnancies with hypertensive disorders and of small-for-gestational-age infants]. Rev Assoc Med Bras 2003; 49: 67–71
351. Russell P. Inflammatory lesions of the human placenta. III. The histopathology of villitis of unknown etiology. Placenta 1980; 1: 227–44
352. Knox WF, Fox H. Villitis of unknown aetiology: its incidence and significance in placentae from a British population. Placenta 1984; 5: 395–402
353. Jacques SM, Qureshi F. Chronic chorioamnionitis: a clinicopathologic and immunohistochemical study. Hum Pathol 1998; 29: 1457–61
354. Altshuler G, Russell P, Ermocilla R. The placental pathology of small-for-gestational age infants. Am J Obstet Gynecol 1975; 121: 351–9
355. Bjoro K Jr, Myhre E. The role of chronic non-specific inflammatory lesions of the placenta in intrauterine growth retardation. Acta Pathol Microbiol Immunol Scand [A] 1984; 92: 133–7
356. Althabe O, Labarrere C. Chronic villitis of unknown aetiology and intrauterine growth-retarded infants of normal and low ponderal index. Placenta 1985; 6: 369–73
357. Agapitos E, Papadopoulou C, Kavantzas N, et al. The contribution of pathological examination of the placenta in the investigation of the causes of foetal mortality. Arch Anat Cytol Pathol 1996; 44: 5–11
358. Redline RW, Abramowsky CR. Clinical and pathologic aspects of recurrent placental villitis. Hum Pathol 1985; 16: 727–31
359. Mallozzi-Eberle A, Levesque D, Vintzileos AM, et al. Placental pathology in discordant twins. Am J Obstet Gynecol 1993; 169: 931–5

360. Jacques SM, Qureshi F. Chronic villitis of unknown etiology in twin gestations. Pediatr Pathol 1994; 14: 575–84
361. Khong TY, Staples A, Moore L, Byard RW. Observer reliability in assessing villitis of unknown aetiology. J Clin Pathol 1993; 46: 208–10
362. Labarrere C, Mullen E. Fibrinoid and trophoblastic necrosis with massive chronic intervillositis: an extreme variant of villitis of unknown etiology. Am J Reprod Immunol Microbiol 1987; 15: 85–91
363. Altemani AM. Immunohistochemical study of the inflammatory infiltrate in villitis of unknown etiology. Path Res Pract 1992; 188: 303–9
364. Greco MA, Wieczorek R, Sachdev R, et al. Phenotype of villous stromal cells in placentas with cytomegalovirus, syphilis, and nonspecific villitis. Am J Pathol 1992; 141: 835–42
365. Labarrere CA, Faulk WP. Maternal cells in chorionic villi from placentae of normal and abnormal human pregnancies. Am J Reprod Immunol 1995; 33: 54–9
366. Labarrere CA, Althabe O, Caletli E, Muscolo D. Deficiency of blocking factors in intrauterine growth retardation and its relationship with chronic villitis. Am J Reprod Immunol Microbiol 1986; 10: 14–19
367. Hasegawa I, Takakuwa K, Adachi S, Kanazawa K. Cytotoxic antibody against trophoblast and lymphocytes present in pregnancy with intrauterine growth retardation and its relation to antiphospholipid antibody. J Reprod Immunol 1990; 17: 127–39
368. Xiao J, Garcia-Loret M, Winkler-Lowen B, et al. ICAM-1-mediated adhesion of peripheral blood monocytes to the maternal surface of placental syncytiotrophoblasts. Implications for placental villitis. Am J Pathol 1997; 150: 1845–60
369. Jacques SM, Qureshi F. Chronic intervillositis of the placenta. Arch Pathol Lab Med 1993; 117: 1032–5
370. Ordi J, Ismail MR, Ventura PJ, et al. Massive chronic intervillositis of the placenta associated with malaria infection. Am J Surg Pathol 1998; 22: 1006–11
371. Ornoy A, Dudai M, Sadovsky E. Placental and fetal pathology in infectious mononucleosis. A possible indicator for Epstein–Barr virus teratogenicity. Diagn Gynecol Obstet 1982; 4: 11–16
372. Wiktor SZ, Ekpini E, Nduati RW. Prevention of mother-to-child transmission of HIV-1 in Africa. AIDS 1997; 11 (Suppl B): S79–87
373. Connor EM, Sperling RS, Gelber R, et al. Reduction of maternal–infant transmission of human immunodeficiency virus type 1 with zidovudine treatment. Pediatric AIDS Clinical Trials Group Protocol 076 Study Group. N Engl J Med 1994; 331: 1173–80
374. Davis SF, Byers RH Jr, Lindegren ML, et al. Prevalence and incidence of vertically acquired HIV infection in the United States. J Am Med Assoc 1995; 274: 952–5
375. De Cock KM, Fowler MG, Mercier E, et al. Prevention of mother-to-child HIV transmission in resource-poor countries: translating research into policy and practice. J Am Med Assoc 2000; 283: 1175–82
376. Dunn DT, Newell ML, Ades AE, Peckham CS. Risk of human immunodeficiency virus type 1 transmission through breastfeeding. Lancet 1992; 340: 585–8
377. Soilleux EJ, Coleman N. Transplacental transmission of HIV: a potential role for HIV binding lectins. Int J Biochem Cell Biol 2003; 35: 283–7
378. Mwanyumba F, Gaillard P, Inion I, et al. Placental inflammation and perinatal transmission of HIV-1. J Acquir Immune Defic Syndr 2002; 29: 262–9
379. Anderson V, Carneiro M, Bulterys M, et al. Perinatal infections: HIV and co-infections in the placenta and therapeutic interventions – a workshop report. Placenta 2001; 22 (Suppl A): S34–7
380. Burgess T. Determinants of transmission of HIV from mother to child. Clin Obstet Gynecol 2001; 44: 198–209
381. Miller RK, Polliotti BM, Laughlin T, et al. Role of the placenta in fetal HIV infection. Teratology 2000; 61: 391–4
382. Temmerman M, Nagelkerke N, Bwayo J, et al. HIV-1 and immunological changes during pregnancy: a comparison between HIV-1-seropositive and HIV-1-seronegative women in Nairobi, Kenya. AIDS 1995; 9: 1057–60
383. Ladner J, Leroy V, Hoffman P, et al. Chorioamnionitis and pregnancy outcome in HIV-infected African women. Pregnancy and HIV Study Group. J Acquir Immune Defic Syndr Hum Retrovirol 1998; 18: 293–8
384. Mofenson LM, Lambert JS, Stiehm ER, et al. Risk factors for perinatal transmission of human immunodeficiency virus type 1 in women treated with zidovudine. Pediatric AIDS Clinical Trials Group Study 185 Team. N Engl J Med 1999; 341: 385–93
385. Van Dyke RB, Korber BT, Popek E, et al. The Ariel Project: a prospective cohort study of maternal–child transmission of human immunodeficiency virus type 1 in the era of maternal antiretroviral therapy. J Infect Dis 1999; 179: 319–28

386. Wabwire-Mangen F, Gray RH, Mmiro FA, et al. Placental membrane inflammation and risks of maternal-to-child transmission of HIV-1 in Uganda. J Acquir Immune Defic Syndr 1999; 22: 379–85
387. Schwartz DA, Sungkarat S, Shaffer N, et al. Placental abnormalities associated with human immunodeficiency virus type 1 infection and perinatal transmission in Bangkok, Thailand. J Infect Dis 2000; 182: 1652–7
388. Lee BN, Hammill H, Popek EJ, et al. Production of interferons and beta-chemokines by placental trophoblasts of HIV-1-infected women. Infect Dis Obstet Gynecol 2001; 9: 95–104
389. Cohen J. Epidemiology. Mothers' malaria appears to enhance spread of AIDS virus. Science 2003; 302: 1311
390. Brahmbhatt H, Kigozi G, Wabwire-Mangen F, et al. The effects of placental malaria on mother-to-child HIV transmission in Rakai, Uganda. AIDS 2003; 17: 2539–41
391. Ayisi JG, van Eijk AM, Newman RD, et al. Maternal malaria and perinatal HIV transmission, western Kenya. Emerg Infect Dis 2004; 10: 643–52
392. Patterson BK, Behbahani H, Kabat WJ, et al. Leukemia inhibitory factor inhibits HIV-1 replication and is upregulated in placentae from nontransmitting women. J Clin Invest 2001; 107: 287–94
393. Fujino T, Iwamoto I, Otsuka H, et al. Apoptosis in placentas from human T-lymphotropic virus type I-seropositive pregnant women: a possible defense mechanism against transmission from mother to fetus. Obstet Gynecol 1999; 94: 279–83
394. Vidricaire G, Tardif MR, Tremblay MJ. The low viral production in trophoblastic cells is due to a high endocytic internalization of the human immunodeficiency virus type 1 and can be overcome by the pro-inflammatory cytokines tumor necrosis factor-alpha and interleukin-1. J Biol Chem 2003; 278: 15832–41
395. Polliotti BM, Gnall-Sazenski S, Laughlin TS, Miller RK. Inhibitory effects of human chorionic gonadotropin (hCG) preparations on HIV infection of human placenta in vitro. Placenta 2002; 23 (Suppl A):S102–6
396. Soilleux EJ, Morris LS, Rushbrook S, et al. Expression of human immunodeficiency virus (HIV)-binding lectin DC-SIGNR: consequences for HIV infection and immunity. Hum Pathol 2002; 33: 652–9
397. Geijtenbeek TB, van Vliet SJ, van Duijnhoven GC, et al. DC-SIGN, a dentritic cell-specific HIV-1 receptor present in placenta that enhances trans-infection of T cells – a review. Placenta 2001; 22 (Suppl A):S19–23
398. Chandwani S, Greco MA, Mittal K, et al. Pathology and human immunodeficiency virus expression in placentas of seropositive women. J Infect Dis 1991; 163: 1134–8
399. Anderson VM. The placental barrier to maternal HIV infection. Obstet Gynecol Clin North Am 1997; 24: 797–820
400. Jauniaux E, Nessmann C, Imbert MC, et al. Morphological aspects of the placenta in HIV pregnancies. Placenta 1988; 9: 633–42
401. Martin AW, Brady K, Smith SI, et al. Immunohistochemical localization of human immunodeficiency virus p24 antigen in placental tissue. Hum Pathol 1992; 23: 411–14
402. Sheikh AU, Polliotti BM, Miller RK. In situ PCR detection of HIV expression in the human placenta. Meth Mol Biol 2000; 137: 75–86
403. Engelhart CM, van de Vijver NM, Nienhuis SJ, Hasaart TH. Fetal Candida sepsis at mid-gestation: a case report. Eur J Obstet Gynecol Reprod Biol 1998; 77: 107–9
404. Bittencourt AL, dos Santos WL, de Oliveira CH. Placental and fetal candidiasis. Presentation of a case of an abortus. Mycopathologia 1984; 87: 181–7
405. Marelli G, Mariani A, Frigerio L, et al. Fetal Candida infection associated with an intrauterine contraceptive device. Eur J Obstet Gynecol Reprod Biol 1996; 68: 209–12
406. Qureshi F, Jacques SM, Bendon RW, et al. Candida funisitis: a clinicopathologic study of 32 cases. Pediatr Dev Pathol 1998; 1: 118–24
407. Segal D, Gohar J, Huleihel M, Mazor M. Fetal death associated with asymptomatic intrauterine Candida albicans infection and a retained intrauterine contraceptive device. Scand J Infect Dis 2001; 33: 77–8
408. Rivasi F, Gasser B, Bagni A, et al. Placental candidiasis: report of four cases, one with villitis. Acta Pathol Microbiol Immunol Scand 1998; 106: 1165–9
409. VanBerger WS, Fleury FJ, Cheatle EL. Fatal maternal coccidioidomycosis in a nonendemic area. Am J Obstet Gynecol 1976; 124: 661–4
410. Blotta MH, Altemani AM, Amaral E, et al. Placental involvement in paracoccidioidomycosis. J Med Vet Mycol 1993; 31: 249–57
411. Lemos LB, Soofi M, Amir E. Blastomycosis and pregnancy. Ann Diagn Pathol 2002; 6: 211–15
412. McGregor JA, Kleinschmidt-DeMasters BK, Ogle J. Meningoencephalitis caused by Histoplasma

capsulatum complicating pregnancy. Am J Obstet Gynecol 1986; 154: 925–31
413. Whitt SP, Koch GA, Fender B, et al. Histoplasmosis in pregnancy: case series and report of transplacental transmission. Arch Intern Med 2004; 164: 454–8
414. Kambham N, Heller DS, Weitzman I. Incidental finding of Zygomyceteslike hyphae in the placenta. A case report. J Reprod Med 1998; 43: 230–2
415. Kida M, Abramowsky CR, Santoscoy C. Cryptococcosis of the placenta in a woman with acquired immunodeficiency syndrome. Hum Pathol 1989; 20: 920–1
416. Molnar-Nadasdy G, Haesly I, Reed J, Altshuler G. Placental cryptococcosis in a mother with systemic lupus erythematosus. Arch Pathol Lab Med 1994; 118: 757–9
417. Klock C, Cerski M, Dargel A, Goldani LZ. Case report. Disseminated aspergillosis complicating pregnancy. Mycoses 2002; 45: 408–10
418. Bittencourt AL. Congenital Chagas disease. Am J Dis Child 1976; 130: 97–103
419. Sugiyama T, Cuevas LE, Bailey W, et al. Expression of intercellular adhesion molecule 1 (ICAM-1) in Plasmodium falciparum-infected placenta. Placenta 2001; 22: 573–9
420. Dische MR, Gooch WM 3rd. Congenital toxoplasmosis. Perspect Pediatr Pathol 1981; 6: 83–113
421. Abbasi M, Kowalewska-Grochowska K, Bahar MA, et al. Infection of placental trophoblasts by Toxoplasma gondii. J Infect Dis 2003; 188: 608–16
422. Benirschke K. Recent trends in chorangiomas, especially those of multiple and recurrent chorangiomas. Pediatr Dev Pathol 1999; 2: 264–9
423. Wallenburg HC. Chorioangioma of the placenta. Thirteen new cases and a review of the literature from 1939 to 1970 with special reference to the clinical complications. Obstet Gynecol Surv 1971; 26: 411–25
424. Guschmann M, Henrich W, Entezami M, Dudenhausen JW. Chorioangioma – new insights into a well-known problem. I. Results of a clinical and morphological study of 136 cases. J Perinat Med 2003; 31: 163–9
425. Sepulveda W, Alcalde JL, Schnapp C, Bravo M. Perinatal outcome after prenatal diagnosis of placental chorioangioma. Obstet Gynecol 2003; 102: 1028–33
426. Drut R, Drut RM, Toulouse JC. Hepatic hemangioendotheliomas, placental chorioangiomas, and dysmorphic kidneys in Beckwith–Wiedemann syndrome. Pediatr Pathol 1992; 12: 197–203
427. Verloes A, Schapps JP, Herens C. Prenatal diagnosis of cystic hygroma and chorangioma in the Wolf–Hirschorn syndrome. Prenat Diagn 1991; 11: 129–32
428. Quintero RA, Reich H, Romero R, et al. In utero endoscopic devascularization of a large chorioangioma. Ultrasound Obstet Gynecol 1996; 8: 48–52
429. Jauniaux E, Ogle R. Color Doppler imaging in the diagnosis and management of chorioangiomas. Ultrasound Obstet Gynecol 2000; 15: 463–7
430. Locham KK, Garg R, Goel S. Hydrops fetalis in placental chorioangioma. Indian Pediatr 2001; 38: 112–13
431. Zalel Y, Weisz B, Gamzu R, et al. Chorioangiomas of the placenta: sonographic and Doppler flow characteristics. J Ultrasound Med 2002; 21: 909–13
432. Batukan C, Holzgreve W, Danzer E, et al. Large placental chorioangioma as a cause of sudden intrauterine fetal death. A case report. Fetal Diagn Ther 2001; 16: 394–7
433. Mara M, Calda P, Zizka Z, et al. Fetal anemia, thrombocytopenia, dilated umbilical vein, and cardiomegaly due to a voluminous placental chorioangioma. A case report. Fetal Diagn Ther 2002; 17: 286–92
434. Arodi J, Auslender R, Atad J, Abramovici H. Case report: giant chorangioma of the placenta. Acta Obstet Gyencol Scand 1985; 64: 91–2
435. Haak MC, Oosterhof H, Mouw RJ, et al. Pathophysiology and treatment of fetal anemia due to placental chorioangioma. Ultrasound Obstet Gynecol 1999; 14: 68–70
436. Makino Y, Horiuchi S, Sonoda M, et al. A case of large placental chorioangioma with non-immunological hydrops fetalis. J Perinat Med 1999; 27: 128–31
437. Mancuso A, D'Anna R, Corrado F, Cannata ML. Large placental chorioangioma. Acta Obstet Gynecol Scand 2001; 80: 965–6
438. Bashiri A, Furman B, Erez O, et al. Twelve cases of placental chorioangioma. Pregnancy outcome and clinical significance. Arch Gynecol Obstet 2002; 266: 53–5
439. Zalel Y, Weisz B, Gamzu R, et al. Chorioangiomas of the placenta: sonographic and Doppler flow characteristics. J Ultrasound Med 2002; 21: 909–13
440. DeLia JE. Surgery of the placenta and the umbilical cord. Clin Obstet Gynecol 1996; 39: 607–25
441. Bhide A, Prefumo F, Sairam S, et al. Ultrasound-guided interstitial laser therapy for the treatment of

placental chorioangioma. Obstet Gynecol 2003; 102: 1189–91
442. Gallot D, Sapin V, Beaufrere AM, et al. [Recurrence of multiple chorioangiomas: a case-report]. Gynecol Obstet Fertil 2003; 31: 943–7
443. Witters I, Van Damme MT, Ramaekers P, et al. Benign multiple diffuse neonatal hemangiomatosis after a pregnancy complicated by polyhydramnios and a placental chorioangioma. Eur J Obstet Gynecol Reprod Biol 2003; 106: 83–5
444. Maymon R, Hermann G, Reish O, et al. Chorioangioma and its severe infantile sequelae: case report. Prenat Diagn 2003; 23: 976–80
445. Bakaris S, Karabiber H, Yuksel M, et al. Case of large placental chorioangioma associated with diffuse neonatal hemangiomatosis. Pediatr Dev Pathol 2004; 7: 258–61
446. Khong TY. Chorangioma with trophoblastic proliferation. Virchows Arch 2000; 436: 167–71
447. Guschmann M, Henrich W, Dudenhausen JW. Chorioangiomas – new insights into a well-known problem. II. An immuno-histochemical investigation of 136 cases. J Perinat Med 2003; 31: 170–5
448. North PE, Waner M, Mizeracki A, et al. A unique microvascular phenotype shared by juvenile hemangiomas and human placenta. Arch Dermatol 2001; 137: 559–70
449. Mesia AF, Mo P, Ylagan LR. Atypical cellular chorangioma. Arch Pathol Lab Med 1999; 123: 536–8
450. Jauniaux E, Zucker M, Meuris S, et al. Chorangiocarcinoma: an unusual tumour of the placenta. The missing link? Placenta 1988; 9: 607–13
451. Trask C, Lage JM, Roberts DJ. A second case of chorangiocarcinoma presenting in a term asymptomatic twin pregnancy: choriocarcinoma in situ with associated villous vascular proliferation. Int J Gynecol Pathol 1994; 13: 87–91
452. Aonahata M, Masuzawa Y, Tsutsui Y. A case of intraplacental choriocarcinoma associated with placental hemangioma. Pathol Int 1998; 48: 897–901
453. Suh YK. Placental pathology casebook. Choriocarcinoma in situ of placenta associated with transplacental hemorrhage. J Perinatol 1999; 19: 153–4
454. Takai N, Miyazaki T, Yoshimatsu J, et al. Intraplacental choriocarcinoma with fetomaternal transfusion. Pathol Int 2000; 50: 258–61
455. Ohyama M, Ijiri R, Tanaka Y, et al. Congenital primitive epithelial tumor of the liver showing focal rhabdoid features, placental involvement, and clinical features mimicking multifocal hemangioma or stage 4S neuroblastoma. Hum Pathol 2000; 31: 259–63
456. Gibson BR, Muir-Padilla J, Champeaux A, Suarez ES. Mesenchymal dysplasia of the placenta. Placenta 2004; 25: 671–2
457. Caldarella A, Buccoliero AM, Taddei GL. Chorangiosis: report of three cases and review of the literature. Pathol Res Pract 2003; 199: 847–50
458. Khalifa MA, Gersell DJ, Hansen CH, Lage JM. Hepatic (hepatocellular) adenoma of the placenta: a study of four cases. Int J Gynecol Pathol 1998; 17: 241–4
459. Meinhard K, Dimitrov S, Nicolov A, et al. Placental teratoma – a case report. Pathol Res Pract 1999; 195: 649–51
460. Ahmed N, Kale V, Thakkar H, et al. Sonographic diagnosis of placental teratoma. J Clin Ultrasound 2004; 32: 98–101
461. Tapia RH, White VA, Ruffolo EH. Leiomyoma of the placenta. South Med J 1985; 78: 863–4
462. Ernst LM, Hui P, Parkash V. Intraplacental smooth muscle tumor: a case report. Int J Gynecol Pathol 2001; 20: 284–8
463. Harirah HM, Jones DC, Donia SE, Bahado-Singh R. Intraplacental smooth muscle tumor. A case report. J Reprod Med 2001; 46: 937–40
464. Misselevich I, Abramovici D, Reiter A, Boss JH. Leiomyoma of the fetal membranes: report of a case. Gynecol Oncol 1989; 33: 108–11
465. Tarim E, Killicadag E, Kayaselcuk F, et al. Submucosal leiomyoma of the uterus incorporated into the fetal membranes and mimicking a placental neoplasm: a case report. Placenta 2003; 24: 706–9
466. Borden EC. Melanoma and pregnancy. Semin Oncol 2000; 27: 654–6
467. Alexander A, Harris RM, Grossman D, et al. Vulvar melanoma: diffuse melanosis and metastasis to the placenta. J Am Acad Dermatol 2004; 50: 293–8
468. Marsh RD, Chu NM. Placental metastasis from primary ocular melanoma: a case report. Am J Obstet Gynecol 1996; 174: 1654–5
469. Eltorky M, Khare VK, Osborne P, Shanklin DR. Placental metastasis from maternal carcinoma. A report of three cases. J Reprod Med 1995; 40: 399–403
470. Ben Brahim E, Mrad K, Driss M, et al. [Placental metastasis of breast cancer]. Gynecol Obstet Fertil 2001; 29: 545–8
471. Kochman AT, Rabczynski JK, Baranowski W, et al. Metastases to the products of conception from a maternal bronchial carcinoma. A case report and review of literature. Pol J Pathol 2001; 52: 137–40

472. Sakurai H, Mitsuhashi N, Ibuki Y, et al. Placental metastasis from maternal primitive neuroectodermal tumor. Am J Clin Oncol 1998; 21: 39–41
473. Gourley C, Monaghan H, Beattie G, et al. Intrauterine death resulting from placental metastases in adenocarcinoma of unknown primary. Clin Oncol (R Coll Radiol) 2002; 14: 213–16
474. Tsujimura T, Matsumoto K, Aozasa K. Placental involvement by maternal non-Hodgkin's lymphoma. Arch Pathol Lab Med 1993; 117: 325–7
475. Honore LH, Brown LB. Intervillous placental metastasis with maternal myeloid leukemia. Arch Pathol Lab Med 1990; 114: 450
476. Lynn AA, Parry SI, Morgan MA, Mennuti MT. Disseminated congenital neuroblastoma involving the placenta. Arch Pathol Lab Med 1997; 121: 741–4
477. Ohyama M, Kobayashi S, Aida N, et al. Congenital neuroblastoma diagnosed by placental examination. Med Pediatr Oncol 1999; 33: 430–1
478. Rivasi F, Gasser B, Collina G, et al. [Congenital fetal neuroblastoma]. Ann Pathol 2001; 21: 76–80
479. Robinson HB Jr, Bolande RP. Case 3. Fetal hepatoblastoma with placental metastases. Pediatr Pathol 1985; 4: 163–7
480. Doss BJ, Jacques SM, Mayes MD, Qureshi F. Maternal scleroderma: placental findings and perinatal outcome. Hum Pathol 1998; 29: 1524–30
481. Leung JC, Mann S, Salafia C, Brion LP. Sacrococcygeal teratoma with vascular placental dissemination. Obstet Gynecol 1999; 93: 856
482. Chin YM, Wan Ariffin A, Lin HP, Chan YS. Concordant childhood acute lymphoblastic leukemia in monozygotic twins. Med J Malaysia 1996; 51: 145–8
483. Boyd TK, Schofield DE. Monozygotic twins concordant for congenital neuroblastoma: case report and review of the literature. Pediatr Pathol Lab Med 1995; 15: 931–40
484. Ford AM, Pombo-de-Oliveira MS, McCarthy KP, et al. Monoclonal origin of concordant T-cell malignancy in identical twins. Blood 1997; 89: 281–5
485. Stron TH, Elliott JP, Radin G. Noncoiled umbilical blood vessels: a new marker for the fetus at risk. Obstet Gynecol 1993; 81: 409–11
486. Lacro RV, Jones KL, Benirschke K. The umbilical cord twist: origin, direction, and relevance. Am J Obstet Gynecol 1987; 157: 833–8
487. Giacoia GP. Body stalk anomaly: congenital absence of the umbilical cord. Obstet Gynecol 1992; 80: 527–9
488. Naeye RL. Umbilical cord length: clinical significance. J Pediatr 1985; 107: 278–81
489. Larson JD, Rayburn WF, Crosby S, Thurnau GR. Multiple nuchal cord entanglements and intrapartum complications. Am J Obstet Gynecol 1995; 173: 1228–31
490. Jauniaux E, Ramsay B, Peellaerts C, Scholler Y. Perinatal features of pregnancies complicated by nuchal cord. Am J Perinatol 1995; 12: 255–8
491. Heifetz SA. The umbilical cord: obstetrically important lesions. Clin Obstet Gynecol 1996; 39: 571–87
492. Bjoro K. Vascular anomalies of the umbilical cord II. Perinatal and pediatric implications. Early Hum Dev 1983; 8: 279–87
493. Sherer DM, Anyaegbunam A. Prenatal ultrasonographic morphologic assessment of the umbilical cord: a review. Part I. Obstet Gynecol Surv 1997; 52: 506–14
494. Rinehart BK, Terrone DA, Taylor CW, et al. Single umbilical artery is associated with an increased incidence of structural and chromosomal anomalies and growth restriction. Am J Perinatol 2000; 17: 229–32
495. Clausen I. Umbilical cord anomalies and antenatal fetal deaths. Obstet Gynecol Surv 1989; 44: 841–5
496. Schinmel MS, Eidelman AI. Supernumerary umbilical vein resulting in a four-vessel cord. Am J Perinatol 1998; 15: 299–301
497. Vandevijver N, Hermans RH, Schrander-Stumpel CC, et al. Aneurysm of the umbilical vein: case report and review of the literature. Eur J Obstet Gynecol Reprod Biol 2000; 89: 85–7
498. Benirschke K. Obstetrically important lesions of the umbilical cord. J Reprod Med 1994; 39: 262–72
499. Seoud M, Aboul-Hosn L, Nassar A, et al. Spontaneous umbilical cord hematoma: a rare cause of acute fetal distress. Am J Perinatol 2001; 18: 99–102
500. Gregora MG, Lai J. Umbilical cord hematoma: a serious pregnancy complication. Aust NZ J Obstet Gynecol 1995; 35: 212–14
501. Jauniaux E, Donner C, Simon P, et al. Pathologic aspects of the umbilical cord after percutaneous umbilical blood sampling. Obstet Gynecol 1989; 73: 215–18
502. Benirschke K, Pekarske SL. Placental pathology casebook. Extensive calcification of the umbilical cord and placenta J Perinatol 1995; 15: 81–3
503. Khong TY, Dilly SA. Calcification of the umbilical artery: two distinct lesions. J Clin Pathol 1989; 42: 931–4
504. Arias U, Heinonen S. Clinical significance of true umbilical knots: a population based analysis. Am J Perinatol 2002; 19: 127–32

505. Blickstein I, Shoam-Schwartz Z, Lancet M. Predisposing factors in the formation of true knots of the umbilical cord: analysis of morphometric and perinatal data. Int J Gynaecol Obstet 1987; 25: 395–8
506. Sornes T. Umbilical cord knots. Acta Obstet Gynecol Scand 2000; 79: 157–9
507. Browne FJ. On abnormalities of umbilical cord which may cause antenatal death. J Obstet Gynecol Br Emp 1925; 32: 17–48
508. Machin GA, Ackerman J, Gilbert-Barness E. Abnormal umbilical cord coiling is associated with adverse perinatal outcome. Pediatr Dev Pathol 2000; 3: 462–71
509. Bakotic BW, Boyd T, Poppiti R, Pfueger S. Recurrent umbilical cord torsion leading to fetal death in 3 subsequent pregnancies. Arch Pathol Lab Med 2000; 124: 1352–5
510. Sun Y, Arbuckle S, Hocking G. Umbilical cord stricture and intrauterine fetal death. Ped Pathol Lab Med 1995; 15: 723–32
511. Coulter JBS, Scott JM, Jordan MM. Edema of the cord and respiratory distress in the newborn. Br J Obstet Gynaecol 1975; 82: 453–9
512. Quartero HWP, Berg WVD, Kolkman PH. A prenatal diagnosis of umbilical cord oedema made by ultrasound; a case report. Eur J Obstet Gynecol Reprod Biol 1984; 17: 409–12
513. Juaniaux E, De Munter C, Vanesse M, et al. Embryonic remnants of the umbilical cord: morphologic and clinical aspects. Hum Pathol 1989; 20: 458–62
514. Blanc WA, Allan GW. Intrafunicular ulceration of persistent omphalomesenteric duct with intra-amniotic hemorrhage and fetal death. Am J Obstet Gynecol 1961; 72: 1392–6
515. Heifetz SA, Rueda-Pedraza E. Omphalomesenteric duct cysts of the umbilical cord. Pediatr Pathol 1983; 1: 325–35
516. Sondergaard G. Hemangioma of the umbilical cord. Acta Obstet Gynecol Scand 1994; 73: 434–6
517. Yavner DL, Redline RW. Angiomyxoma of the umbilical cord with massive cystic degeneration of Wharton's jelly. Arch Pathol Lab Med 1989; 113: 935–7
518. Usta IM, Mercer BM, Sibai BM. Current obstetrical practice and umbilical cord prolapse. Am J Perinatol 1999; 16: 479–84
519. Uygur D, Kis S, Tuncer R, et al. Risk factors and infant outcomes associated with umbilical cord prolapse. Int J Gynecol Obstet 2002; 78: 127–30
520. Heifetz SA. Strangulation of the umbilical cord by amniotic bands: report of 6 cases and literature review. Pediatr Pathol 1984; 2: 285–304
521. Kaplan C, Lowell DM, Salafia C. College of American Pathologists Conference XIX on the Examination of the Placenta: report of the Working Group on the Definition of Structural Changes Associated with Abnormal Function in the Maternal/Fetal/Placental Unit in the Second and Third Trimesters. Arch Pathol Lab Med 1991; 115: 709–16
522. Dimmick J, Kalousek DK. Developmental Pathology of the Embryo and Fetus. Philadelphia: JB Lippincott, 1992
523. Torpin R. Fetal Malformation Caused by Amnion Rupture During Gestation. Springfield, IL: Charles C Thomas, 1968
524. Colpaert C, Bogers J, Hertveldt K, et al. Limb–body wall complex: 4 new cases illustrating the importance of examining placenta and umbilical cord. Pathol Res Pract 2000; 196: 783–90
525. Pumberger W, Schaller A, Bernaschek G. Limb–body wall complex: a compound anomaly pattern in body-wall defects. Pediatr Surg Int 2001; 17: 486–90
526. Lockwood L, Ghidini A, Romero R, Hobbins JC. Amniotic band syndrome: re-evaluation of its pathogenesis. Am J Obstet Gynecol 1989; 160: 1030–3
527. Young ID, Lindenbaum RH, Thompson EM, Pembrey ME. Amniotic bands in connective tissue disorders. Arch Dis Child 1985; 60: 1061–3
528. Mahony BS, Filly RA, Callen PW, Golbus MS. The amniotic band syndrome: antenatal sonographic diagnosis and potential pitfalls. Am J Obstet Gynecol 1985; 152: 63–8
529. Perlman M, Tennenbaum A, Menashi M, et al. Extramembranous pregnancy: maternal, placental, and perinatal implications. Obstet Gynecol 1980; 55: 34S–7S
530. Sienko A, Altshuler G. Meconium-induced umbilical vascular necrosis in abortuses and fetuses: a histopathologic study for cytokines. Obstet Gynecol 1999; 94: 415–20
531. Holeberg G, Huleihel M, Katz M, et al. Vasoconstrictive activity of meconium stained amniotic fluid in the human placental vasculature. Eur J Obstet Gynecol Reprod Biol 1999; 87: 147–50
532. Altshuler G, Arizawa M, Molnar-Nadascy G. Meconium-induced umbilical cord vascular necrosis and ulcerations: a potential link between the placenta and poor pregnancy outcome. Obstet Gynecol 1992; 79: 760–6
533. King EL, Redline RW, Smith SD, et al. Myocytes of chorionic vessels from placentas with meconium-associated vascular necrosis exhibit apoptotic markers. Hum Pathol 2004; 35: 412–17

534. Miller PW, Coen RW, Benirschke K. Dating the time interval from meconium passage to birth. Obstet Gynecol 1985; 66: 459–62
535. Morhaime L, Park K, Benirschke K, Baergen RN. Disappearance of meconium pigment in placental specimens on exposure to light. Arch Pathol Lab Med 2003; 127: 711–14
536. Naeye RL. Functionally important disorders of the placenta, umbilical cord, and fetal membranes. Hum Pathol 1987; 18: 680–91
537. DePaepe ME, Friedman RM, Gundogan F, et al. The histologic fetoplacental inflammatory response in fatal perinatal group B-streptococcus infection. J Perinatol 2004; 24: 441–5
538. Dammann O, Leviton A. Maternal intrauterine infection, cytokines, and brain damage in the preterm newborn. Pediatr Res 1997; 42: 1–8
539. Goncalves LF, Chaiworapongsa T, Romero R. Intrauterine infection and prematurity. Ment Retard Dev Disabil Res Rev 2002; 8: 3–13
540. Lauweryns J, Bernat R, Lerut A, Detournay G. Intrauterine pneumonia. Biol Neonate 1972; 22: 301–18
541. Schlievert P, Larsen B, Johnson W, Galask RP. Bacterial growth inhibition by amniotic fluid. Am J Obstet Gynecol 1975; 122: 809–19
542. Lamont RF, Fisk N. The role of infection in the pathogenesis of preterm labour. Prog Obstet Gynecol 1993; 10: 135–58
543. Scott RJ, Peat D, Rhodes CA. Investigation of the fetal pulmonary inflammatory reaction in chorioamnionitis, using an in situ Y chromosome marker. Pediatr Pathol 1994; 14: 997–1003
544. Blanc WA. Pathology of the placenta, membranes, and umbilical cord in bacterial, fungal, and viral infections in man. Monogr Pathol 1981; 22: 67–132
545. Redline RW, Faye-Petersen O, Heller D, et al. Society for Pediatric Pathology, Perinatal Section, Amniotic Fluid Infection Nosology Committee. Amniotic infection syndrome: nosology and reproducibility of placental reaction patterns. Pediatr Dev Pathol 2003; 6: 435–48
546. Redline RW, Wilson-Costello D, Borawski E, et al. Placental lesions associated with neurologic impairment and cerebral palsy in very low-birth-weight infants. Arch Pathol Lab Med 1998; 122: 1091–8
547. Dashe JS, Rogers BB, McIntire DD, Leveno KJ. Epidural analgesia and intrapartum fever: placental findings. Obstet Gynecol 1999; 93: 341–4
548. Romero R, Chaiworapongsa T, Espinoza J. Micronutrients and intrauterine infection, preterm birth and the fetal inflammatory response syndrome. J Nutr 2003; 133: 1668S–73S
549. Hillier SL, Martius J, Krohn M, et al. A case control study of chorioamniotic infection and histologic chorioamnionitis in prematurity. N Engl J Med 1988; 319: 972–8
550. Pacora P, Chaiworapongsa T, Maymon E, et al. Funisitis and chorionic vasculitis: the histological counterpart of the fetal inflammatory response syndrome. J Matern Fetal Neonatal Med 2002; 11: 18–25
551. Mittendorf R, Montag AG, MacMillan W, et al. Components of the systemic fetal inflammatory response syndrome as predictors of impaired neurologic outcomes in children. Am J Obstet Gynecol 2003; 188: 1438–44; discussion 1444–6
552. Yoon BH, Romero R, Kim KS, et al. A systemic fetal inflammatory response and the development of bronchopulmonary dysplasia. Am J Obstet Gynecol 1999; 181: 773–9
553. Miyano A, Miyamichi T, Nakayama M, et al. Differences among acute, subacute, and chronic chorioamnionitis based on levels of inflammation-associated proteins in cord blood. Pediatr Dev Pathol 1998; 1: 513–21
554. Ohyama M, Itani Y, Yamanaka M, et al. Re-evaluation of chorioamnionitis and funisitis with a special reference to subacute chorioamnionitis. Hum Pathol 2002; 33: 183–90
555. Fraser RB, Wright JR Jr. Eosinophilic/T-cell chorionic vasculitis. Ped Dev Pathol 2002; 5: 350–5
556. Grether JK, Nelson KB, Walsh E, et al. Intrauterine exposure to infection and risk of cerebral palsy in very preterm infants. Arch Pediatr Adolesc Med 2003; 157: 26–32
557. Macaubas C, de Klerk NH, Holt BJ, et al. Association between antenatal cytokine production and the development of atopy and asthma at age 6 years. Lancet 2003; 362: 1192–7
558. Torres AR. Is fever suppression involved in the etiology of autism and neurodevelopmental disorders? BMC Pediatr 2003; 3: 9
559. Wilkerson DS, Volpe AG, Dean RS, Titus JB. Perinatal complications as predictors of infantile autism. Int J Neurosci 2002; 112: 1085–98
560. Juul-Dam N, Townsend J, Courchesne E. Prenatal, perinatal, and neonatal factors in autism, pervasive developmental disorder-not otherwise specified, and the general population. Pediatrics 2001; 107: E63
561. Pletnikov MV, Rubin SA, Moran TH, Carbone KM. Exploring the cerebellum with a new tool: neonatal

Borna disease virus (BDV) infection of the rat's brain. Cerebellum 2003; 2: 62–70
562. Hornig M, Weissenbock H, Horscroft N, Lipkin WI. An infection-based model of neurodevelopmental damage. Proc Natl Acad Sci USA 1999; 96: 12102–7
563. Navarro C, Blanc WA. Chronic viral funisitis. J Pediatr 1977; 91: 967–73
564. Navarro C, Blanc WA. Subacute necrotizing funisitis. A variant of cord inflammation with a high rate of perinatal infection. J Pediatr 1974; 85: 689–97
565. Fojaco RM, Hensley GT, Moskowitz L. Congenital syphilis and necrotizing funisitis. J Am Med Assoc 1989; 261: 1788–90
566. Genest DR, Granter S, Pinkus GS. Umbilical cord 'pseudovasculitis' following second trimester fetal death: a clinicopathological and immunohistochemical study of 13 cases. Histopathology 1997; 30: 563–9
567. Clark SL, Pavlova Z, Greenspoon J, et al. Squamous cells in the maternal pulmonary circulation. Am J Obstet Gynecol 1986; 154: 104–6
568. Lee W, Ginsburg KA, Cotton DB, Kaufman RH. Squamous and trophoblastic cells in the maternal pulmonary circulation identified by invasive hemodynamic monitoring during the peripartum period. Am J Obstet Gynecol 1986; 155: 999–1001
569. Khong TY. Expression of endothelin-1 in amniotic fluid embolism and possible pathophysiological mechanism. Br J Obstet Gynaecol 1998; 105: 802–4
570. Case Records of the Massachusetts General Hospital Weekly Clinicopathologic Exercises, Case 9–1998. Cardiovascular collapes after vaginal delivery in a patient with history of Cesareans section. N Engl J Med 1998; 338: 821–6
571. Jacques SM, Qureshi F. Subamnionic vernix caseosa. Pediatr Pathol 1994; 14: 585–93
572. Keski-Nisula L, Aalto ML, Katila ML, Kirkinen P. Intrauterine inflammation at term: a histopathologic study. Hum Pathol 2000; 31: 841–6
573. Locatelli A, Patane L, Ghidini A, et al. Pathology findings in preterm placentas of women with autoantibodies: a case–control study. J Matern Fetal Neonatal Med 2002; 11: 339–44
574. American College of Obstetricians and Gynecologists. Diagnosis and Management of Preeclampsia and Eclampsia, ACOG Practice Bulletin 33. Washington, DC: ACOG, January 2002
575. Leung DN, Smith SC, To KF, et al. Increased placental apoptosis in pregnancies complicated by preeclampsia. Am J Obstet Gynecol 2002; 184: 1249–50
576. DeWolf F, Brosens I, Renaer M. Fetal growth retardation and maternal arterial supply of the human placenta in the absence of sustained hypertension. Br J Obstet Gynaecol 1980; 87: 678–85
577. Kitzmiller JS, Watt N, Driscoll SG. Decidual arteriopathy in hypertension and diabetes in pregnancy. Immunofluorescent studies. Am J Obstet Gynecol 1981; 141: 773–9
578. Weinstein L. Preeclampsia/eclampsia with hemolysis, elevated liver enzymes, and thrombocytopenia. Obstet Gynecol 1985; 66: 657–60
579. Labarrere C, Althabe O. Chronic villitis of unknown etiology and decidual maternal vasculopathies in sustained chronic hypertension. Eur J Obstet Gynecol Reprod Biol 1986; 21: 27–32
580. White P. Classification of obstetric diabetes. Am J Obstet Gynecol 1978; 130: 228–30
581. Diamant YZ. The human placenta in diabetes mellitus. Isr J Med Sci 1991; 27: 493–7
582. Morriss FH Jr. Infants of diabetic mothers: fetal and neonatal pathophysiology. Perspect Pediatr Pathol 1984; 8: 223–34
583. Zumkeller W. Current topic: the role of growth hormone and insulin-like growth factors for placental growth and development. Placenta 2000; 21: 451–67
584. Mayhew TM. Enhanced fetoplacental angiogenesis in pre-gestational diabetes mellitus: the extra growth is exclusively longitudinal and not accompanied by microvascular remodelling. Diabetologia 2002; 45: 1434–9
585. Jirkovska M, Kubinova L, Janacek J, et al. Topological properties and spatial organization of villous capillaries in normal and diabetic placentas. J Vasc Res 2002; 39: 268–78
586. Singer DB. The placenta in pregnancies complicated by diabetes mellitus. Perspect Pediatr Pathol 1984; 8: 199–212
587. Teasdale F. Histomorphometry of the human placenta in class C diabetes mellitus. Placenta 1984; 5: 69–86
588. McFadden DE, Pantzar JT. Placental pathology of triploidy. Hum Pathol 1996; 27: 1018–20
589. Keep D, Zaragoza MV, Hassold T, Redline RW. Very early complete hydatidiform mole. Hum Pathol 1996; 27: 708–13
590. Genest DR, Dorfman DM, Castrillon DH. Ploidy and imprinting in hydatidiform moles. Complementary use of flow cytometry and

immunohistochemistry of the imprinted gene product p57KIP2 to assist molar classification. J Reprod Med 2002; 47: 342–6
591. Redline RW, Zaragoza M, Hassold T. Prevalence of developmental and inflammatory lesions in nonmolar first-trimester spontaneous abortions. Hum Pathol 1999; 30: 93–100
592. Kohut KG, Anthony MA, Salafia CM. Decidual and placental histologic findings in patients experiencing spontaneous abortions in relation to pregnancy order. Am J Reprod Immunol 1997; 37: 257–61
593. Ghidini A, Pezzullo JC, Sylyestre G, et al. Antenatal corticosteroids and placental histopathology in preterm birth. Placenta 2001; 22: 412–17
594. Polzin WJ. Brady K. The etiology of premature rupture of the membranes. Clin Obstet Gynecol 1998; 41: 810–16
595. Arias F, Rodriquez L, Rayne SC, Kraus FT. Maternal placental vasculopathy and infections: two distinct subgroups among patients with preterm labor and preterm ruptured membranes. Am J Obstet Gynecol 1993; 168: 585–91
596. Smulian JC, Bhandari V, Vintzileos AM, et al. Intrapartum fever at term: serum and histological markers of inflammation. Am J Obstet Gynecol 2003; 188: 269–74
597. Gilbert WM, Lafferty CM, Benirschke K, Resnik R. Lack of specific placental abnormality associated with cocaine use. Am J Obstet Gynecol 1990; 163: 998–9
598. Mastrogiannis DS, Decavalas GO, Verma U, Tejani N. Perinatal outcome after recurrent cocaine usage. Obstet Gynecol 1990; 76: 8–11
599. Cejtin HE, Young SA, Ungaretti J, et al. Effects of cocaine on the placenta. Pediatr Dev Pathol 1999; 2: 143–7
600. Baldwin VJ, MacLeod PM, Benirschke K. Placental findings in alcohol abuse in pregnancy. Birth Defects 1982; 18: 89–94
601. Asmussen I. Ultrastructure of the villi and fetal capillaries in placentas from smoking and nonsmoking mothers. Br J Obstet Gynaecol 1980; 87: 239–45
602. Teasdale F, Ghislaine JJ. Morphologic changes in the placentas of smoking mothers: a histomorphometric study. Biol Neonate 1989; 55: 251–9
603. Naeye RL, Blanc W, Leblanc W, Khatamee MA. Fetal complications of maternal heroin addiction: abnormal growth, infections, and episodes of stress. J Pediatr 1973; 83: 1055–61
604. Ogishima D, Matsumoto T, Nakamura Y, et al. Placental pathology in systemic lupus erythematosis with antiphospholipid antibodies. Pathol Int 2000; 50: 224–9
605. Levy RA, Ayyad E, Oliveira J, Porto LC. Placental pathology in antiphospholipid syndrome. Lupus 1998; 7 (Suppl 2): S81–5
606. Labarrere CA, Catoggio LJ, Mullen EG, Althabe OH. Placental lesions in maternal autoimmune diseases. Am J Reprod Immunol 1986; 12: 78–86
607. Sebire NJ, Backos M, Goldin RD, Regan L. Placental massive perivillous fibrin deposition associated with antiphospholipid syndrome. Br J Obstet Gynaecol 2002; 109: 570–3
608. Alonso A, Soto I, Urgelles MF, et al. Acquired and inherited thrombophilia in women with unexplained fetal losses. Am J Obstet Gynecol 2002; 187: 1337–42
609. Arias F, Romero R, Joist H, Kraus FT. Thrombophilia: a mechanism of disease in women with adverse pregnancy outcome and thrombotic lesions in the placenta. J Matern Fetal Med 1998; 7: 277–86
610. Baldwin VJ. Pathology of Multiple Pregnancy. New York: Springer-Verlag, 1994
611. Redline RW. Nonidentical twins with a single placenta – disproving dogma in perinatal pathology. N Engl J Med 2003; 349: 111–14
612. Bernirschke K, Masliah E. The placenta in multiple pregnancy; outstanding issues. Reprod Fertil Dev 2001; 13: 615–22
613. Sherer DM. Adverse perinatal outcome of twin pregnancies according to chorionicity: review of the literature. Am J Perinatol 2001; 18: 23–37
614. Powers WF, Kiely JL. The risks confronting twins: a national perspective. Am J Obstet Gynecol 1994; 170: 456–61
615. Redline RW, Shah D, Sakar H, et al. Placental lesions associated with abnormal growth in twins. Pediatr Dev Pathol 2001; 4: 473–81
616. Gaziano EP, De Lia JE, Kuhlmann RS. Diamnionic monochorionic twin gestations: an overview. J Matern Fetal Med 2000; 9: 89–96
617. DeLia JE, Cruickshank DP, Keye WR, Jr. Fetoscopic neodymium–YAG laser occlusion of placental vessels in severe twin-twin transfusion syndromes. Obstet Gynecol 1990; 75: 1046–53
618. DeLia J, Fisk N, Hecher K, et al. Twin-to-twin transfusion syndrome – debates on the etiology, natural history and management. Ultrasound Obstet Gynecol 2000; 16: 210–13
619. DePaepe ME, Burke S, Luks FI, et al. Demonstration of placental vascular anatomy in mono-

chorionic twin gestations. Pediatr Dev Pathol 2002; 5: 37–44
620. Mahieu-Caputo D, Muller F, Joly D, et al. Pathogenesis of twin–twin transfusion syndrome: the rennin–angiotensin system hypothesis. Fetal Diagn Ther 2001; 16: 241–4
621. Tan TY, Denbow ML, Cox PM, et al. Occlusion of arterioarterial anastomosis manifesting as acute twin–twin transfusion syndrome. Placenta 2004; 25: 238–42
622. Banek CS, Hecher K, Hackeloer BJ, Bartmann P. Long-term neurodevelopmental outcome after intrauterine laser treatment for severe twin–twin transfusion syndrome. Am J Obstet Gynecol 2003; 188: 876–80
623. DeLia JE, Kuhlmann RS, Lopez KP. Treating previable twin–twin transfusion syndrome with fetoscopic laser surgery: outcomes following the learning curve. J Perinat Med 1999; 27: 61–7
624. Tummers P, De Sutter P, Dhont M. Risk of spontaneous abortion in singleton and twin pregnancies after IVF/ICSI. Hum Reprod 2003; 18: 1720–3
625. Sampson A, de Crespigny LC. Vanishing twins: the frequency of spontaneous fetal reduction of a twin pregnancy. Ultrasound Obstet Gynecol 1992; 2: 107–9
626. Jauniaux E, Elkazen N, Leroy F, et al. Clinical and morphologic aspects of the vanishing twin phenomenon. Obstet Gynecol 1988; 72: 577–81
627. Wu ML, Jones VA. Images in pathology: placenta: 6 – 4 = 2. Arch Pathol Lab Med 2000; 124: 1564
628. Gimenez-Scherer JA, Davies BR. Malformations in acardiac twins are consistent with reversed blood flow: liver as a clue to their pathogenesis. Pediatr Dev Pathol 2003; 6: 520–30
629. Emery SC, Vaux KK, Pretorius D, et al. Acardiac twin with externalized intestine adherent to placenta: unusual manifestation of omphalocele. Pediatr Dev Pathol 2004; 7: 81–5
630. Machin GA. Conjoined twins; implications for blastogenesis. Birth Defects 1993; 29: 141–79
631. Garite TJ, Clark RH, Elliott JP, Thorp JA. Twins and triplets: the effect of plurality and growth on neonatal outcome compared with singleton infants. Am J Obstet Gynecol 2004; 191: 700–7
632. Cetin I, Foidart JM, Miozzo M, et al. Fetal growth restriction: a workshop report. Placenta 2004; 25: 753–7
633. Brenner B, Grabowski EF, Hellgren M, et al. Thrombophilia and pregnancy complications. Thromb Haemost 2004; 92: 678–81
634. Gilbert-Barness E, Opitz JM. Congenital anomalies and malformation syndromes. In Stocker JT, Dehner LP, eds. Pediatric Pathology. Philadelphia: JB Lippincott, 1992; 1: 104–6
635. Keeling JW. Fetal hydrops. In Keeling JW, ed. Fetal and Neonatal Pathology, 2nd edn. New York: Springer-Verlag, 1993: 253–71
636. Santolaya J, Alley D, Jaffe R, Warsof SL. Antenatal classification of hydrops fetalis. Obstet Gynecol 1992; 79: 256–9
637. Ismail KM, Martin WL, Ghosh S, et al. Etiology and outcome of hydrops fetalis. J Matern Fetal Med 2001; 10: 175–81
638. Rodriguez MM, Chaves F, Romaguera RL, et al. Value of autopsy in non-immune hydrops fetalis: series of 51 stillborn fetuses. Pediatr Dev Pathol 2002; 5: 365–74
639. Kuhlmann RS, Werner AL, Abramowicz J, et al. Placental histology in fetuses between 18 and 23 weeks' gestation with abnormal karyotype. Am J Obstet Gynecol 1990; 163: 1264–70
640. Genest DR, Roberts D, Boyd T, Bieber FR. Fetoplacental histology as a predictor of karyotype: a controlled study of spontaneous first trimester abortions. Hum Pathol 1995; 26: 201–9
641. Roberts DJ, Ampola MG, Lage JM. Diagnosis of unsuspected fetal metabolic storage disease by routine placental examination. Pediatr Pathol 1991; 11: 647–56
642. Jones CJ, Lendon M, Chawner LE, Jauniaux E. Ultrastructure of the human placenta in metabolic storage disease. Placenta 1990; 11: 395–411
643. Johnson A, Wapner RJ. Mosaicism: implications for postnatal outcome. Curr Opin Obstet Gynecol 1997; 9: 126–35
644. Lestou VS, Kalousek DK. Confined placental mosaicism and intrauterine fetal growth. Arch Dis Child Fetal Neonatal Ed 1998; 79: F223–6
645. Kalousek DK, Vekemans M. Confined placental mosaicism and genomic imprinting. Baillière's Best Pract Res Clin Obstet Gynaecol 2000; 14: 723–30
646. Stipoljev F, Latin V, Kos M, et al. Correlation of confined placental mosaicism with fetal intrauterine growth retardation. A case control study of placentas at delivery. Fetal Diagn Ther 2001; 16: 4–9
647. Altemani AM. Thrombosis of fetal placental vessels. A quantitative study in placentas of stillbirths. Pathol Res Pract 1987; 182: 685–9
648. Jacques SM, Qureshi F, Johnson A, et al. Estimation of time of fetal death in the second trimester by

placental histopathological examination. Pediatr Dev Pathol 2003; 6: 226–32
649. Sikovanyecz J, Horvath E, Sallay E, et al. Fetomaternal transfusion and pregnancy outcome after cordocentesis. Fetal Diagn Ther 2001; 16: 83–9
650. Lane PL. Traumatic fetal deaths. J Emerg Med 1989; 7: 433–5
651. Fisher M. Acute Rh isoimmunization following abdominal trauma associated with late abruption placenta. Acta Obstet Gynecol Scand 1989; 68: 657–9
652. Daniel Y, Schreiber L, Geva E, et al. Do placentae of term singleton pregnancies obtained by assisted reproductive technologies differ from those of spontaneously conceived pregnancies? Hum Reprod 1999; 14: 1107–10
653. Gavrill P, Jauniaux E, Leroy F. Pathologic examination of placentas from singleton and twin pregnancies obtained after in vitro fertilization and embryo transfer. Pediatr Pathol 1993; 13: 453–62
654. Sutcliffe AG, Sebire NJ, Pigott AJ, et al. Outcome for children born after in utero laser ablation therapy for severe twin-to-twin transfusion syndrome. Br J Obstet Gynaecol 2001; 108: 1246–50

Index